Also by Joyce Brabner

Animal Rights Comics
Activists!
Our Cancer Year (with Harvey Pekar)
Brought to Light (with Alan Moore)
Real War Stories

Second Avenue Caper

Second Avenue Caper

When Goodfellas, Divas, and Dealers Plotted Against the Plague

Joyce Brabner

Illustrated by Mark Zingarelli

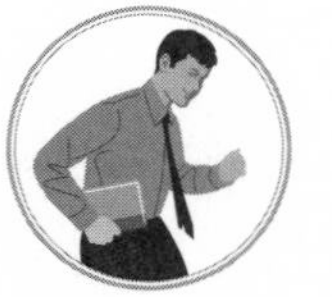

A Novel Graphic from Hill and Wang
A division of Farrar, Straus and Giroux • New York

Hill and Wang
A division of Farrar, Straus and Giroux
18 West 18th Street, New York 10011

Library of Congress Cataloging-in-Publication Data
Brabner, Joyce.
    Second Avenue caper : when goodfellas, divas, and dealers plotted against
the plague / Joyce Brabner ; illustrated by Mark Zingarelli.
        pages cm
    ISBN 978-0-8090-3553-3 (hardback) -- ISBN 978-1-4299-5615-4 (e-book)
    1. AIDS (Disease)--New York (State)--New York--Comic books, strips,
etc. 2. AIDS (Disease)--Political aspects--New York (State)--New York--Comic
books, strips, etc. 3. AIDS (Disease)--Social aspects--New York (State)--New
York--Comic books, strips, etc. I. Zingarelli, Mark, illustrator. II. Title.

RA643.84.N7 B73 2014
362.19697'9200207--dc23

                                                                2014015571

Designed by Mark Zingarelli

Hill and Wang books may be purchased for educational, business, or promotional
use. For information on bulk purchases, please contact the Macmillan
Corporate and Premium Sales Department at 1-800-221-7945, extension 5442,
or write to specialmarkets@macmillan.com.

www.fsgbooks.com
www.twitter.com/fsgbooks • www.facebook.com/fsgbooks

1   3   5   7   9   10   8   6   4   2

**For everyone who should
have been there at the finish**

My friend Raymond left 25th and Lorain here in Cleveland for New York City, to take care of sick people and write very funny drag revues for Lower East Side music halls.

—Joyce Brabner

SECOND AVENUE CAPER

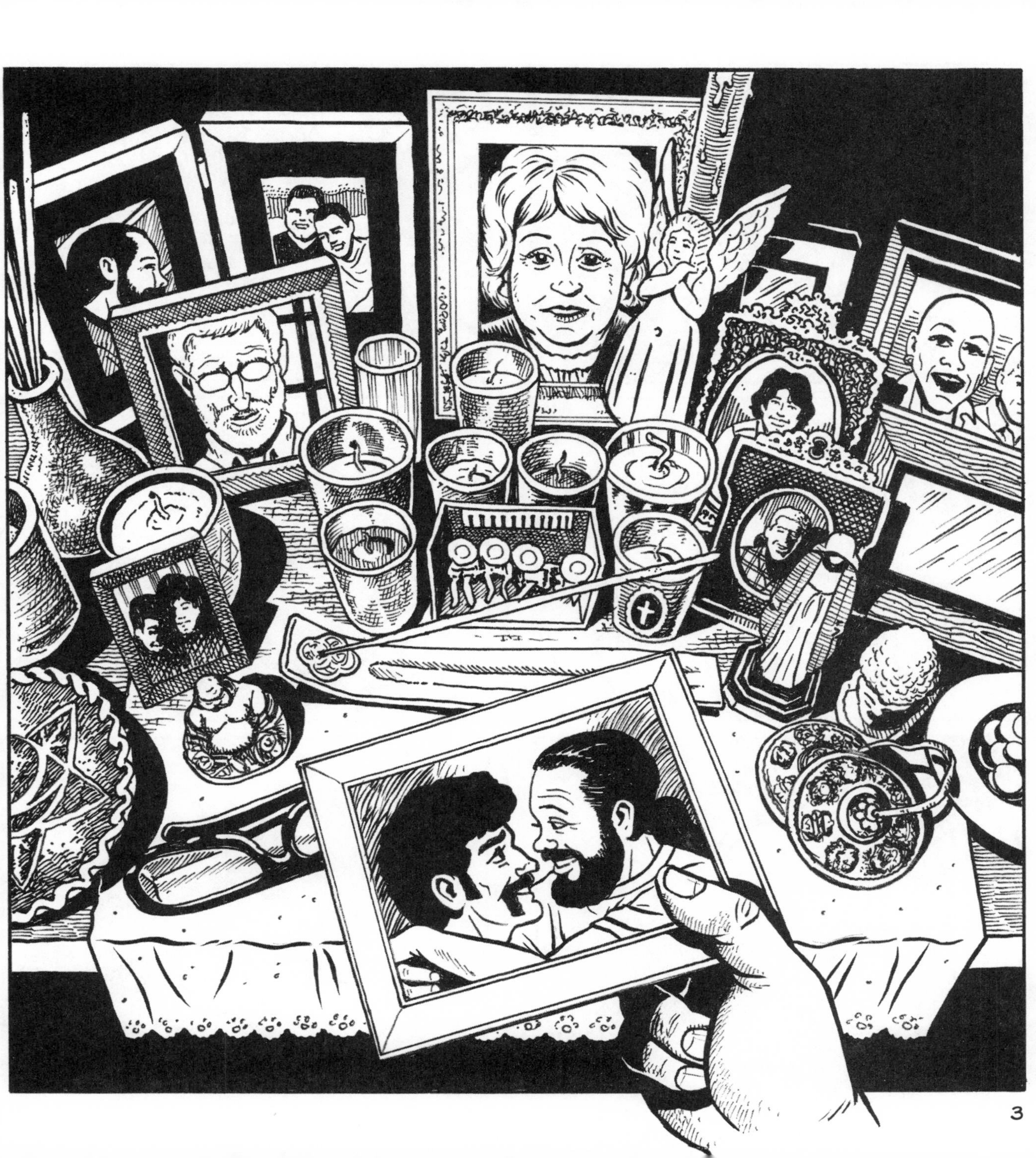

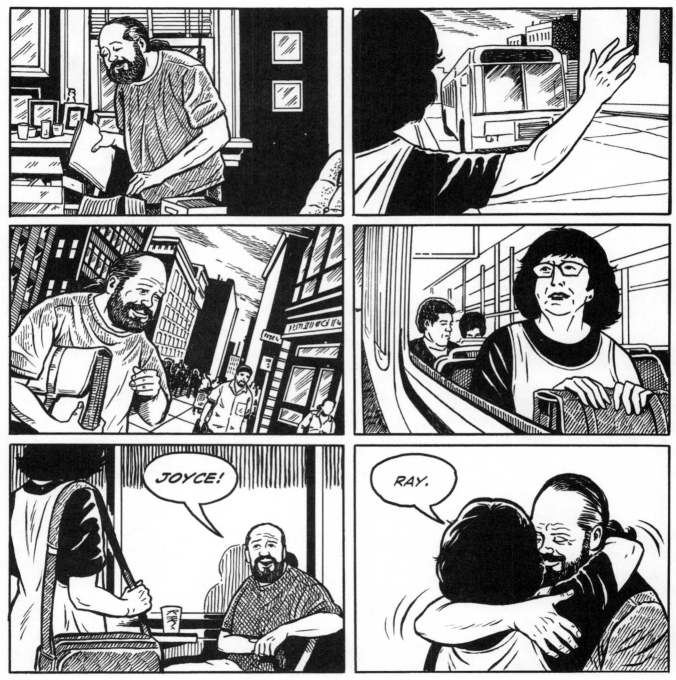

JOYCE!

RAY.

4

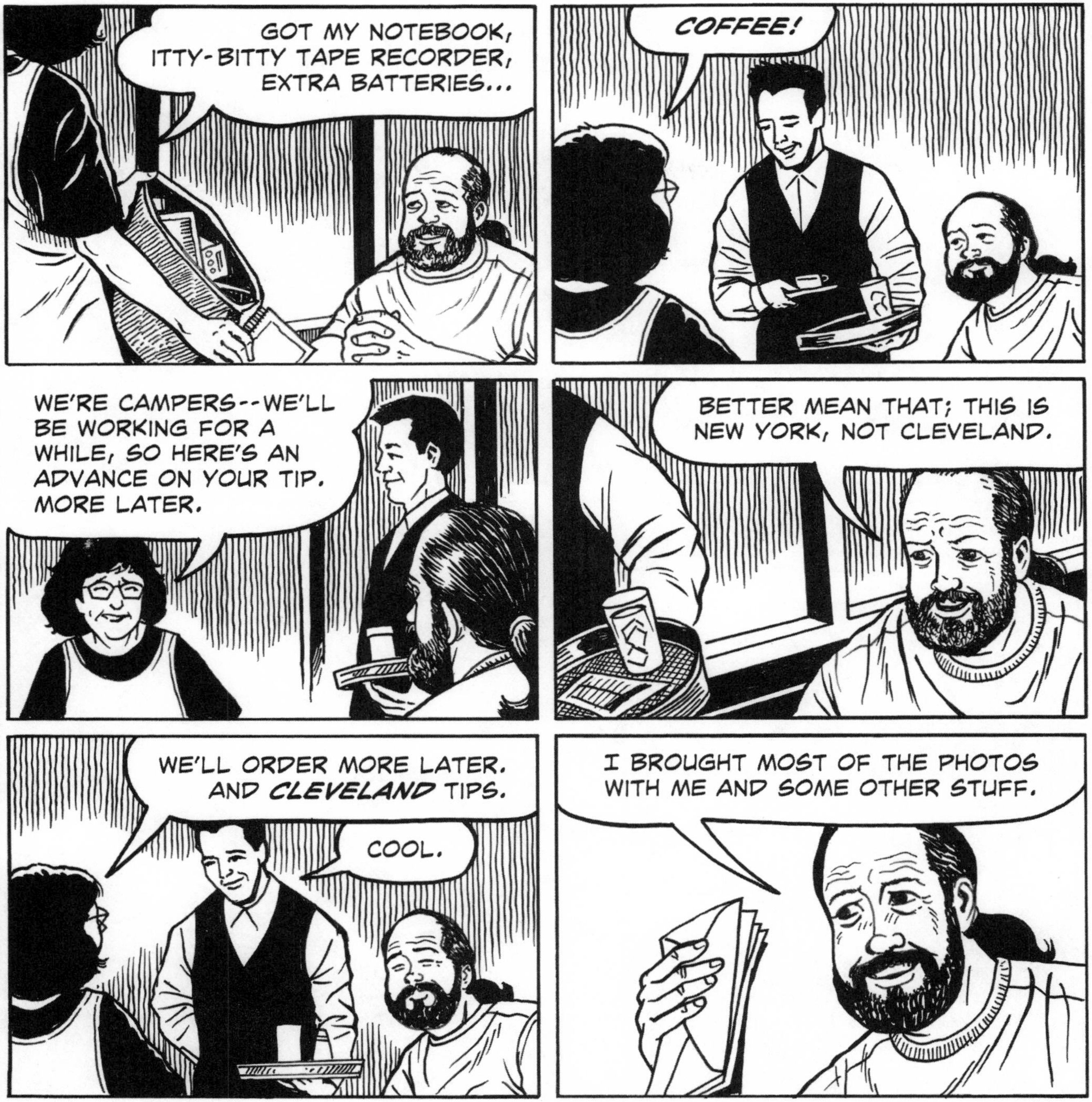
GOT MY NOTEBOOK, ITTY-BITTY TAPE RECORDER, EXTRA BATTERIES...
COFFEE!
WE'RE CAMPERS--WE'LL BE WORKING FOR A WHILE, SO HERE'S AN ADVANCE ON YOUR TIP. MORE LATER.
BETTER MEAN THAT; THIS IS NEW YORK, NOT CLEVELAND.
WE'LL ORDER MORE LATER. AND CLEVELAND TIPS.
COOL.
I BROUGHT MOST OF THE PHOTOS WITH ME AND SOME OTHER STUFF.

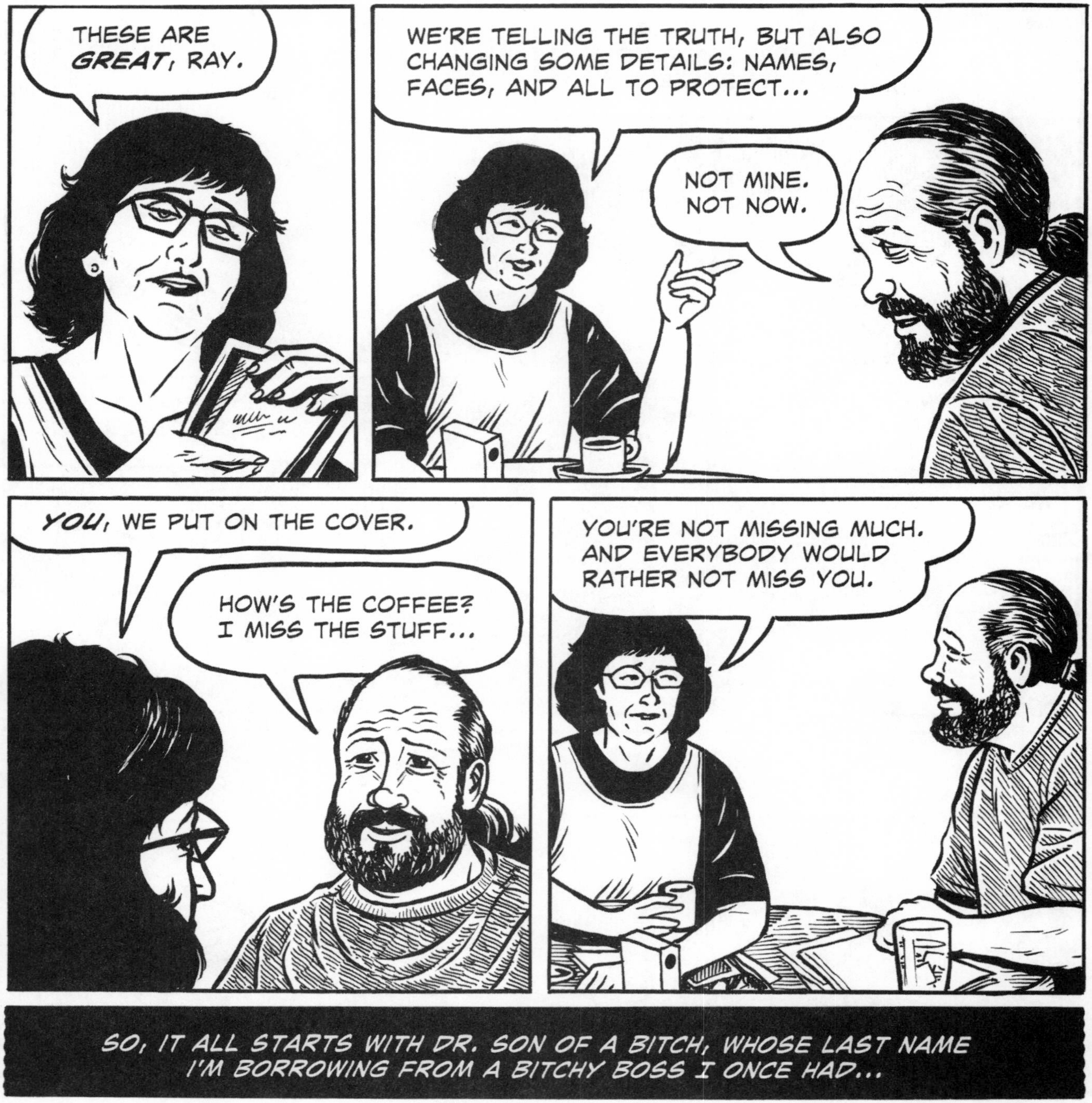
THESE ARE GREAT, RAY.
WE'RE TELLING THE TRUTH, BUT ALSO CHANGING SOME DETAILS: NAMES, FACES, AND ALL TO PROTECT...
NOT MINE. NOT NOW.
YOU, WE PUT ON THE COVER.
HOW'S THE COFFEE? I MISS THE STUFF...
YOU'RE NOT MISSING MUCH. AND EVERYBODY WOULD RATHER NOT MISS YOU.
SO, IT ALL STARTS WITH DR. SON OF A BITCH, WHOSE LAST NAME I'M BORROWING FROM A BITCHY BOSS I ONCE HAD...

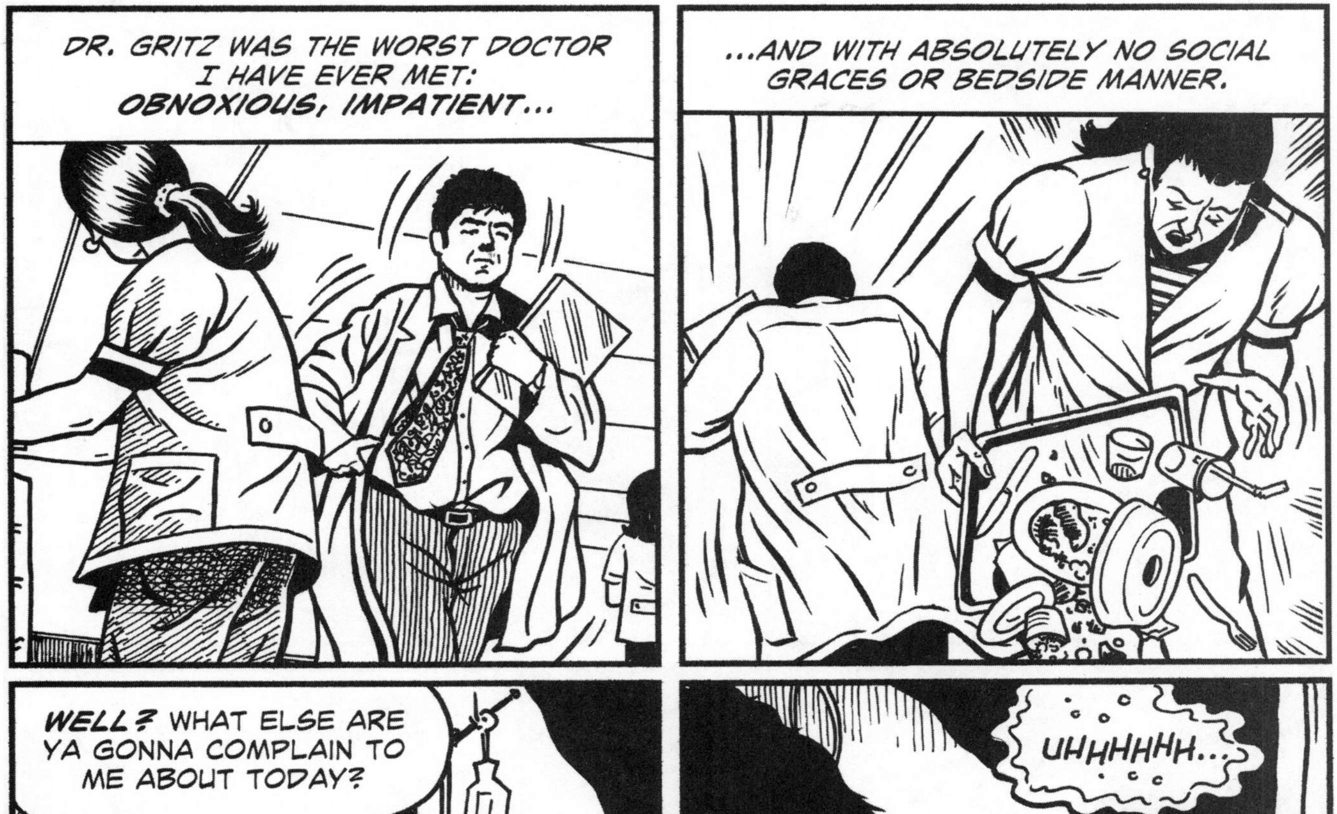
DR. GRITZ WAS THE WORST DOCTOR I HAVE EVER MET: OBNOXIOUS, IMPATIENT...
...AND WITH ABSOLUTELY NO SOCIAL GRACES OR BEDSIDE MANNER.
WELL? WHAT ELSE ARE YA GONNA COMPLAIN TO ME ABOUT TODAY?
UHHHHHH...

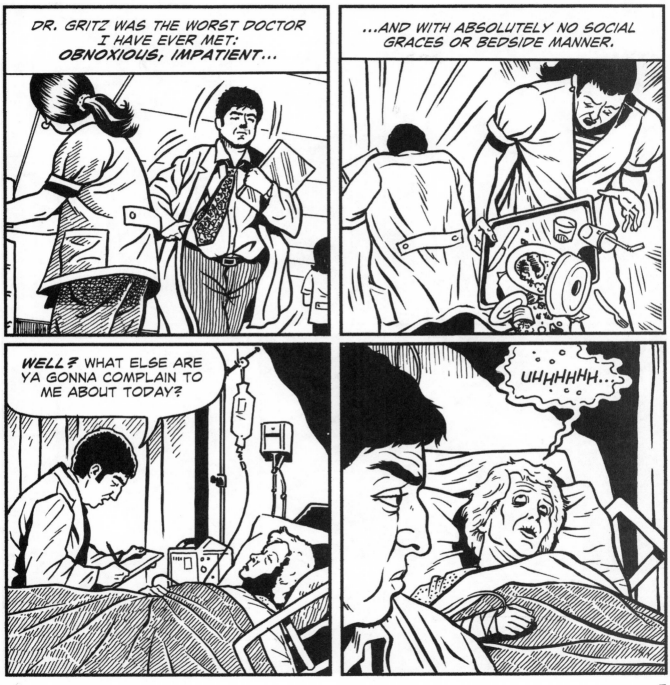

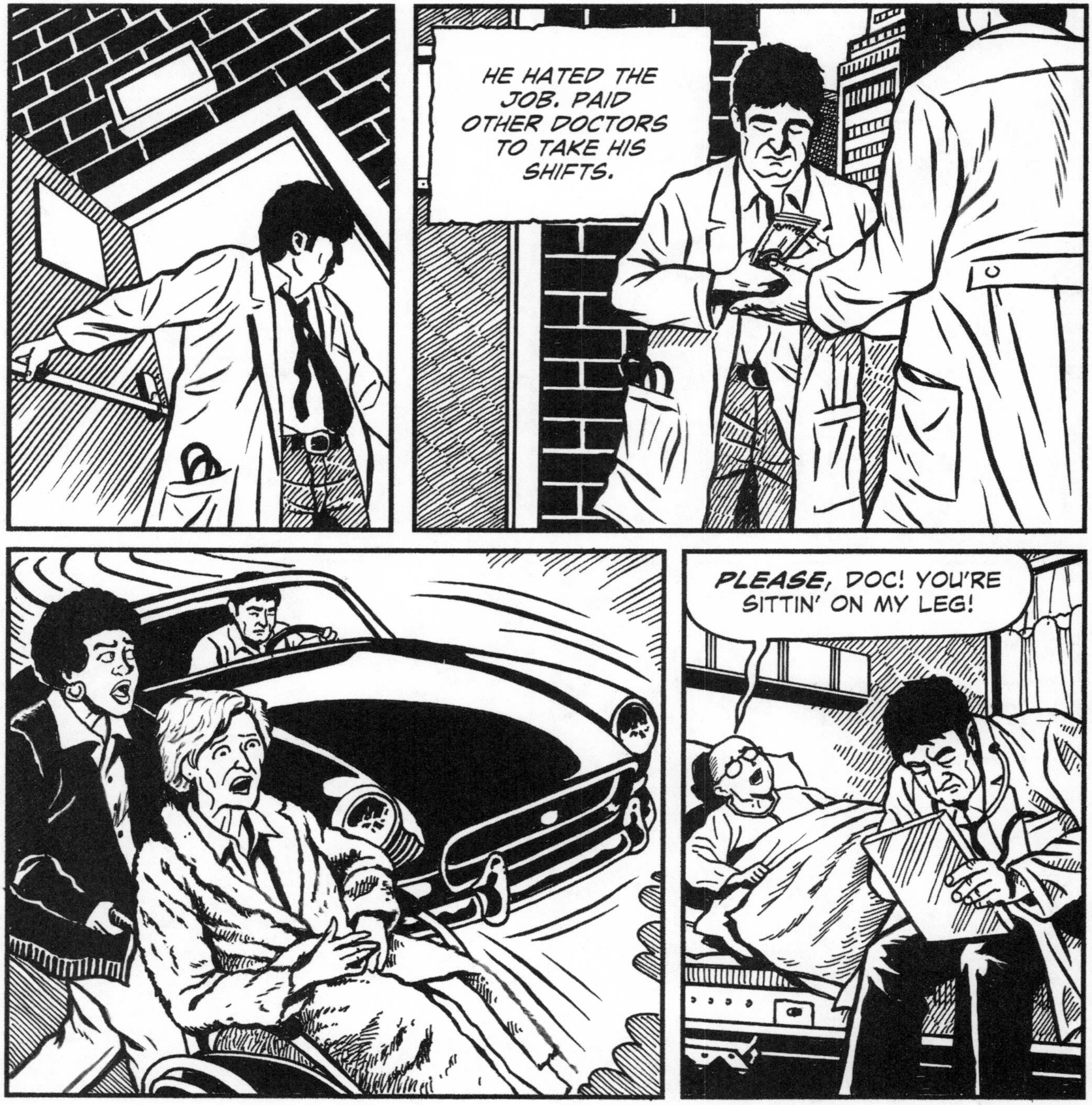
HE HATED THE JOB. PAID OTHER DOCTORS TO TAKE HIS SHIFTS.
PLEASE, DOC! YOU'RE SITTIN' ON MY LEG!

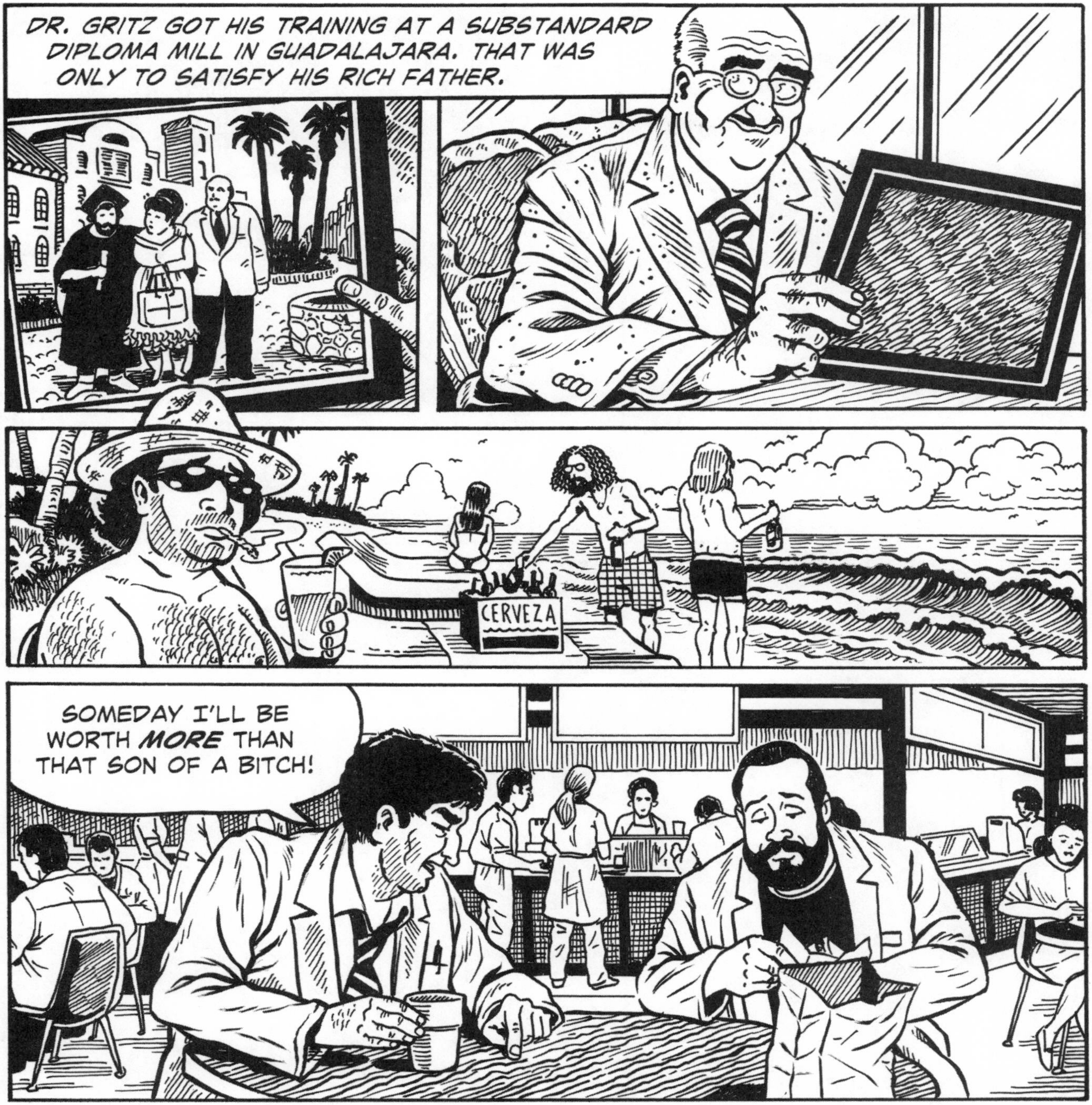
DR. GRITZ GOT HIS TRAINING AT A SUBSTANDARD DIPLOMA MILL IN GUADALAJARA. THAT WAS ONLY TO SATISFY HIS RICH FATHER.
CERVEZA
SOMEDAY I'LL BE WORTH *MORE* THAN THAT SON OF A BITCH!

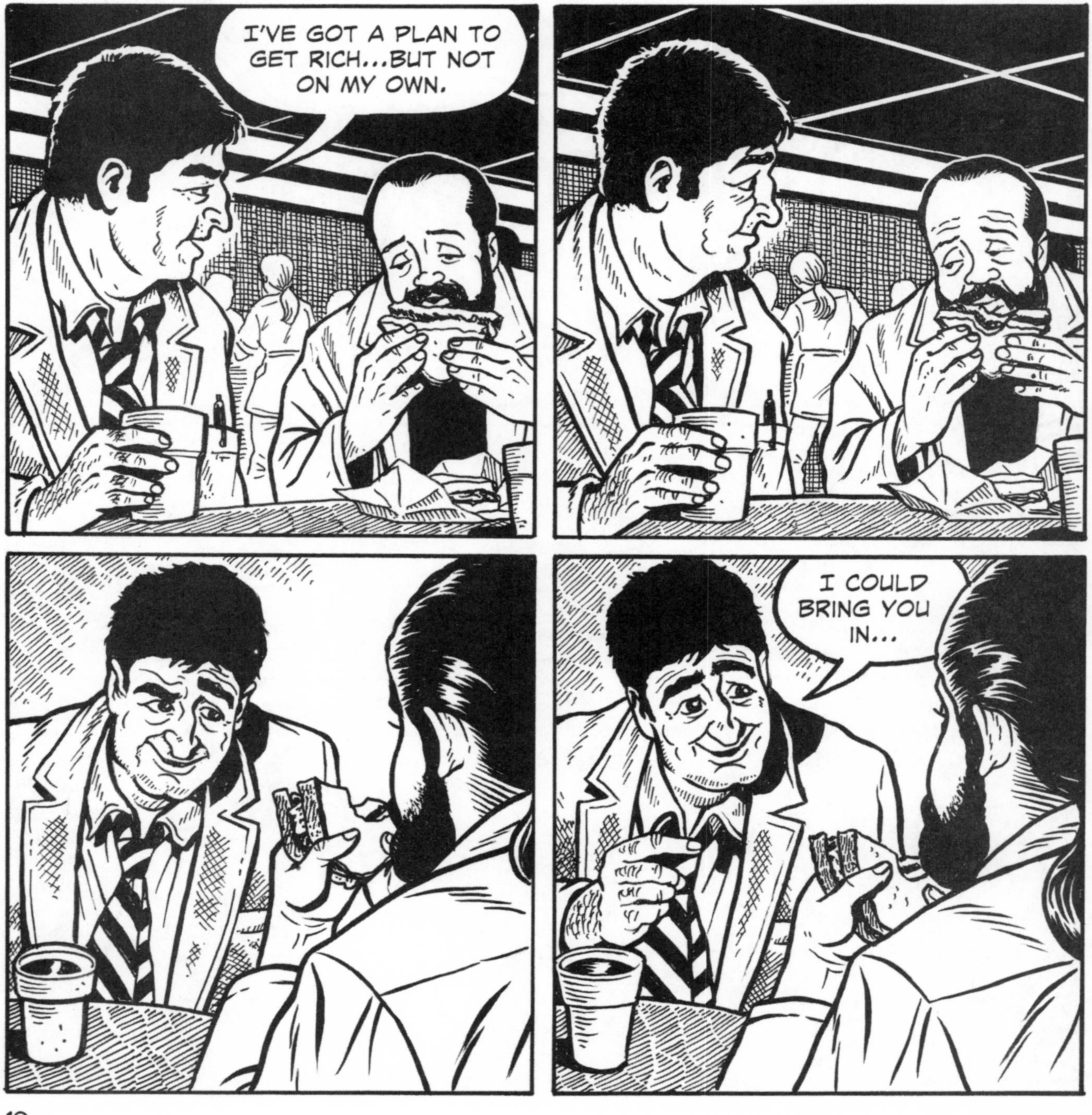
I'VE GOT A PLAN TO GET RICH...BUT NOT ON MY OWN.
I COULD BRING YOU IN...

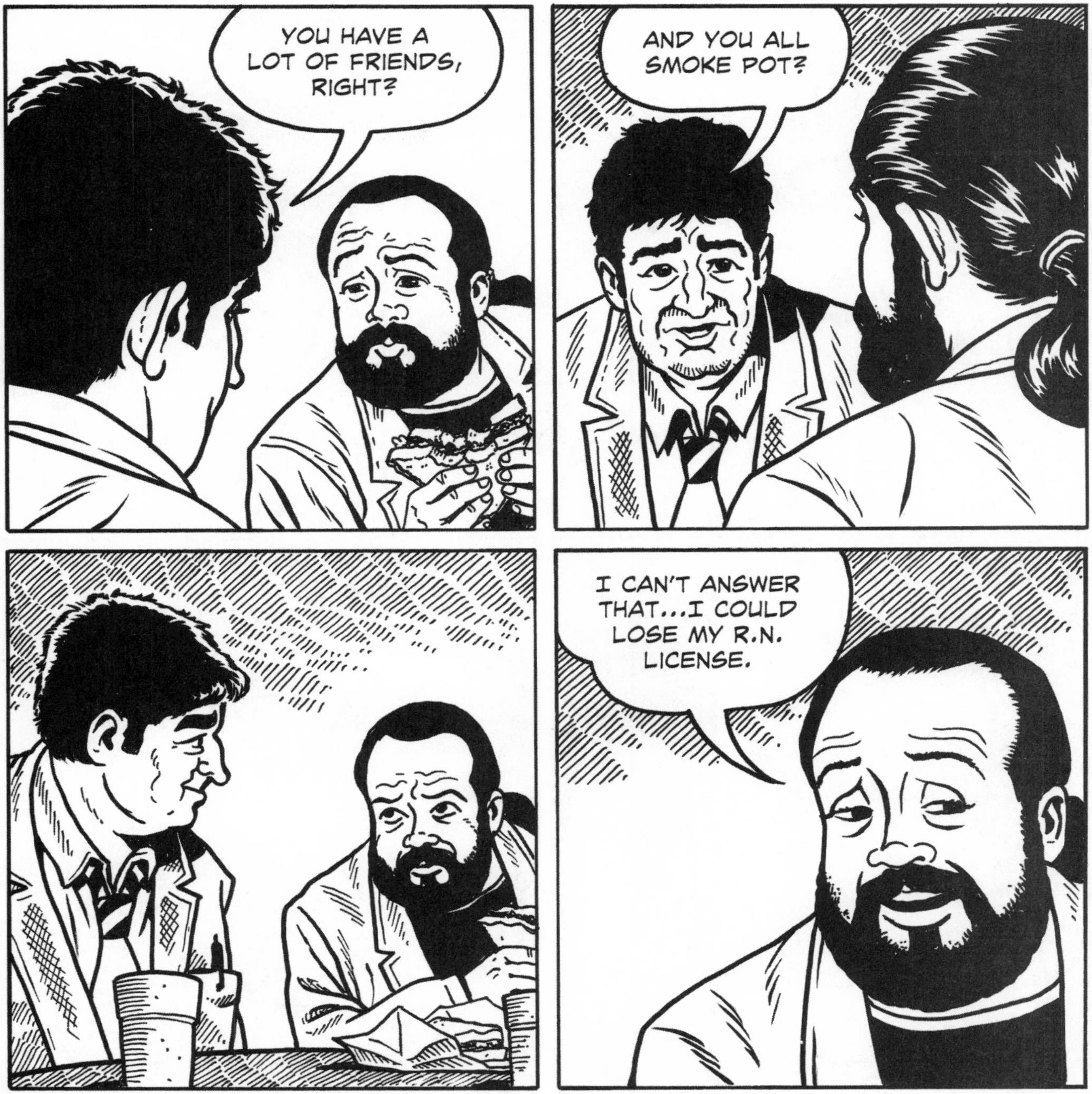
YOU HAVE A LOT OF FRIENDS, RIGHT?
AND YOU ALL SMOKE POT?
I CAN'T ANSWER THAT...I COULD LOSE MY R.N. LICENSE.

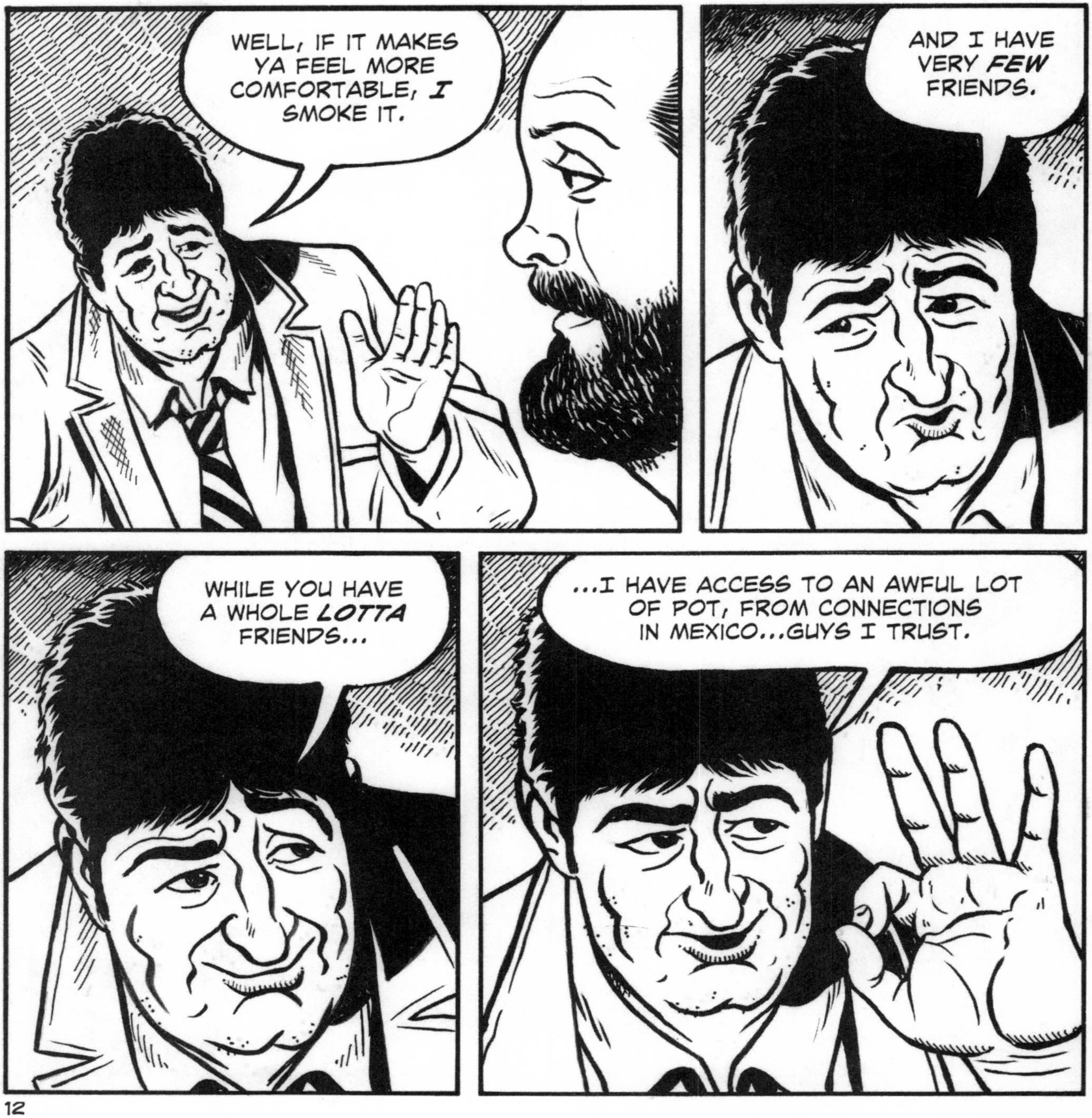
WELL, IF IT MAKES YA FEEL MORE COMFORTABLE, *I* SMOKE IT.
AND I HAVE VERY *FEW* FRIENDS.
WHILE YOU HAVE A WHOLE *LOTTA* FRIENDS...
...I HAVE ACCESS TO AN AWFUL LOT OF POT, FROM CONNECTIONS IN MEXICO...GUYS I TRUST.

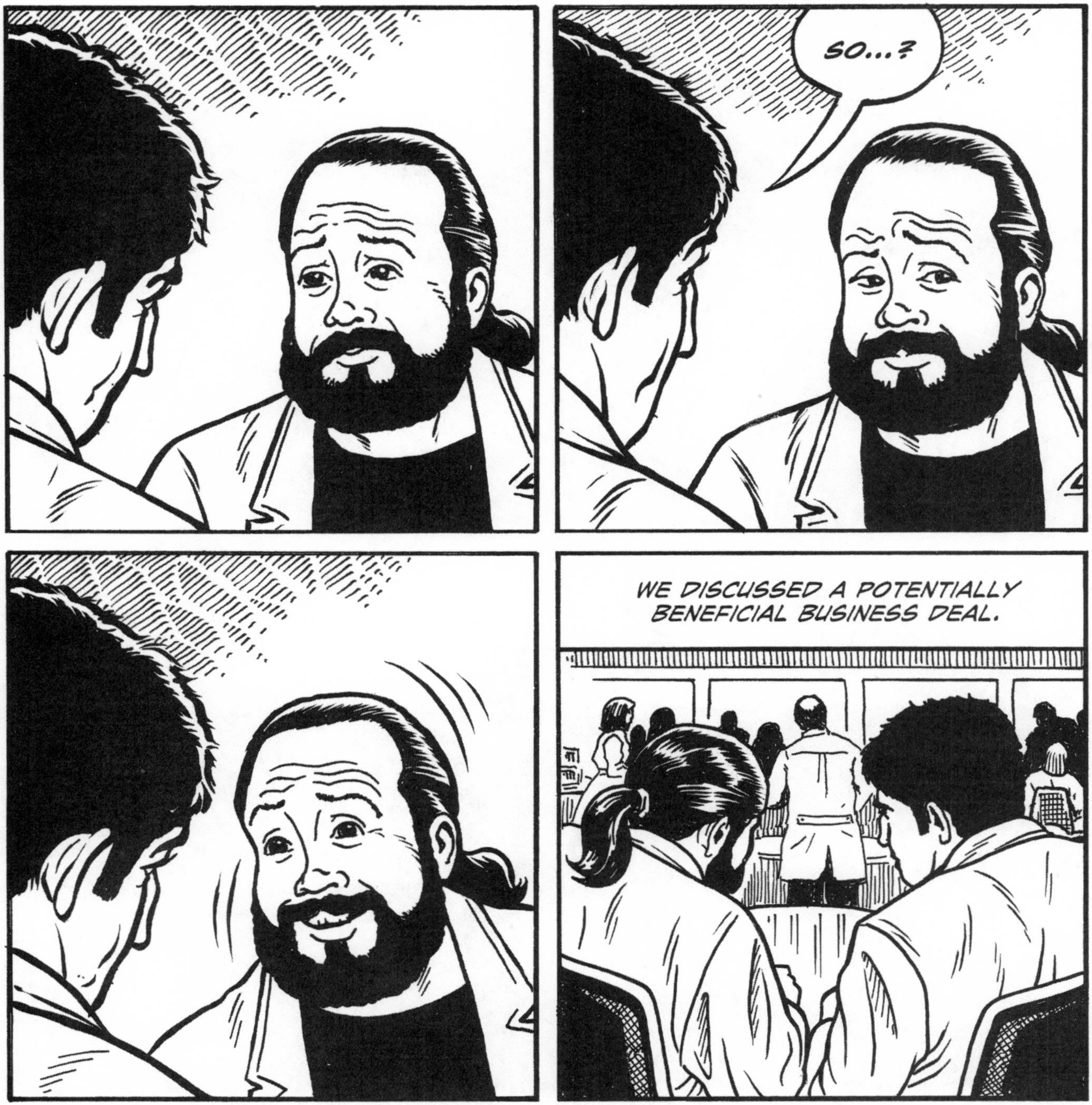
SO...?
WE DISCUSSED A POTENTIALLY BENEFICIAL BUSINESS DEAL.

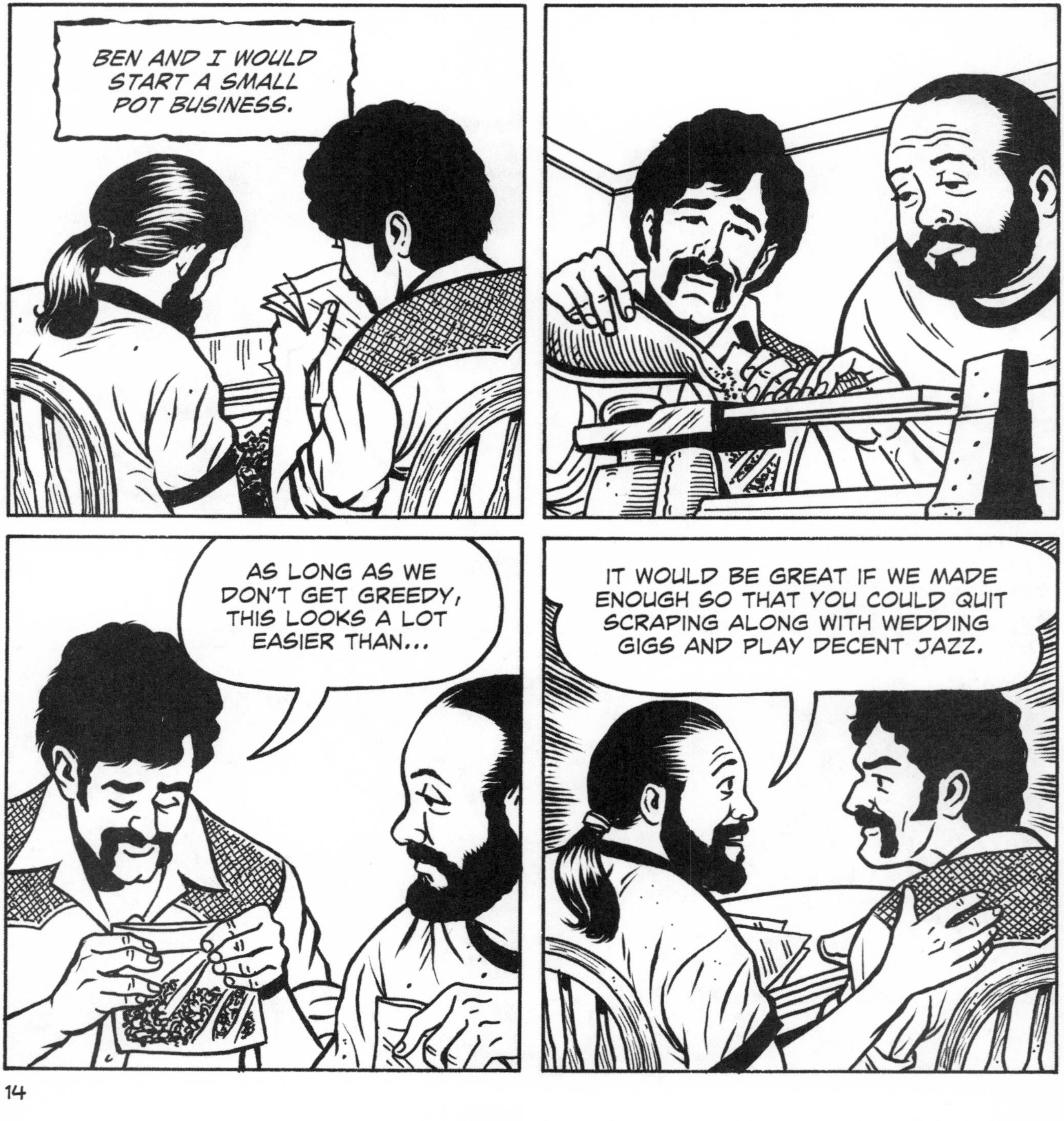
BEN AND I WOULD START A SMALL POT BUSINESS.
AS LONG AS WE DON'T GET GREEDY, THIS LOOKS A LOT EASIER THAN...
IT WOULD BE GREAT IF WE MADE ENOUGH SO THAT YOU COULD QUIT SCRAPING ALONG WITH WEDDING GIGS AND PLAY DECENT JAZZ.

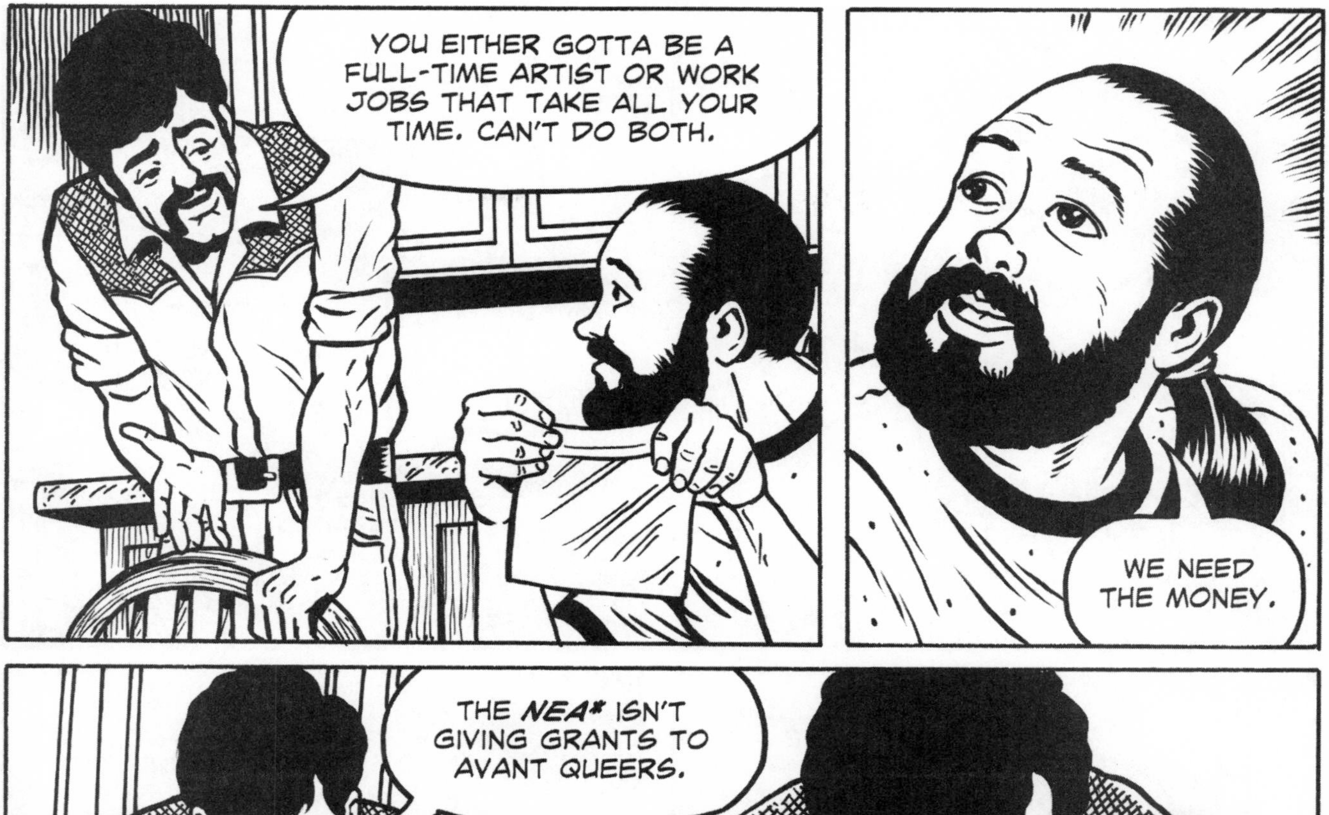

YOU EITHER GOTTA BE A FULL-TIME ARTIST OR WORK JOBS THAT TAKE ALL YOUR TIME. CAN'T DO BOTH.
WE NEED THE MONEY.
THE *NEA** ISN'T GIVING GRANTS TO AVANT QUEERS.
*NATIONAL ENDOWMENT FOR THE ARTS.
BE SERIOUS FOR A MINUTE. WHAT IF WE GET BUSTED?

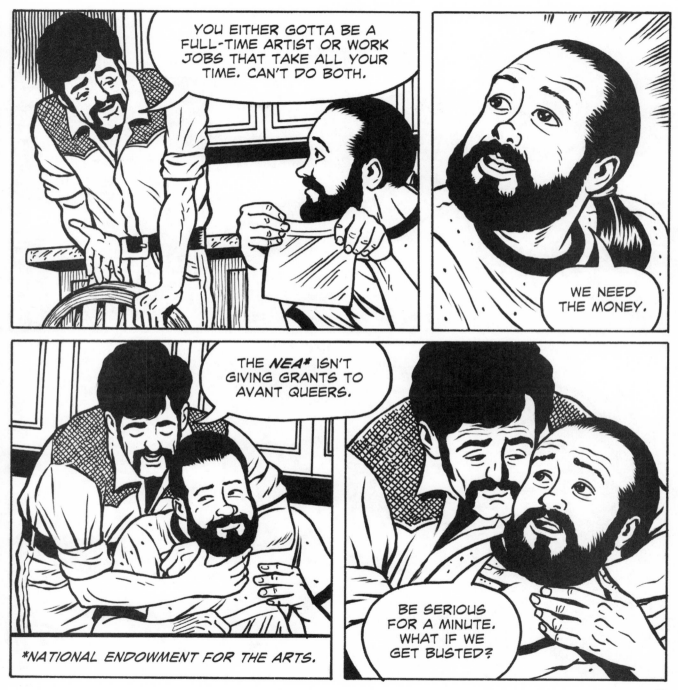

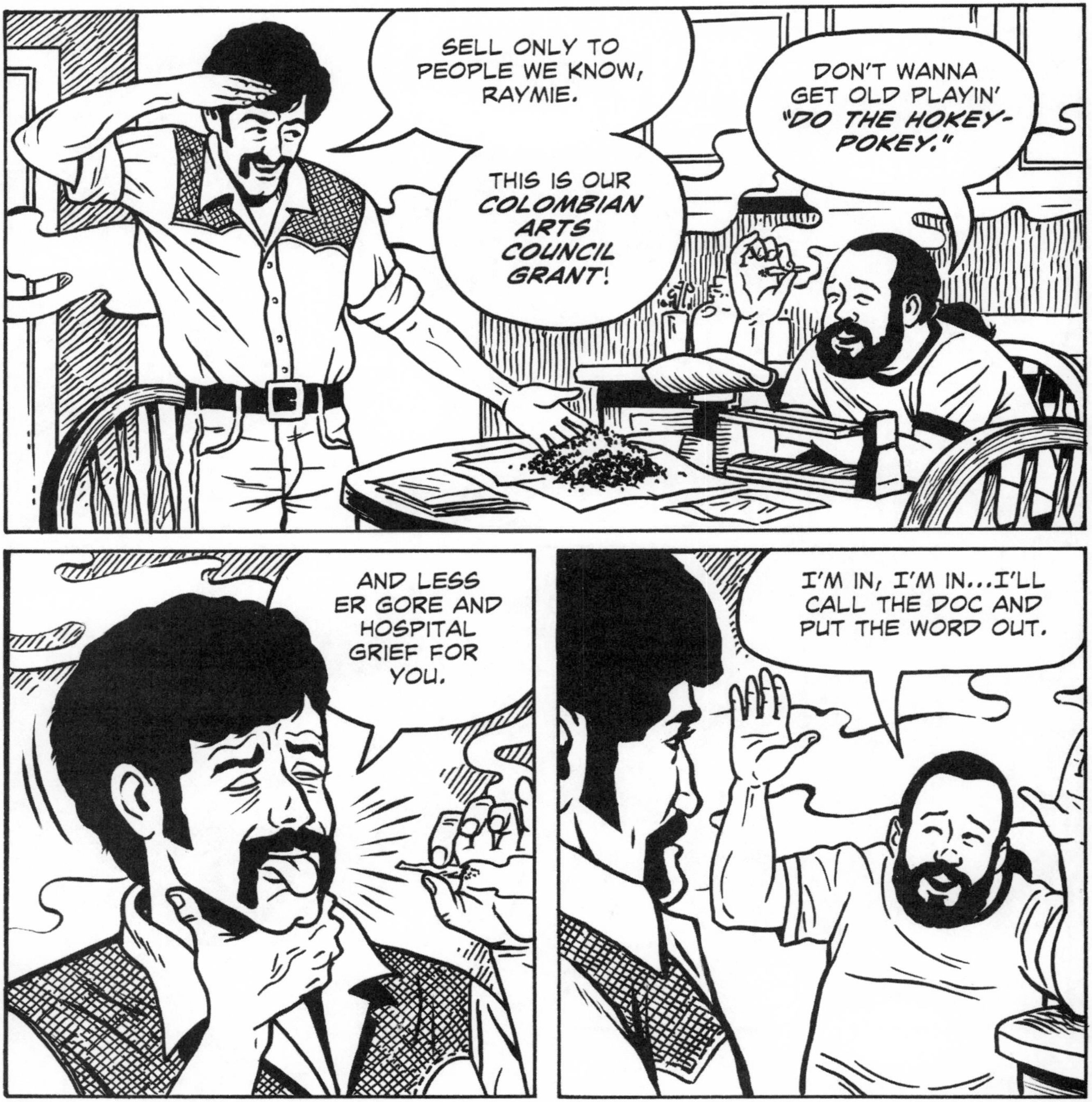
SELL ONLY TO PEOPLE WE KNOW, RAYMIE.
THIS IS OUR *COLOMBIAN ARTS COUNCIL GRANT*!
DON'T WANNA GET OLD PLAYIN' *"DO THE HOKEY-POKEY."*
AND LESS ER GORE AND HOSPITAL GRIEF FOR YOU.
I'M IN, I'M IN...I'LL CALL THE DOC AND PUT THE WORD OUT.

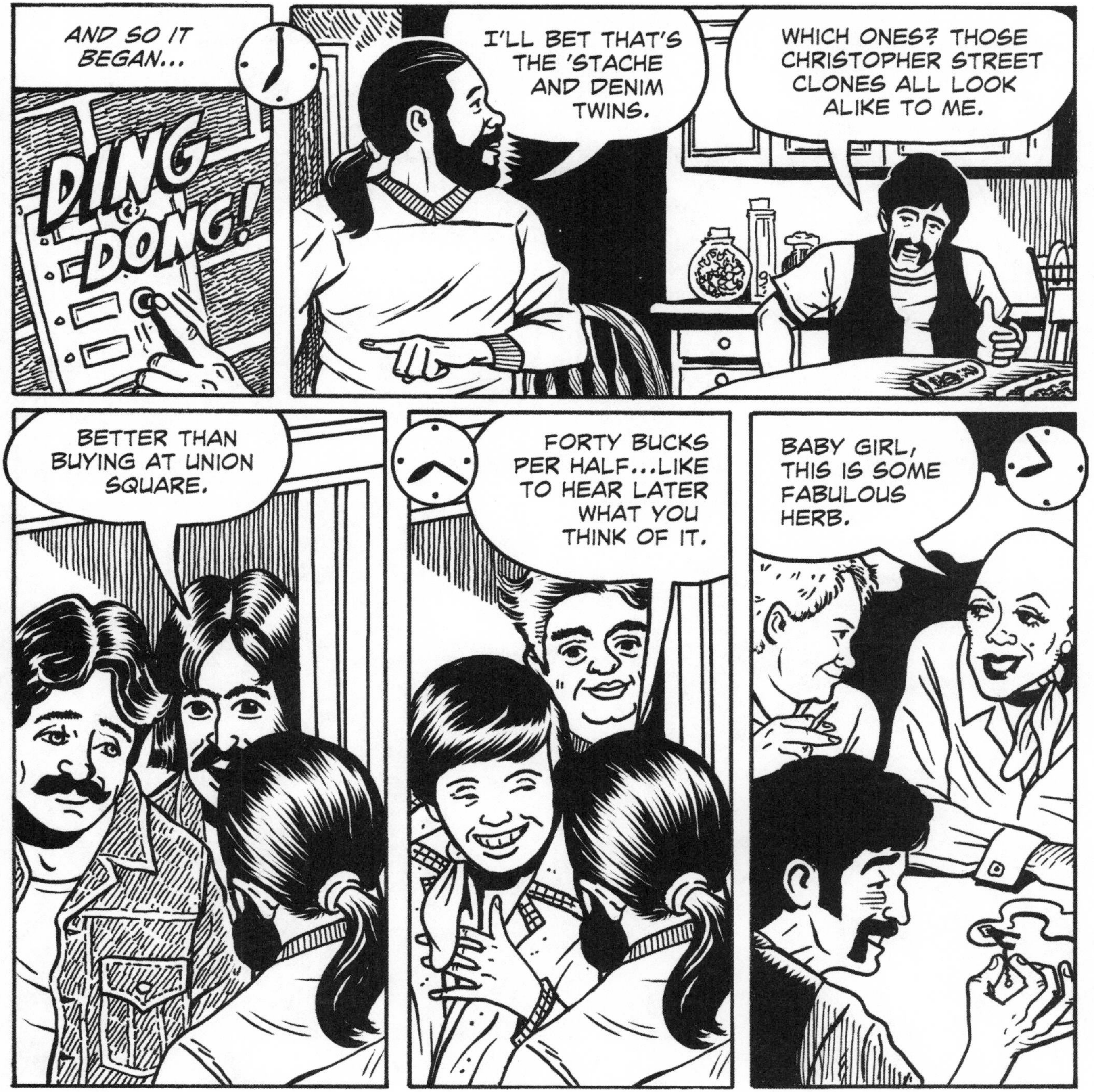
AND SO IT BEGAN...
DING DONG!
I'LL BET THAT'S THE 'STACHE AND DENIM TWINS.
WHICH ONES? THOSE CHRISTOPHER STREET CLONES ALL LOOK ALIKE TO ME.
BETTER THAN BUYING AT UNION SQUARE.
FORTY BUCKS PER HALF...LIKE TO HEAR LATER WHAT YOU THINK OF IT.
BABY GIRL, THIS IS SOME FABULOUS HERB.

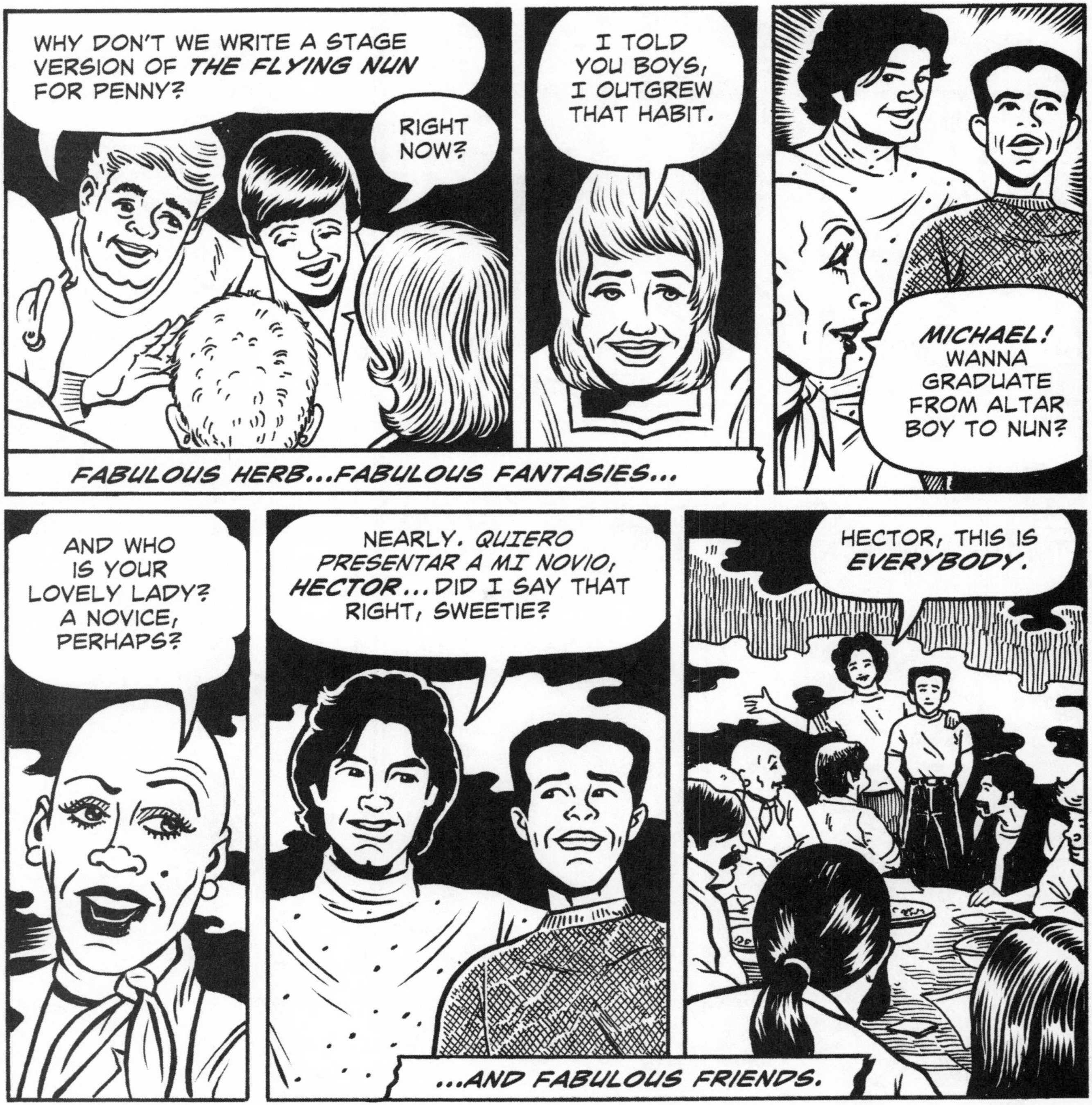
WHY DON'T WE WRITE A STAGE VERSION OF *THE FLYING NUN* FOR PENNY?
RIGHT NOW?
I TOLD YOU BOYS, I OUTGREW THAT HABIT.
FABULOUS HERB...FABULOUS FANTASIES...
MICHAEL! WANNA GRADUATE FROM ALTAR BOY TO NUN?
AND WHO IS YOUR LOVELY LADY? A NOVICE, PERHAPS?
NEARLY. *QUIERO PRESENTAR A MI NOVIO, HECTOR*... DID I SAY THAT RIGHT, SWEETIE?
HECTOR, THIS IS *EVERYBODY.*
...AND FABULOUS FRIENDS.

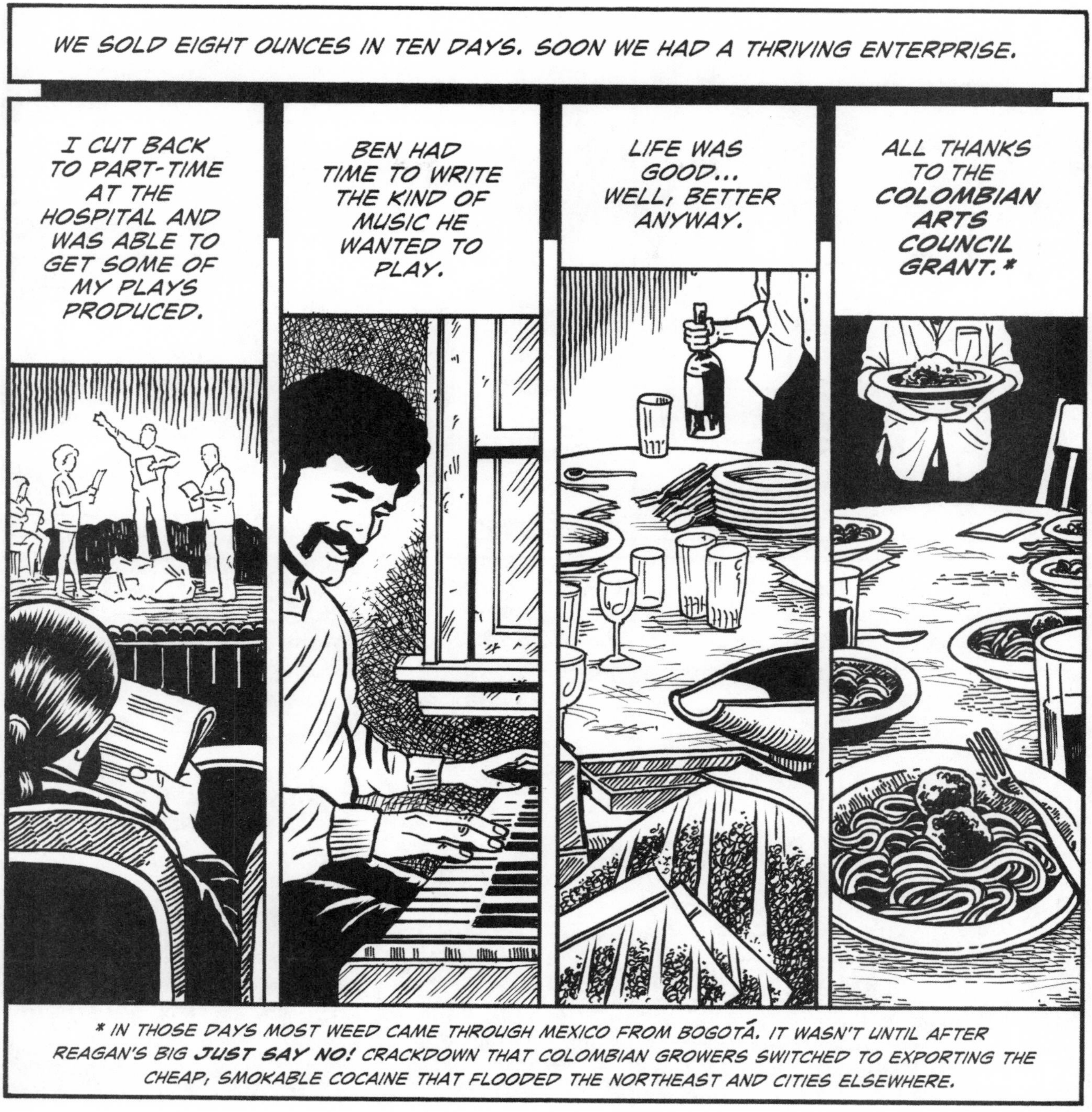
WE SOLD EIGHT OUNCES IN TEN DAYS. SOON WE HAD A THRIVING ENTERPRISE.
I CUT BACK TO PART-TIME AT THE HOSPITAL AND WAS ABLE TO GET SOME OF MY PLAYS PRODUCED.
BEN HAD TIME TO WRITE THE KIND OF MUSIC HE WANTED TO PLAY.
LIFE WAS GOOD... WELL, BETTER ANYWAY.
ALL THANKS TO THE COLOMBIAN ARTS COUNCIL GRANT.*
* IN THOSE DAYS MOST WEED CAME THROUGH MEXICO FROM BOGOTÁ. IT WASN'T UNTIL AFTER REAGAN'S BIG JUST SAY NO! CRACKDOWN THAT COLOMBIAN GROWERS SWITCHED TO EXPORTING THE CHEAP, SMOKABLE COCAINE THAT FLOODED THE NORTHEAST AND CITIES ELSEWHERE.

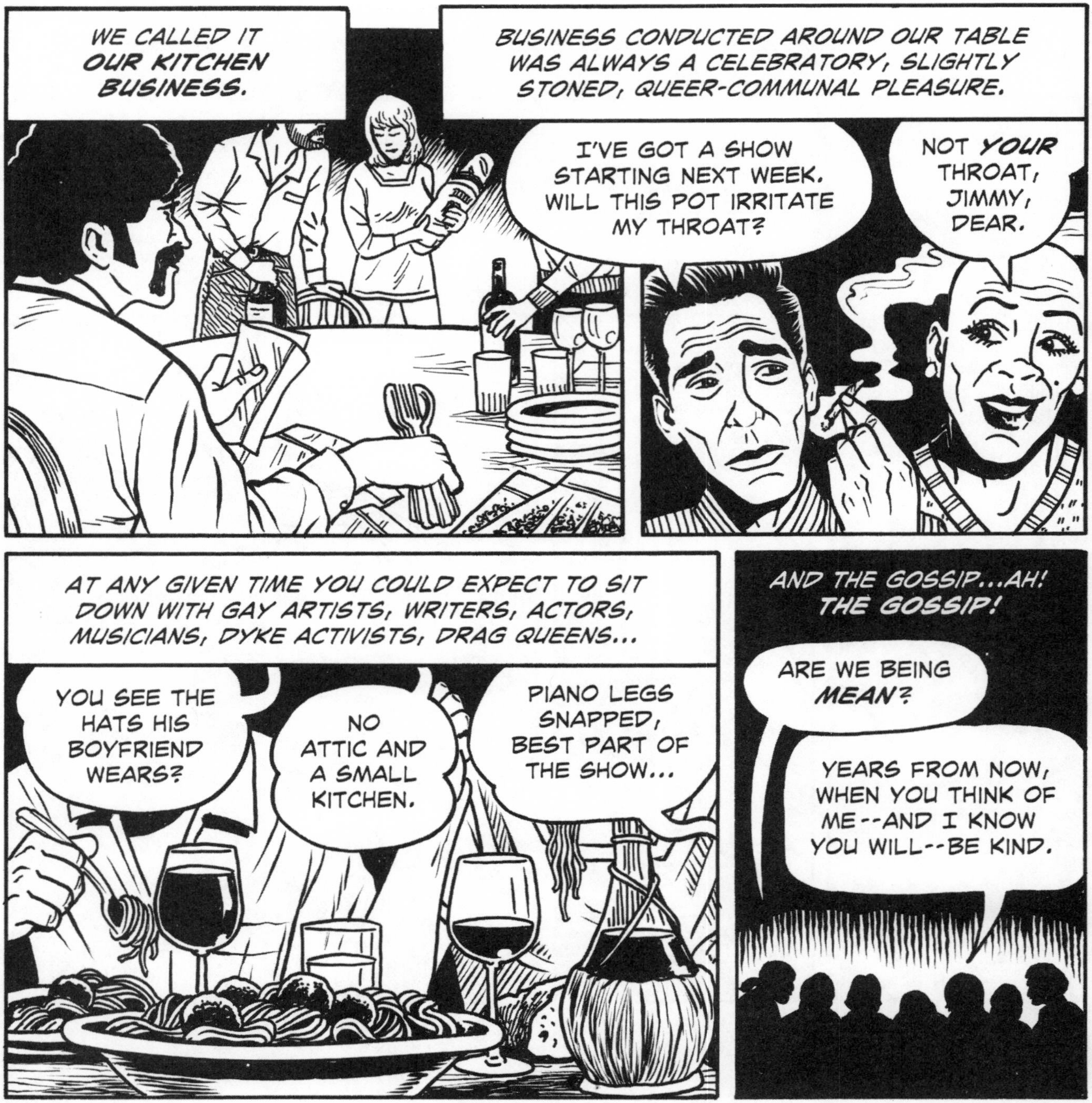
WE CALLED IT OUR KITCHEN BUSINESS.
BUSINESS CONDUCTED AROUND OUR TABLE WAS ALWAYS A CELEBRATORY, SLIGHTLY STONED, QUEER-COMMUNAL PLEASURE.
I'VE GOT A SHOW STARTING NEXT WEEK. WILL THIS POT IRRITATE MY THROAT?
NOT YOUR THROAT, JIMMY, DEAR.
AT ANY GIVEN TIME YOU COULD EXPECT TO SIT DOWN WITH GAY ARTISTS, WRITERS, ACTORS, MUSICIANS, DYKE ACTIVISTS, DRAG QUEENS...
YOU SEE THE HATS HIS BOYFRIEND WEARS?
NO ATTIC AND A SMALL KITCHEN.
PIANO LEGS SNAPPED, BEST PART OF THE SHOW...
AND THE GOSSIP...AH! THE GOSSIP!
ARE WE BEING MEAN?
YEARS FROM NOW, WHEN YOU THINK OF ME--AND I KNOW YOU WILL--BE KIND.

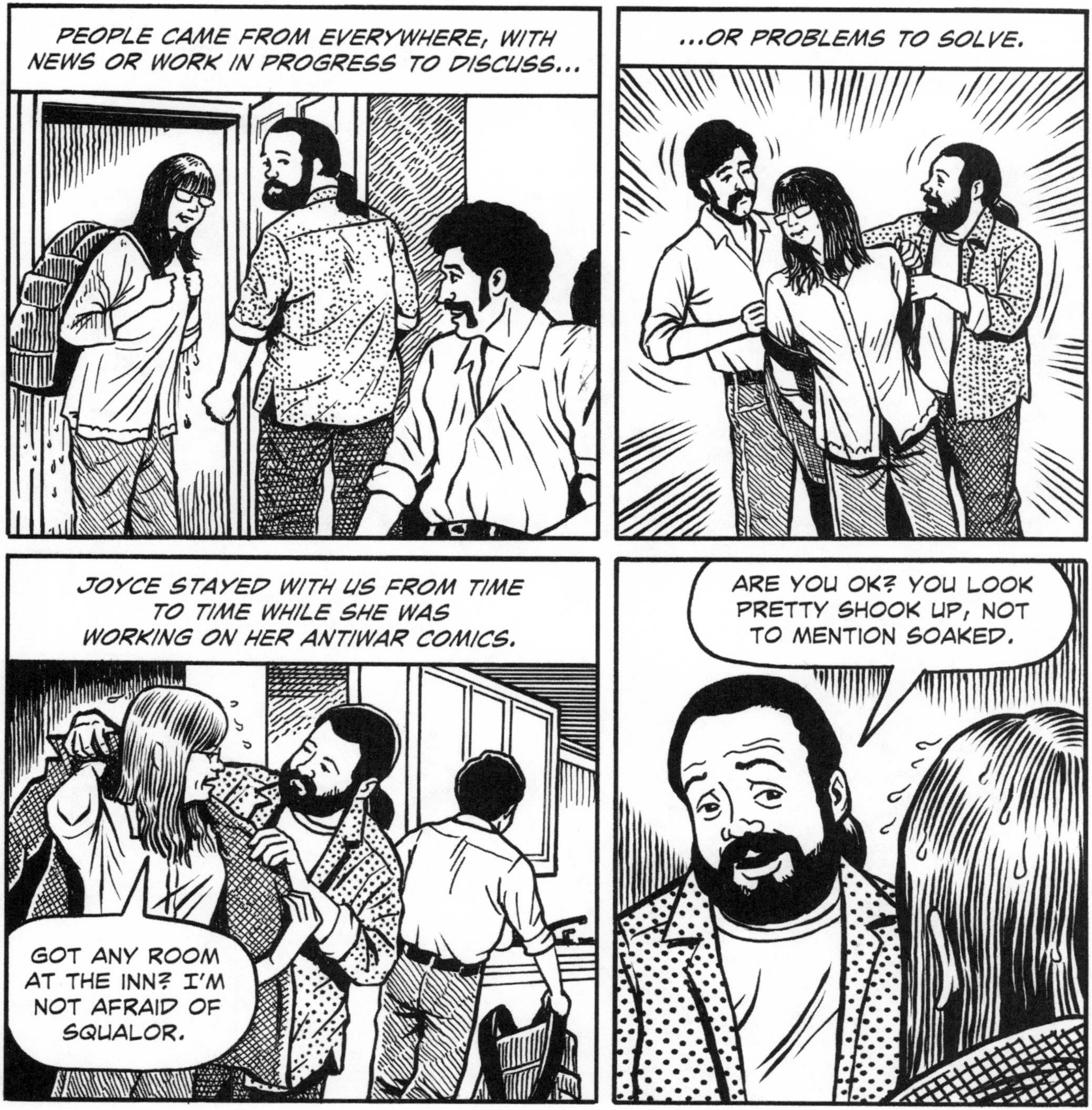
PEOPLE CAME FROM EVERYWHERE, WITH NEWS OR WORK IN PROGRESS TO DISCUSS...
...OR PROBLEMS TO SOLVE.
JOYCE STAYED WITH US FROM TIME TO TIME WHILE SHE WAS WORKING ON HER ANTIWAR COMICS.
GOT ANY ROOM AT THE INN? I'M NOT AFRAID OF SQUALOR.
ARE YOU OK? YOU LOOK PRETTY SHOOK UP, NOT TO MENTION SOAKED.

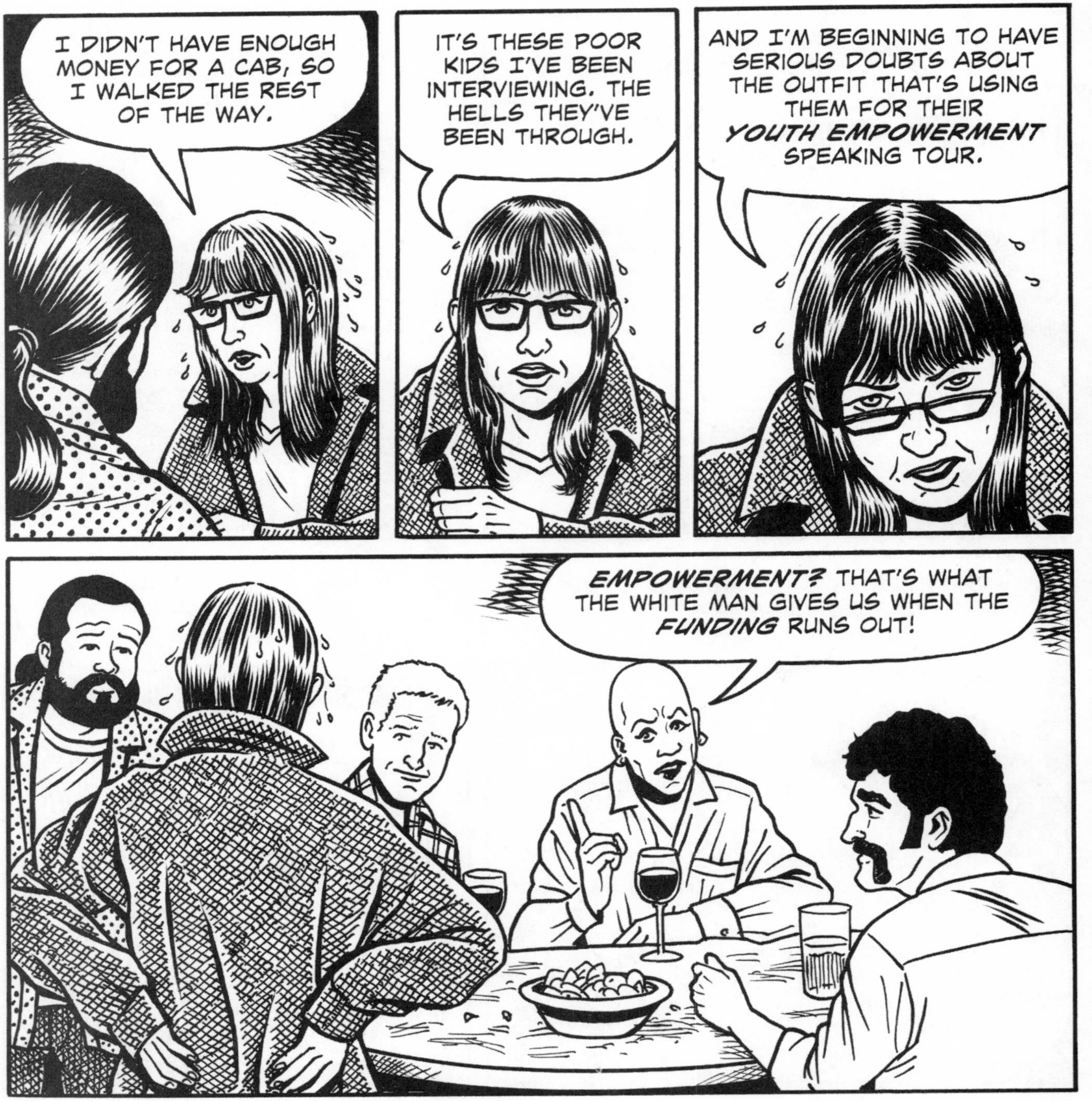
I DIDN'T HAVE ENOUGH MONEY FOR A CAB, SO I WALKED THE REST OF THE WAY.
IT'S THESE POOR KIDS I'VE BEEN INTERVIEWING. THE HELLS THEY'VE BEEN THROUGH.
AND I'M BEGINNING TO HAVE SERIOUS DOUBTS ABOUT THE OUTFIT THAT'S USING THEM FOR THEIR *YOUTH EMPOWERMENT* SPEAKING TOUR.
EMPOWERMENT? THAT'S WHAT THE WHITE MAN GIVES US WHEN THE *FUNDING* RUNS OUT!

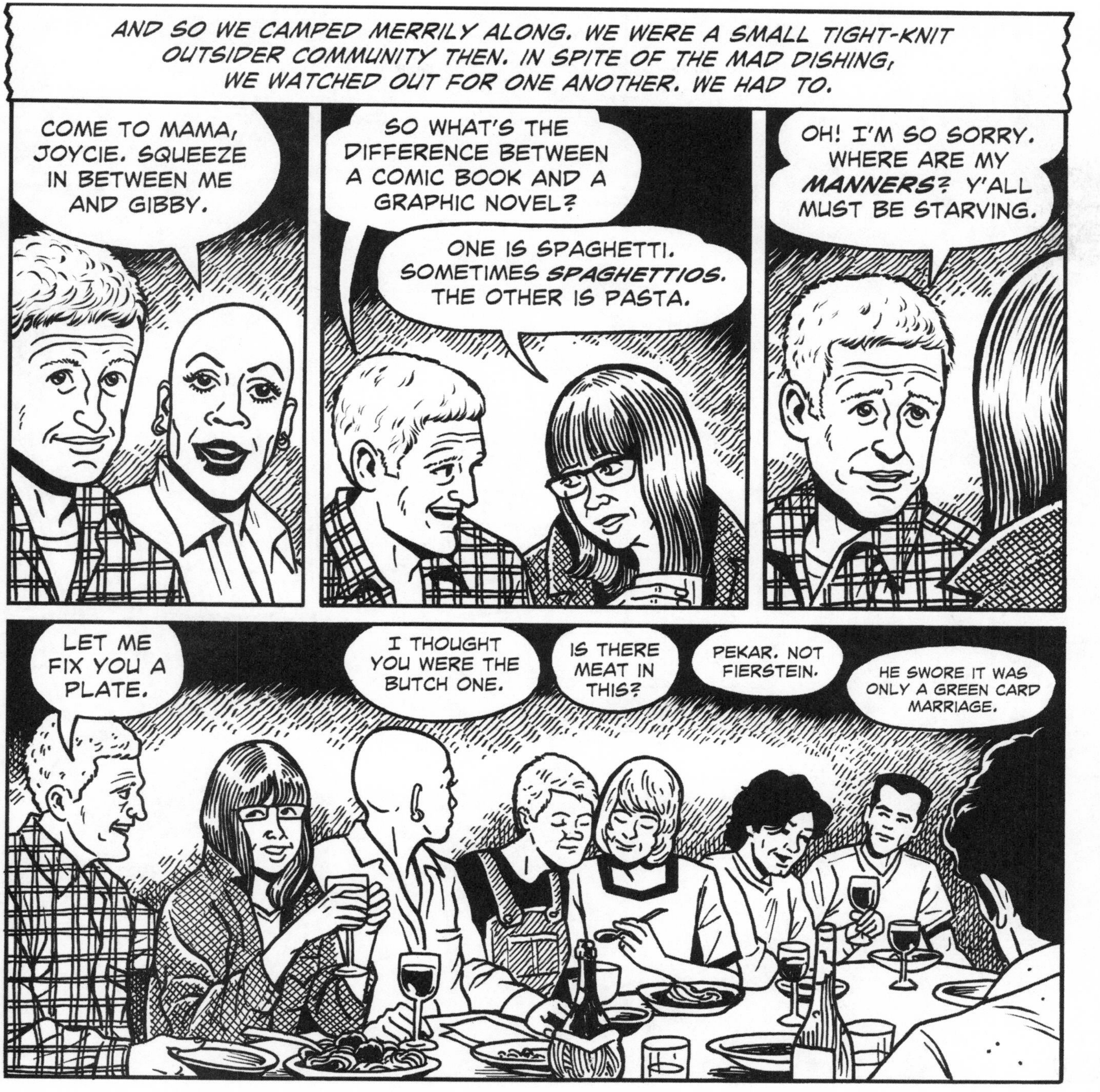
AND SO WE CAMPED MERRILY ALONG. WE WERE A SMALL TIGHT-KNIT OUTSIDER COMMUNITY THEN. IN SPITE OF THE MAD DISHING, WE WATCHED OUT FOR ONE ANOTHER. WE HAD TO.
COME TO MAMA, JOYCIE. SQUEEZE IN BETWEEN ME AND GIBBY.
SO WHAT'S THE DIFFERENCE BETWEEN A COMIC BOOK AND A GRAPHIC NOVEL?
ONE IS SPAGHETTI. SOMETIMES *SPAGHETTIOS*. THE OTHER IS PASTA.
OH! I'M SO SORRY. WHERE ARE MY ***MANNERS***? Y'ALL MUST BE STARVING.
LET ME FIX YOU A PLATE.
I THOUGHT YOU WERE THE BUTCH ONE.
IS THERE MEAT IN THIS?
PEKAR. NOT FIERSTEIN.
HE SWORE IT WAS ONLY A GREEN CARD MARRIAGE.

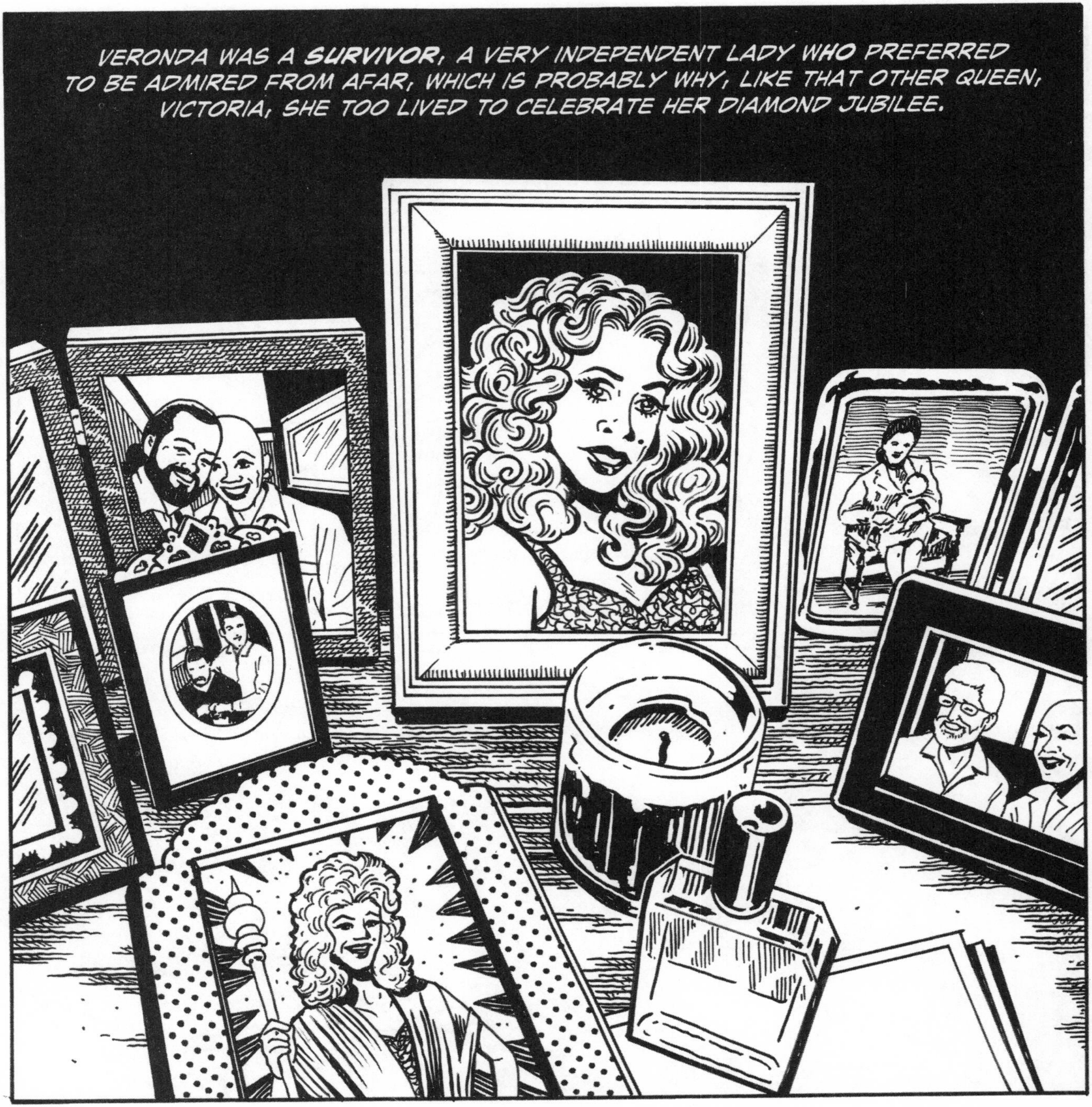
VERONDA WAS A **SURVIVOR**, A VERY INDEPENDENT LADY WHO PREFERRED TO BE ADMIRED FROM AFAR, WHICH IS PROBABLY WHY, LIKE THAT OTHER QUEEN, VICTORIA, SHE TOO LIVED TO CELEBRATE HER DIAMOND JUBILEE.

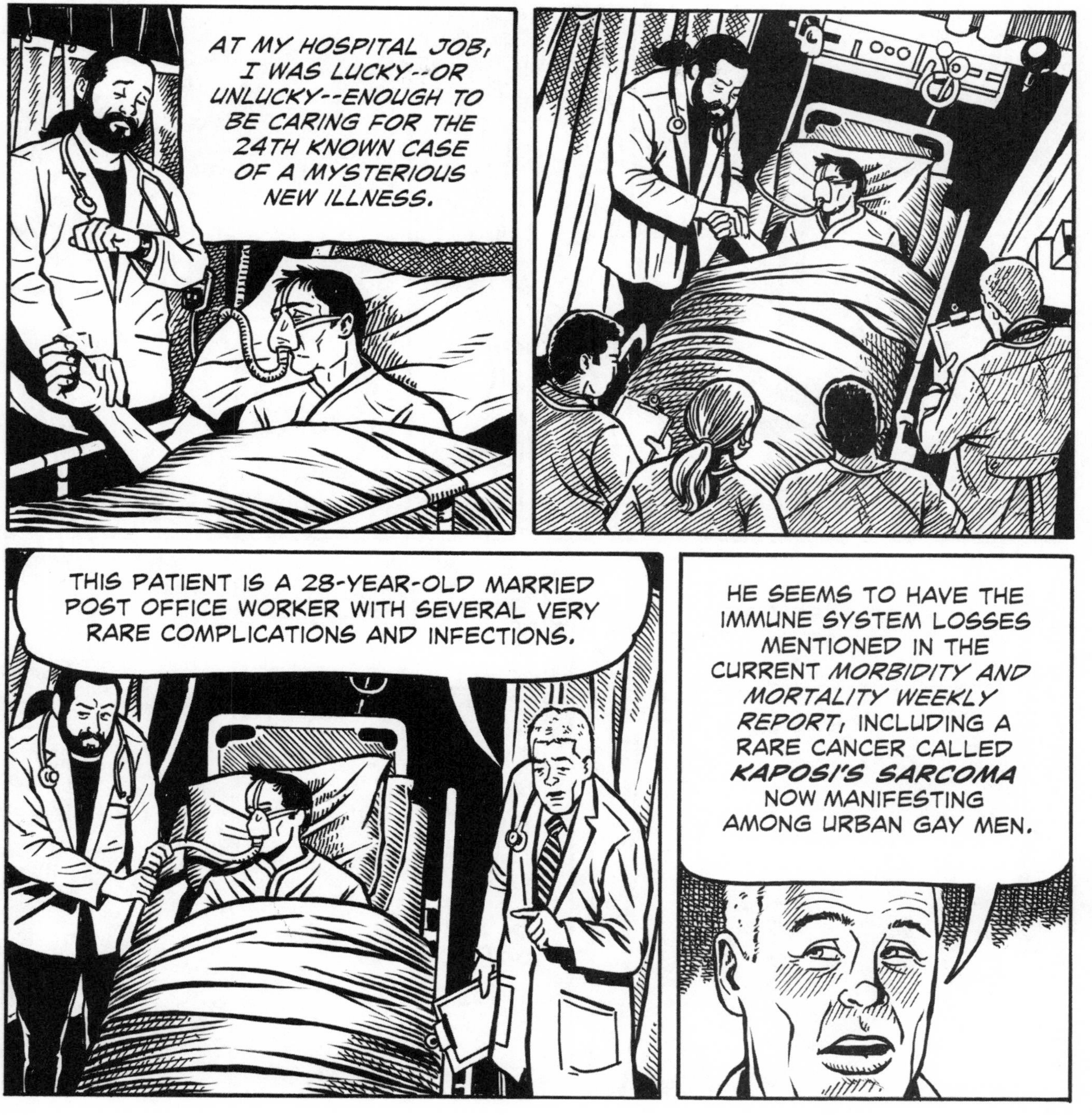
AT MY HOSPITAL JOB, I WAS LUCKY--OR UNLUCKY--ENOUGH TO BE CARING FOR THE 24TH KNOWN CASE OF A MYSTERIOUS NEW ILLNESS.
THIS PATIENT IS A 28-YEAR-OLD MARRIED POST OFFICE WORKER WITH SEVERAL VERY RARE COMPLICATIONS AND INFECTIONS.
HE SEEMS TO HAVE THE IMMUNE SYSTEM LOSSES MENTIONED IN THE CURRENT *MORBIDITY AND MORTALITY WEEKLY REPORT*, INCLUDING A RARE CANCER CALLED **KAPOSI'S SARCOMA** NOW MANIFESTING AMONG URBAN GAY MEN.

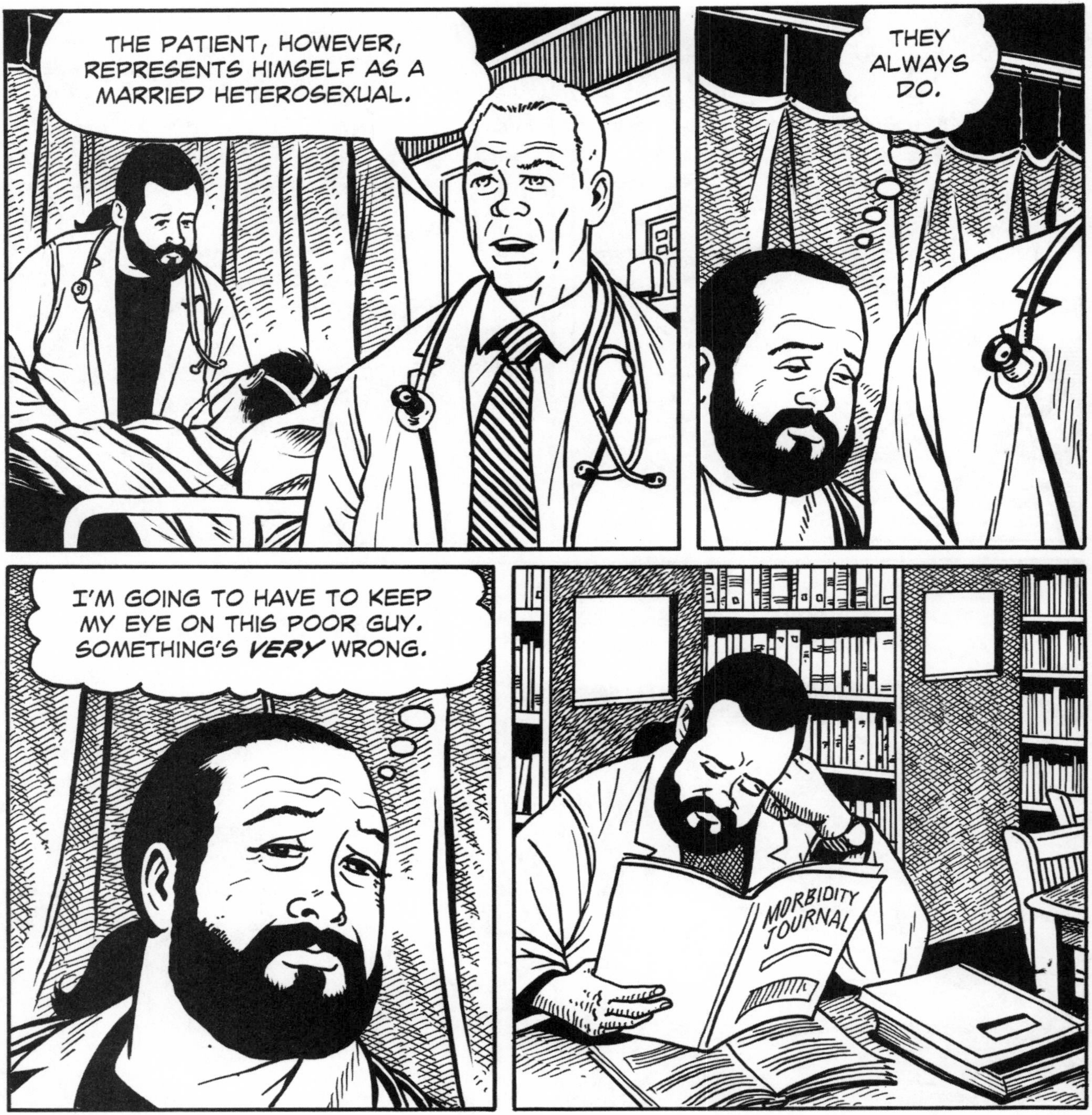
THE PATIENT, HOWEVER, REPRESENTS HIMSELF AS A MARRIED HETEROSEXUAL.
THEY ALWAYS DO.
I'M GOING TO HAVE TO KEEP MY EYE ON THIS POOR GUY. SOMETHING'S *VERY* WRONG.
MORBIDITY JOURNAL

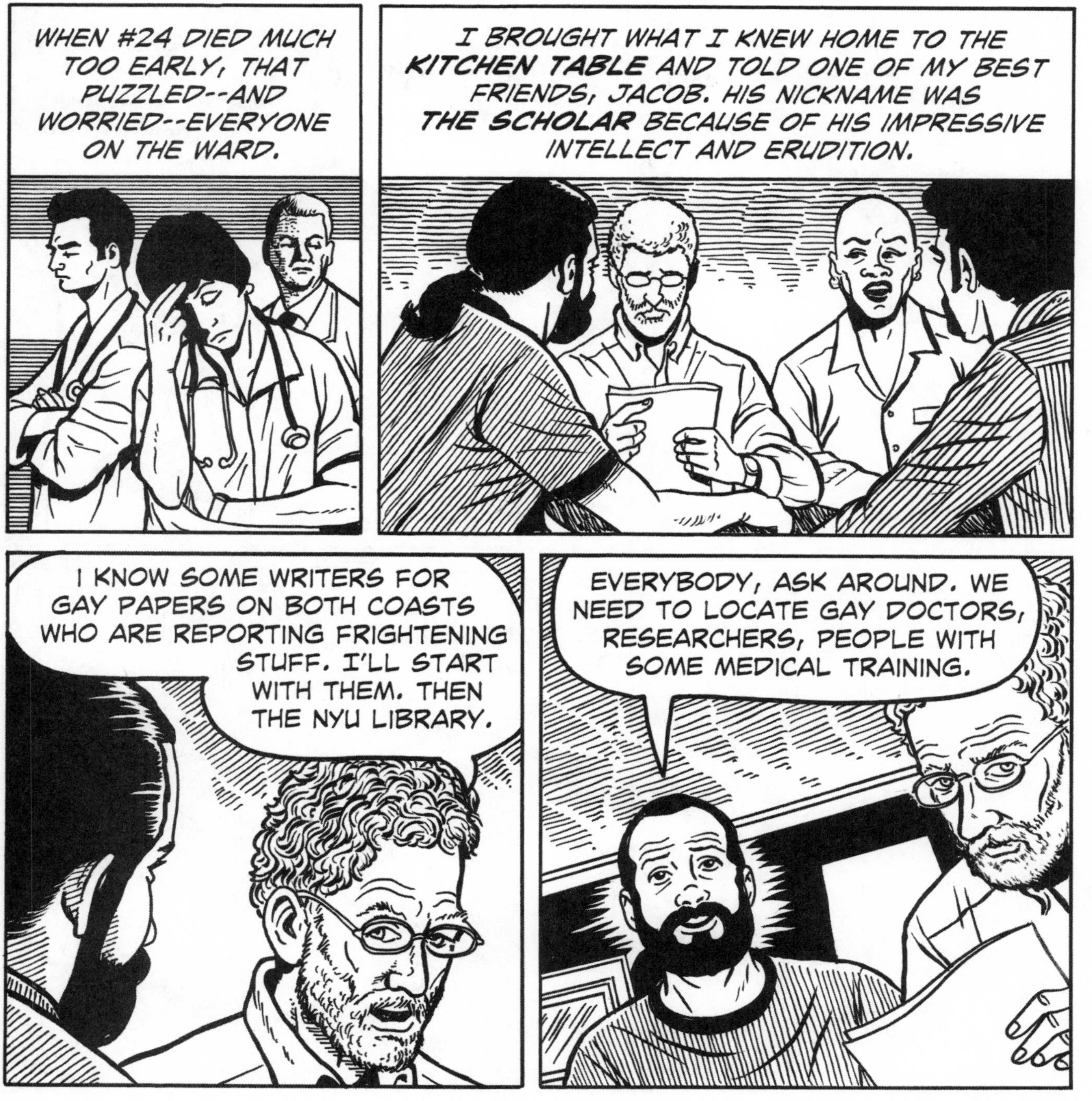

WHEN #24 DIED MUCH TOO EARLY, THAT PUZZLED--AND WORRIED--EVERYONE ON THE WARD.
I BROUGHT WHAT I KNEW HOME TO THE KITCHEN TABLE AND TOLD ONE OF MY BEST FRIENDS, JACOB. HIS NICKNAME WAS THE SCHOLAR BECAUSE OF HIS IMPRESSIVE INTELLECT AND ERUDITION.
I KNOW SOME WRITERS FOR GAY PAPERS ON BOTH COASTS WHO ARE REPORTING FRIGHTENING STUFF. I'LL START WITH THEM. THEN THE NYU LIBRARY.
EVERYBODY, ASK AROUND. WE NEED TO LOCATE GAY DOCTORS, RESEARCHERS, PEOPLE WITH SOME MEDICAL TRAINING.

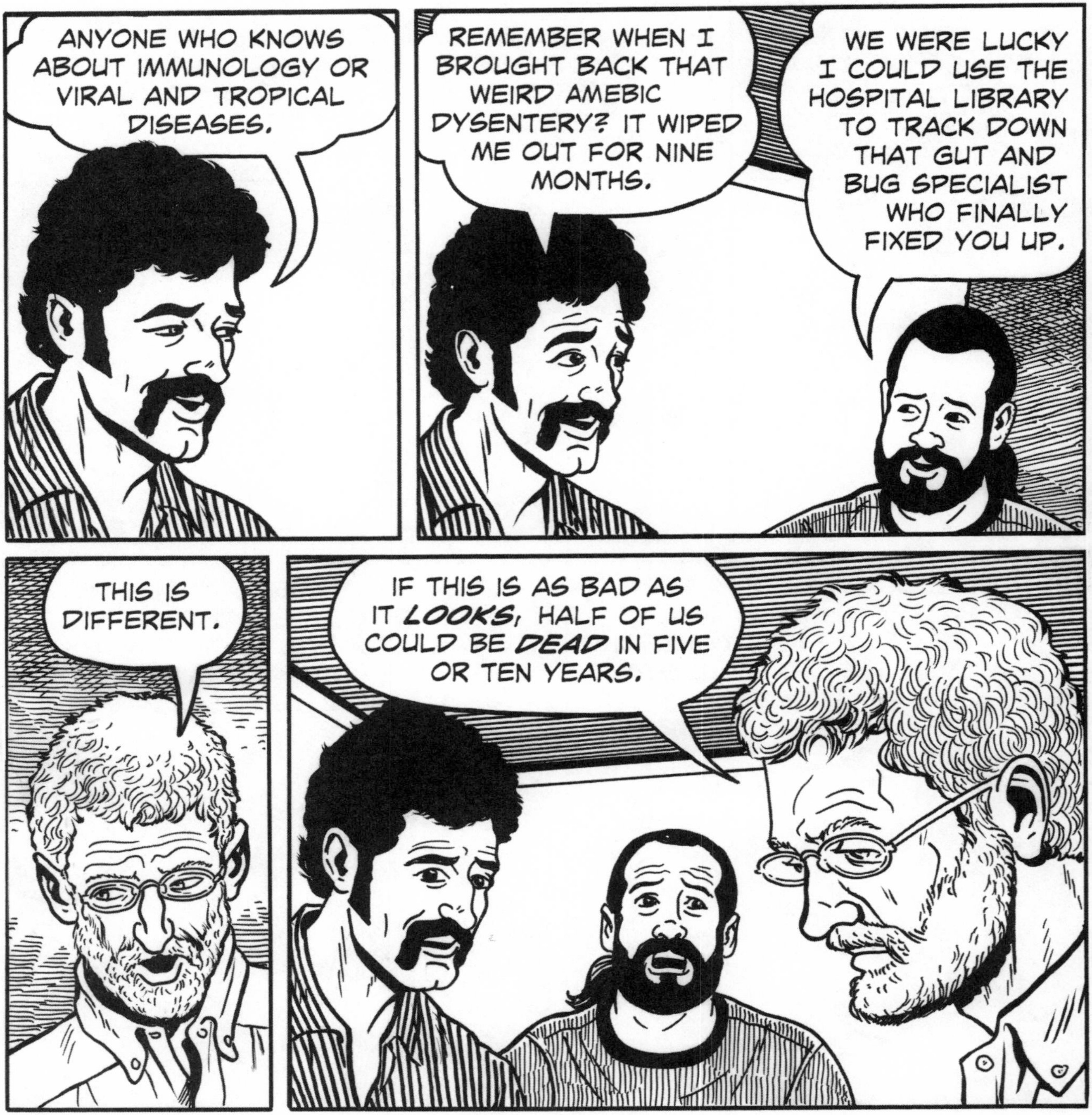
ANYONE WHO KNOWS ABOUT IMMUNOLOGY OR VIRAL AND TROPICAL DISEASES.
REMEMBER WHEN I BROUGHT BACK THAT WEIRD AMEBIC DYSENTERY? IT WIPED ME OUT FOR NINE MONTHS.
WE WERE LUCKY I COULD USE THE HOSPITAL LIBRARY TO TRACK DOWN THAT GUT AND BUG SPECIALIST WHO FINALLY FIXED YOU UP.
THIS IS DIFFERENT.
IF THIS IS AS BAD AS IT *LOOKS*, HALF OF US COULD BE *DEAD* IN FIVE OR TEN YEARS.

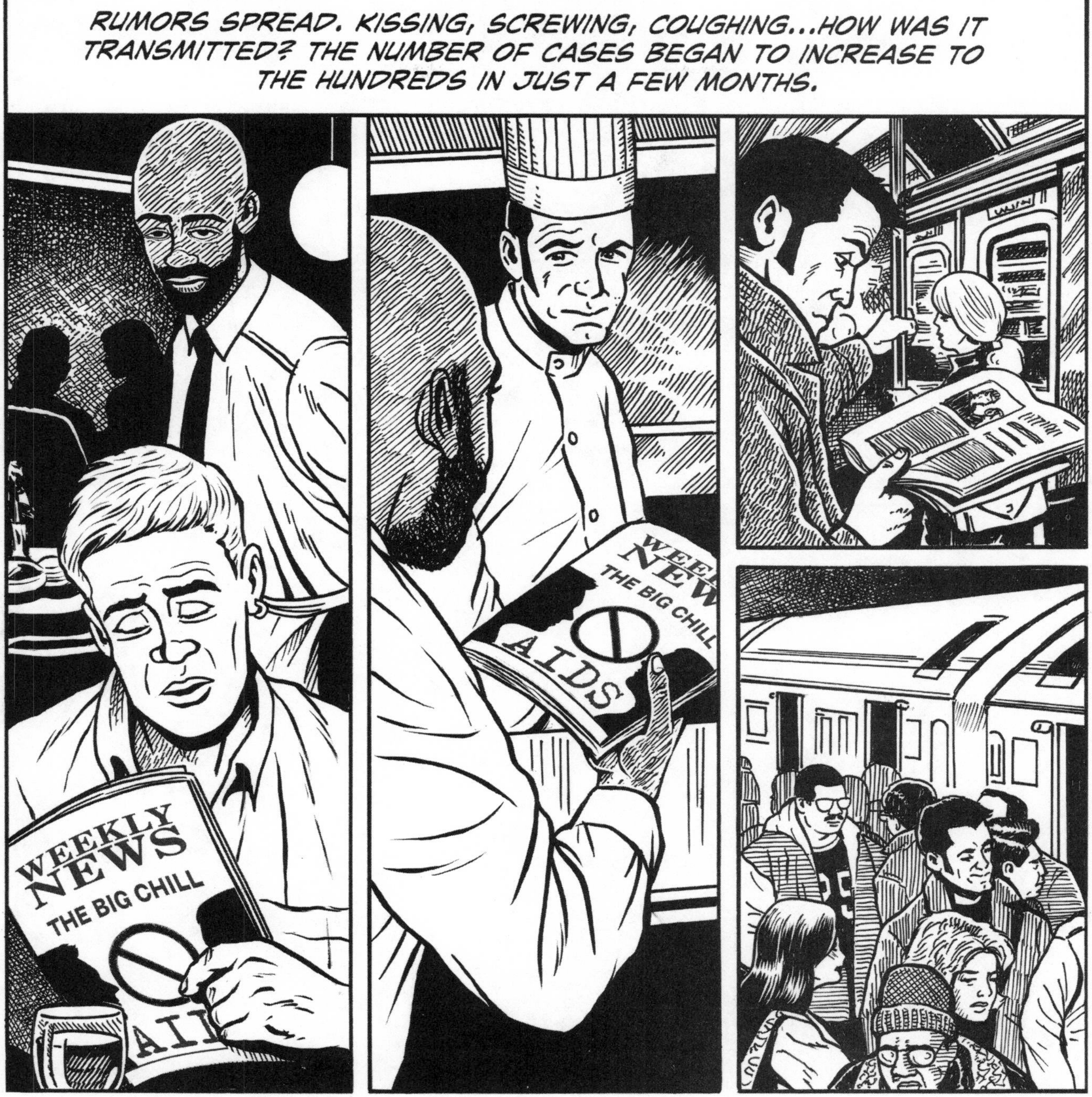
RUMORS SPREAD. KISSING, SCREWING, COUGHING...HOW WAS IT TRANSMITTED? THE NUMBER OF CASES BEGAN TO INCREASE TO THE HUNDREDS IN JUST A FEW MONTHS.
WEEKLY NEWS
THE BIG CHILL
THE BIG CHILL
AIDS

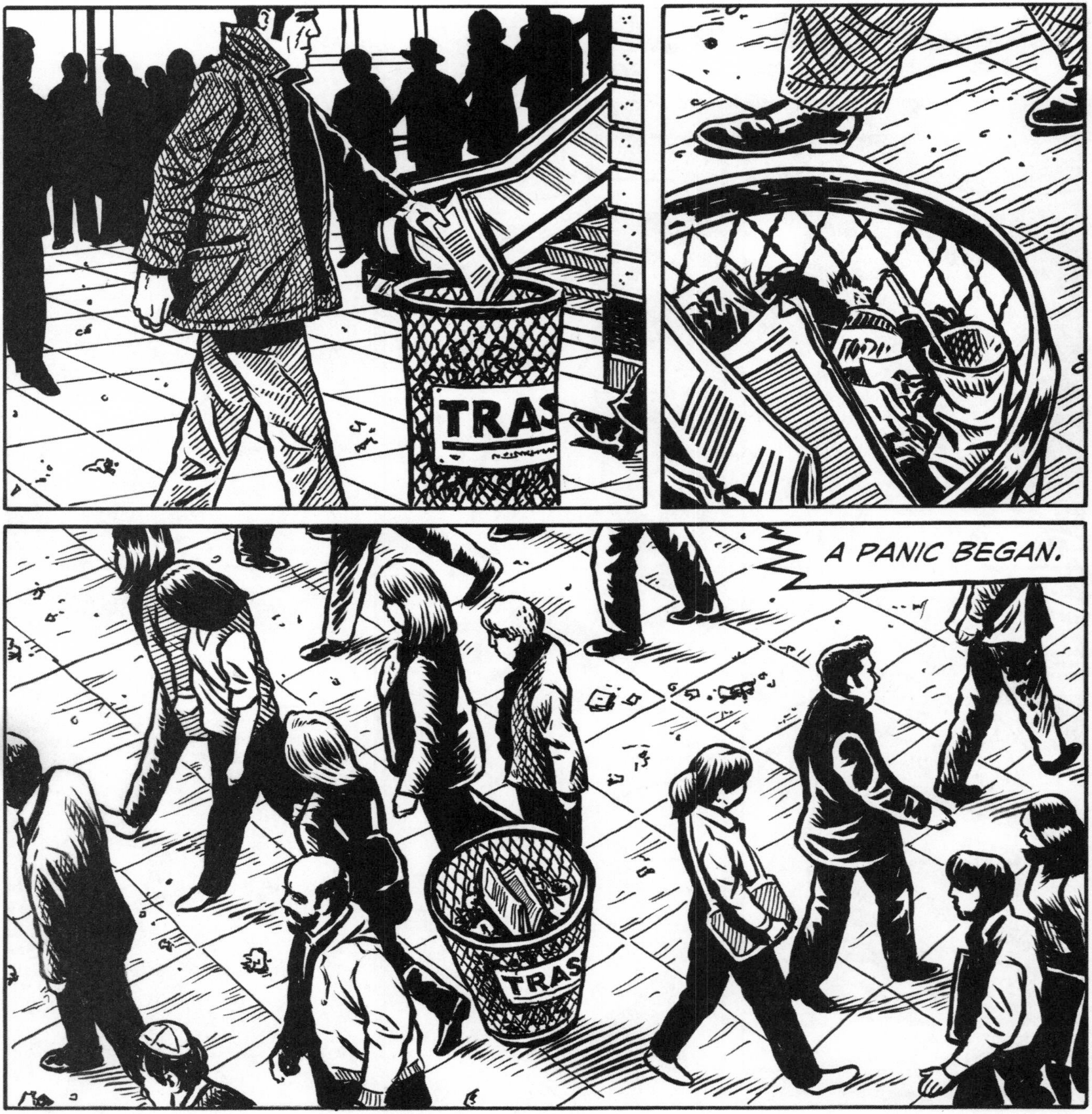
TRAS
TRAS
A PANIC BEGAN.
TRAS

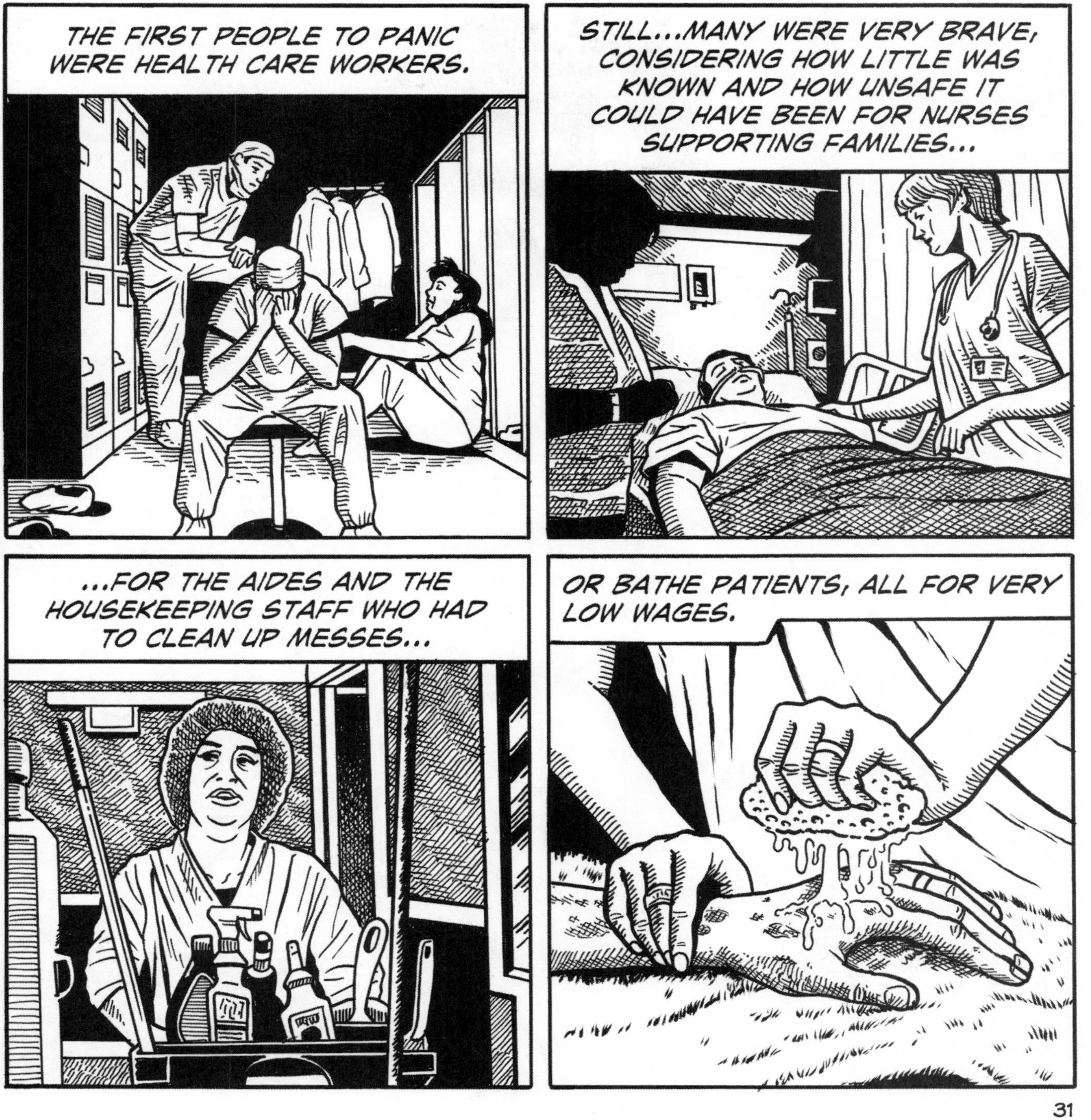
THE FIRST PEOPLE TO PANIC WERE HEALTH CARE WORKERS.
STILL...MANY WERE VERY BRAVE, CONSIDERING HOW LITTLE WAS KNOWN AND HOW UNSAFE IT COULD HAVE BEEN FOR NURSES SUPPORTING FAMILIES...
...FOR THE AIDES AND THE HOUSEKEEPING STAFF WHO HAD TO CLEAN UP MESSES...
OR BATHE PATIENTS, ALL FOR VERY LOW WAGES.

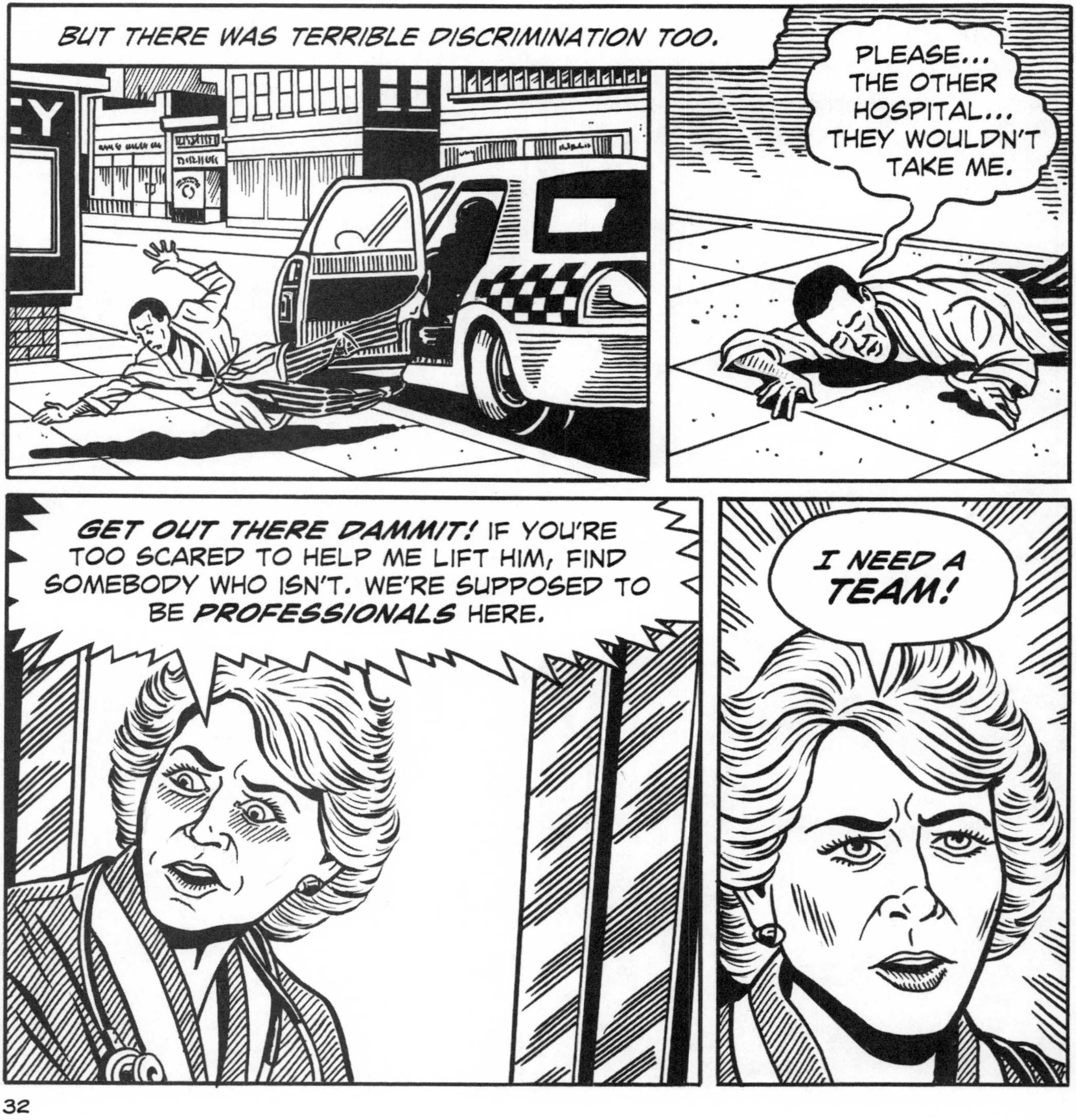
BUT THERE WAS TERRIBLE DISCRIMINATION TOO.
PLEASE... THE OTHER HOSPITAL... THEY WOULDN'T TAKE ME.
GET OUT THERE DAMMIT! IF YOU'RE TOO SCARED TO HELP ME LIFT HIM, FIND SOMEBODY WHO ISN'T. WE'RE SUPPOSED TO BE PROFESSIONALS HERE.
I NEED A TEAM!

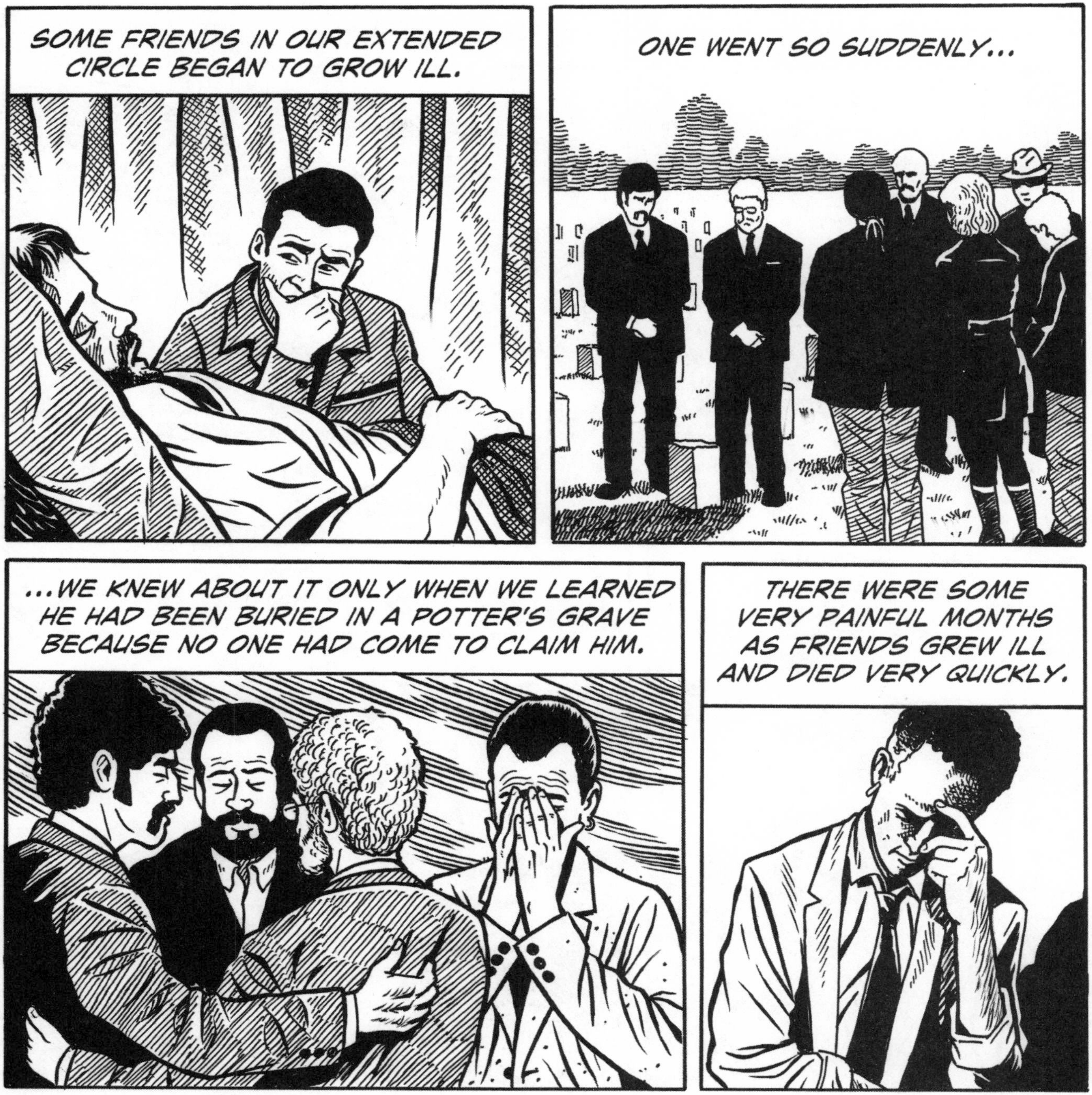
SOME FRIENDS IN OUR EXTENDED CIRCLE BEGAN TO GROW ILL.
ONE WENT SO SUDDENLY...
...WE KNEW ABOUT IT ONLY WHEN WE LEARNED HE HAD BEEN BURIED IN A POTTER'S GRAVE BECAUSE NO ONE HAD COME TO CLAIM HIM.
THERE WERE SOME VERY PAINFUL MONTHS AS FRIENDS GREW ILL AND DIED VERY QUICKLY.

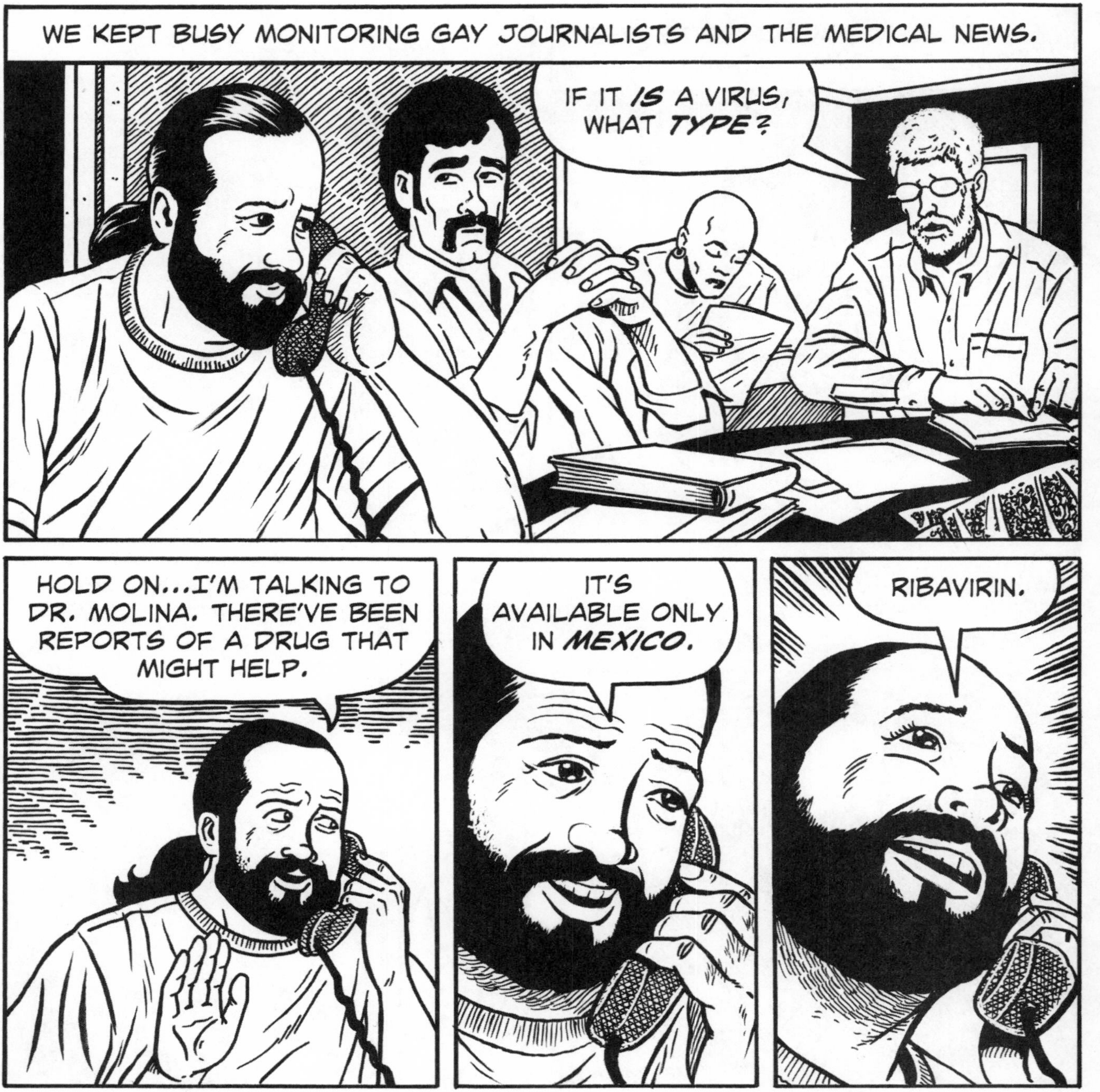
WE KEPT BUSY MONITORING GAY JOURNALISTS AND THE MEDICAL NEWS.
IF IT *IS* A VIRUS, WHAT *TYPE*?
HOLD ON...I'M TALKING TO DR. MOLINA. THERE'VE BEEN REPORTS OF A DRUG THAT MIGHT HELP.
IT'S AVAILABLE ONLY IN *MEXICO*.
RIBAVIRIN.

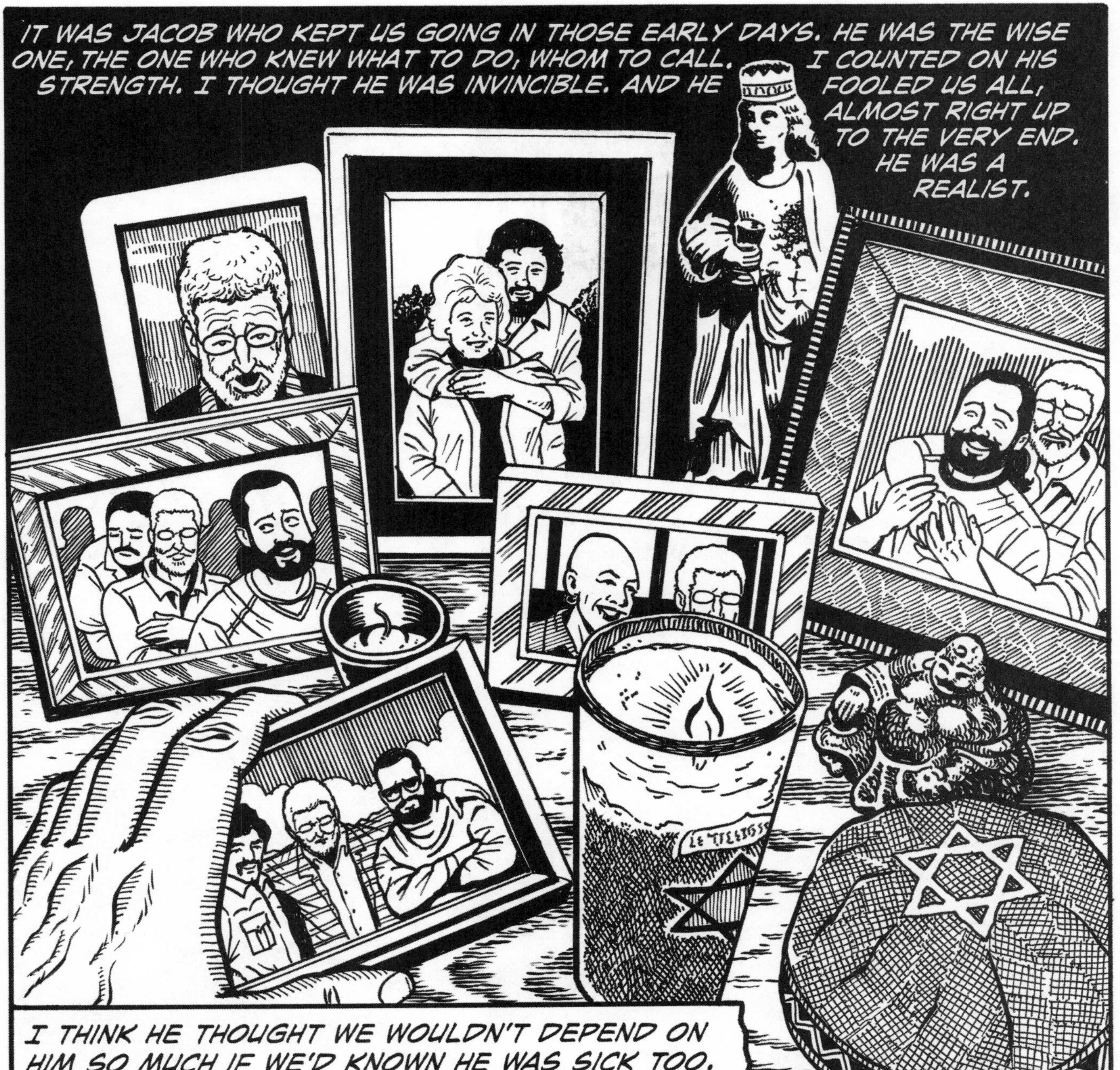
IT WAS JACOB WHO KEPT US GOING IN THOSE EARLY DAYS. HE WAS THE WISE ONE, THE ONE WHO KNEW WHAT TO DO, WHOM TO CALL. I COUNTED ON HIS STRENGTH. I THOUGHT HE WAS INVINCIBLE. AND HE FOOLED US ALL, ALMOST RIGHT UP TO THE VERY END. HE WAS A REALIST.
I THINK HE THOUGHT WE WOULDN'T DEPEND ON HIM SO MUCH IF WE'D KNOWN HE WAS SICK TOO. HE JUST KEPT WORKING UNTIL ONE DAY...GONE.

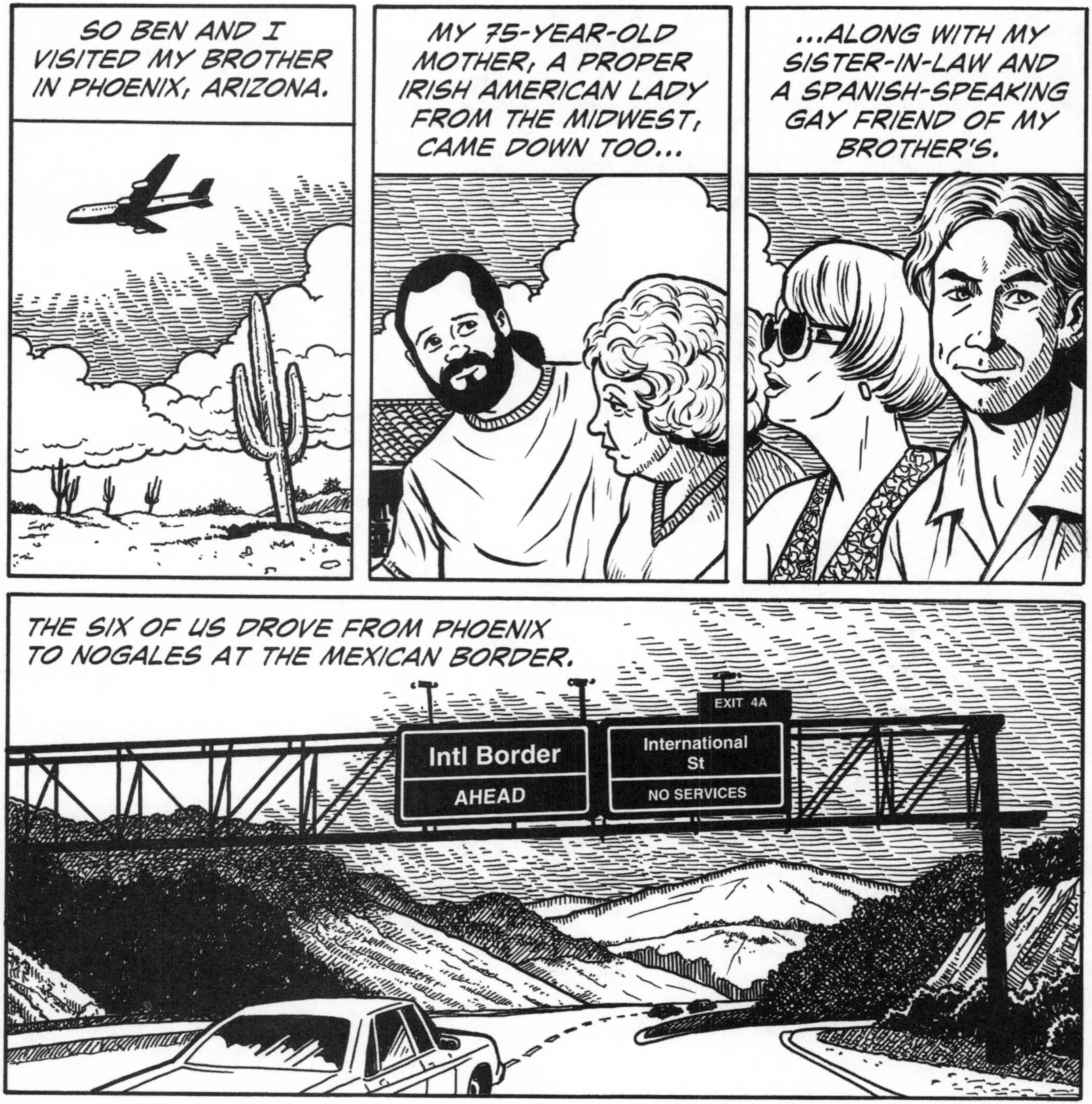
SO BEN AND I VISITED MY BROTHER IN PHOENIX, ARIZONA.
MY 75-YEAR-OLD MOTHER, A PROPER IRISH AMERICAN LADY FROM THE MIDWEST, CAME DOWN TOO...
...ALONG WITH MY SISTER-IN-LAW AND A SPANISH-SPEAKING GAY FRIEND OF MY BROTHER'S.
THE SIX OF US DROVE FROM PHOENIX TO NOGALES AT THE MEXICAN BORDER.
EXIT 4A
Intl Border
AHEAD
International
St
NO SERVICES

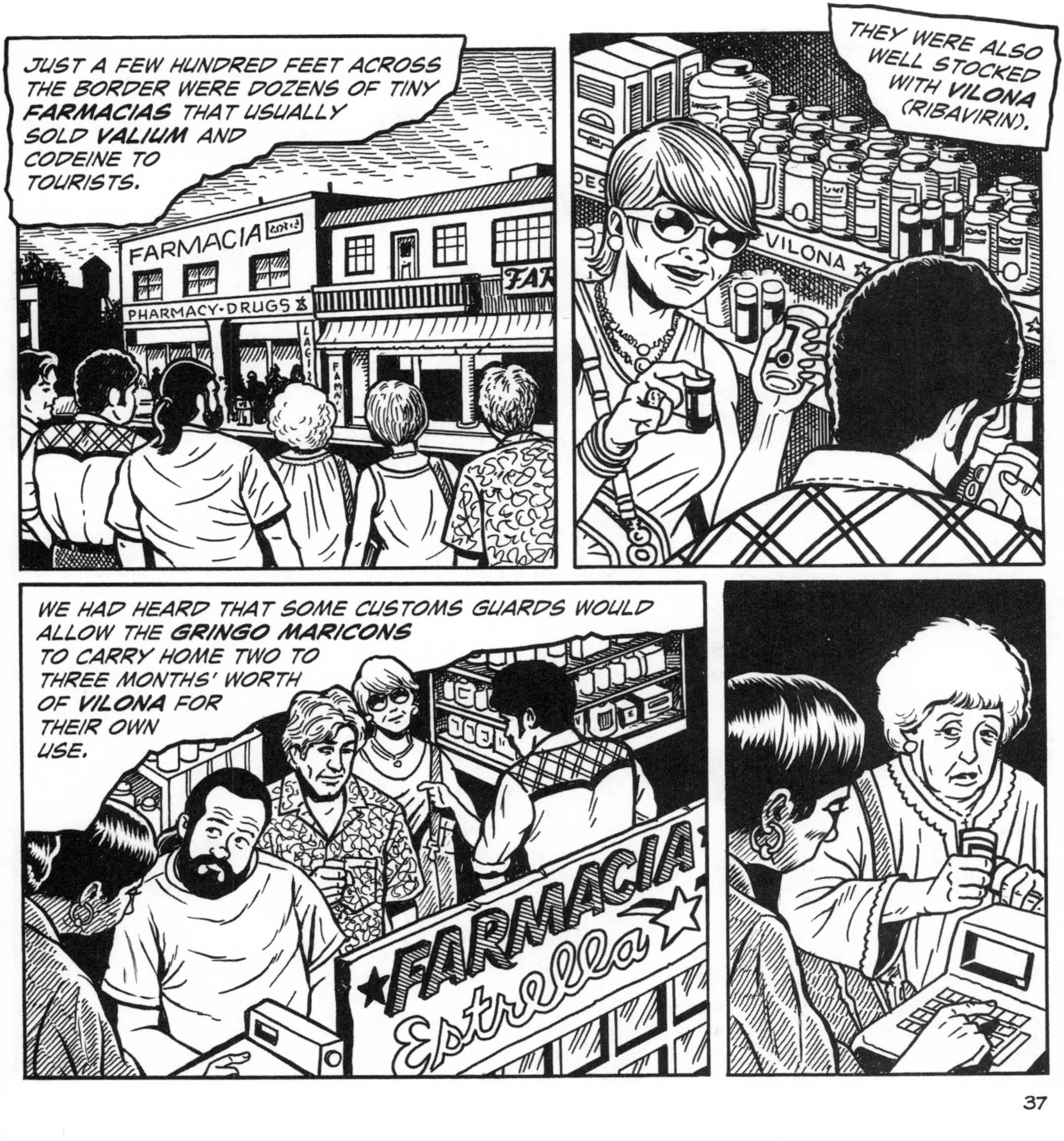
JUST A FEW HUNDRED FEET ACROSS THE BORDER WERE DOZENS OF TINY **FARMACIAS** THAT USUALLY SOLD **VALIUM** AND CODEINE TO TOURISTS.
FARMACIA
PHARMACY·DRUGS
THEY WERE ALSO WELL STOCKED WITH **VILONA** (RIBAVIRIN).
VILONA
WE HAD HEARD THAT SOME CUSTOMS GUARDS WOULD ALLOW THE **GRINGO MARICONS** TO CARRY HOME TWO TO THREE MONTHS' WORTH OF **VILONA** FOR THEIR OWN USE.
FARMACIA
Estrella

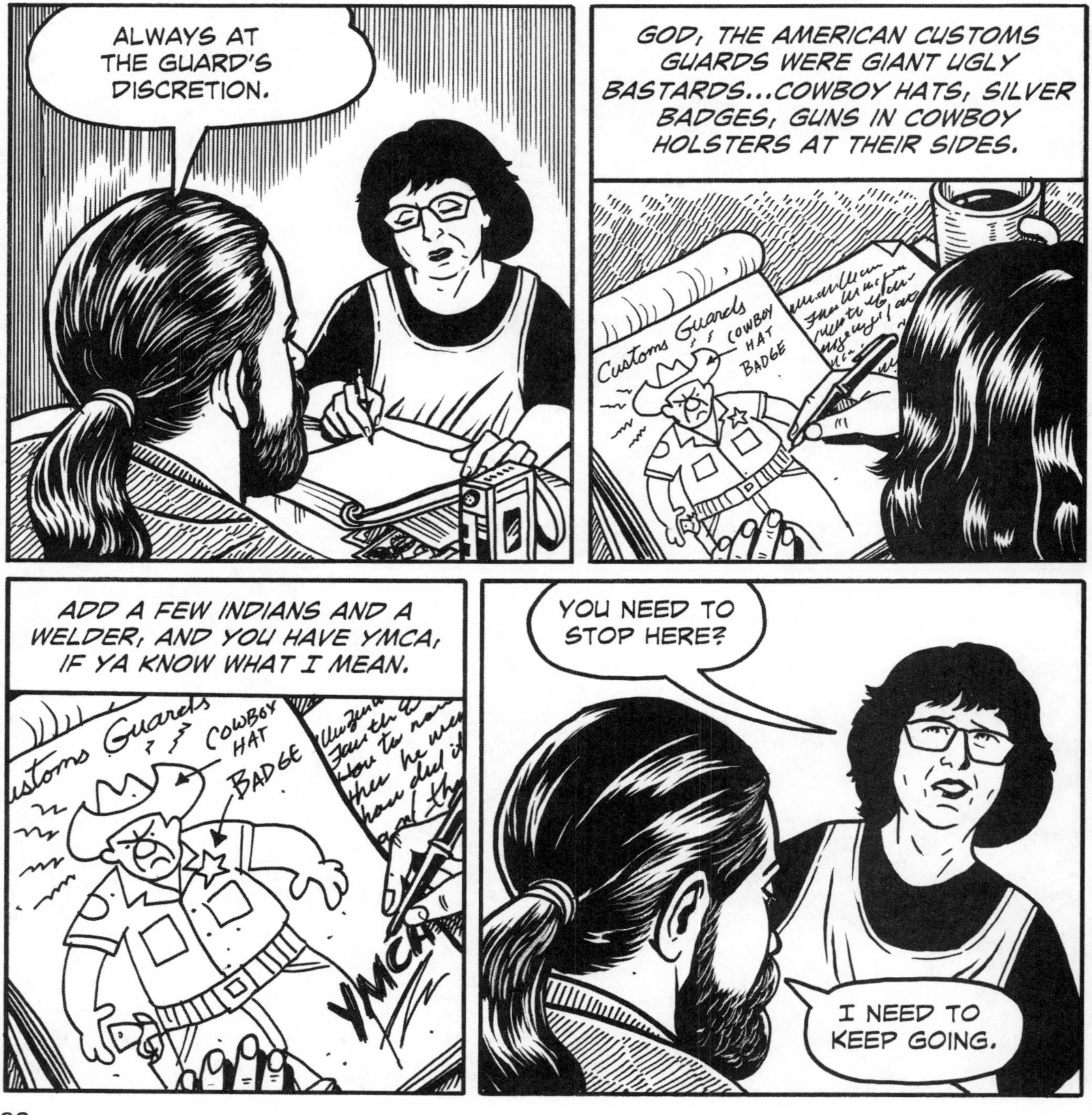
ALWAYS AT THE GUARD'S DISCRETION.
GOD, THE AMERICAN CUSTOMS GUARDS WERE GIANT UGLY BASTARDS...COWBOY HATS, SILVER BADGES, GUNS IN COWBOY HOLSTERS AT THEIR SIDES.
Customs Guards
COWBOY HAT
BADGE
ADD A FEW INDIANS AND A WELDER, AND YOU HAVE YMCA, IF YA KNOW WHAT I MEAN.
Customs Guards
COWBOY HAT
BADGE
YMCA
YOU NEED TO STOP HERE?
I NEED TO KEEP GOING.

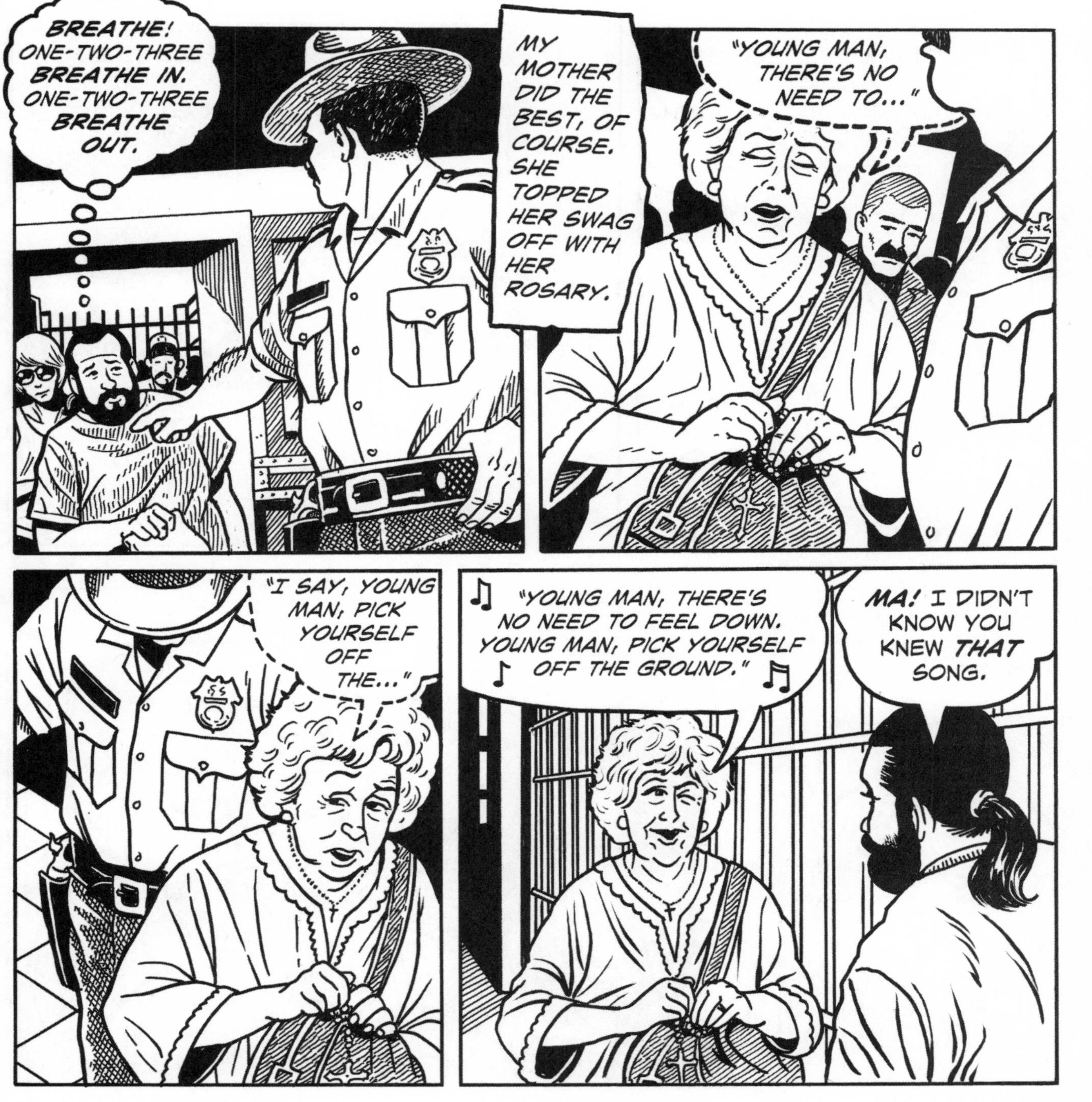
BREATHE! ONE-TWO-THREE BREATHE IN. ONE-TWO-THREE BREATHE OUT.
MY MOTHER DID THE BEST, OF COURSE. SHE TOPPED HER SWAG OFF WITH HER ROSARY.
"YOUNG MAN, THERE'S NO NEED TO..."
"I SAY, YOUNG MAN, PICK YOURSELF OFF THE..."
♫ "YOUNG MAN, THERE'S NO NEED TO FEEL DOWN. YOUNG MAN, PICK YOURSELF ♪ OFF THE GROUND." ♫
MA! I DIDN'T KNOW YOU KNEW THAT SONG.

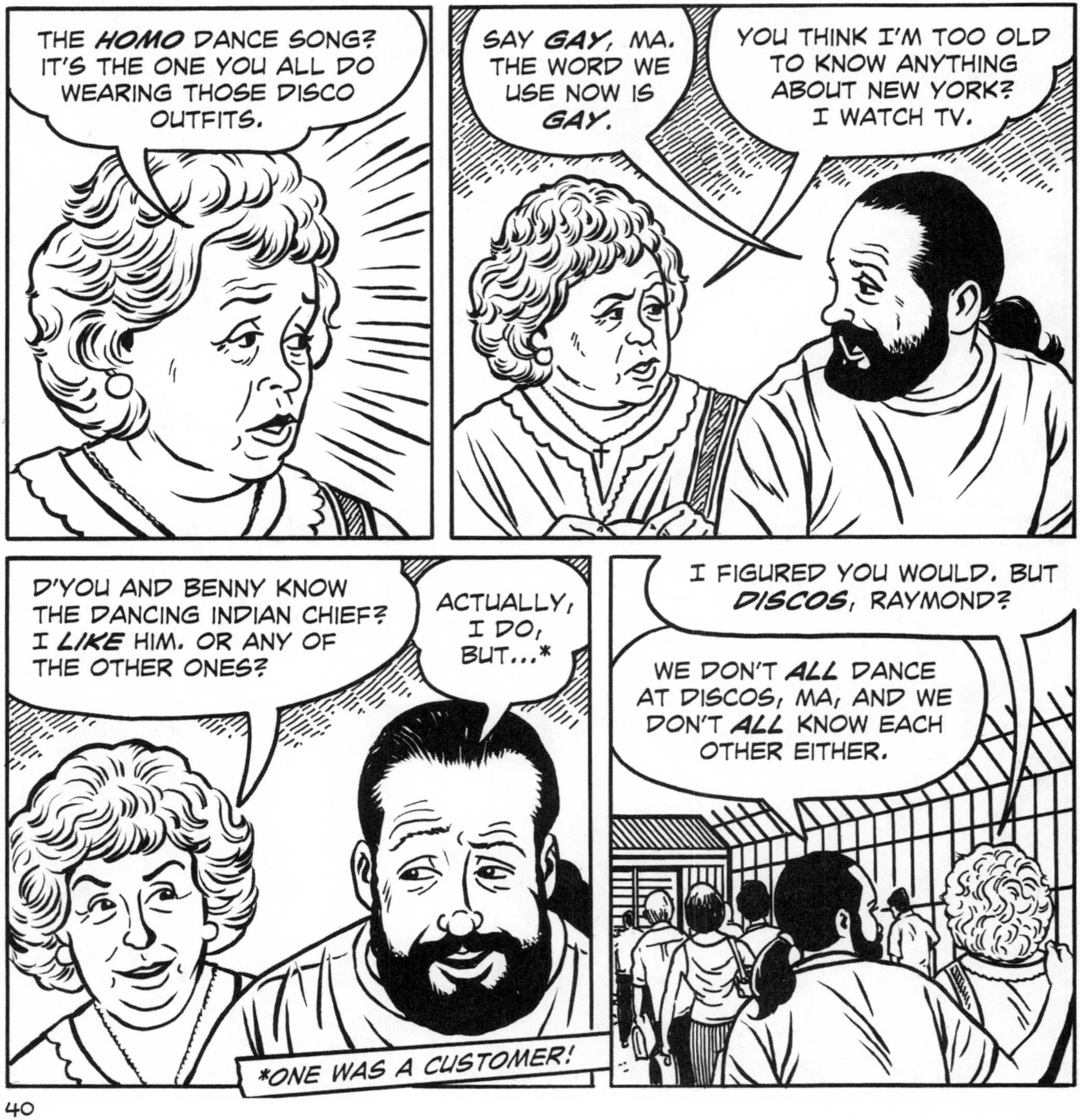
THE HOMO DANCE SONG? IT'S THE ONE YOU ALL DO WEARING THOSE DISCO OUTFITS.
SAY GAY, MA. THE WORD WE USE NOW IS GAY.
YOU THINK I'M TOO OLD TO KNOW ANYTHING ABOUT NEW YORK? I WATCH TV.
D'YOU AND BENNY KNOW THE DANCING INDIAN CHIEF? I LIKE HIM. OR ANY OF THE OTHER ONES?
ACTUALLY, I DO, BUT...*
*ONE WAS A CUSTOMER!
WE DON'T ALL DANCE AT DISCOS, MA, AND WE DON'T ALL KNOW EACH OTHER EITHER.
I FIGURED YOU WOULD. BUT DISCOS, RAYMOND?

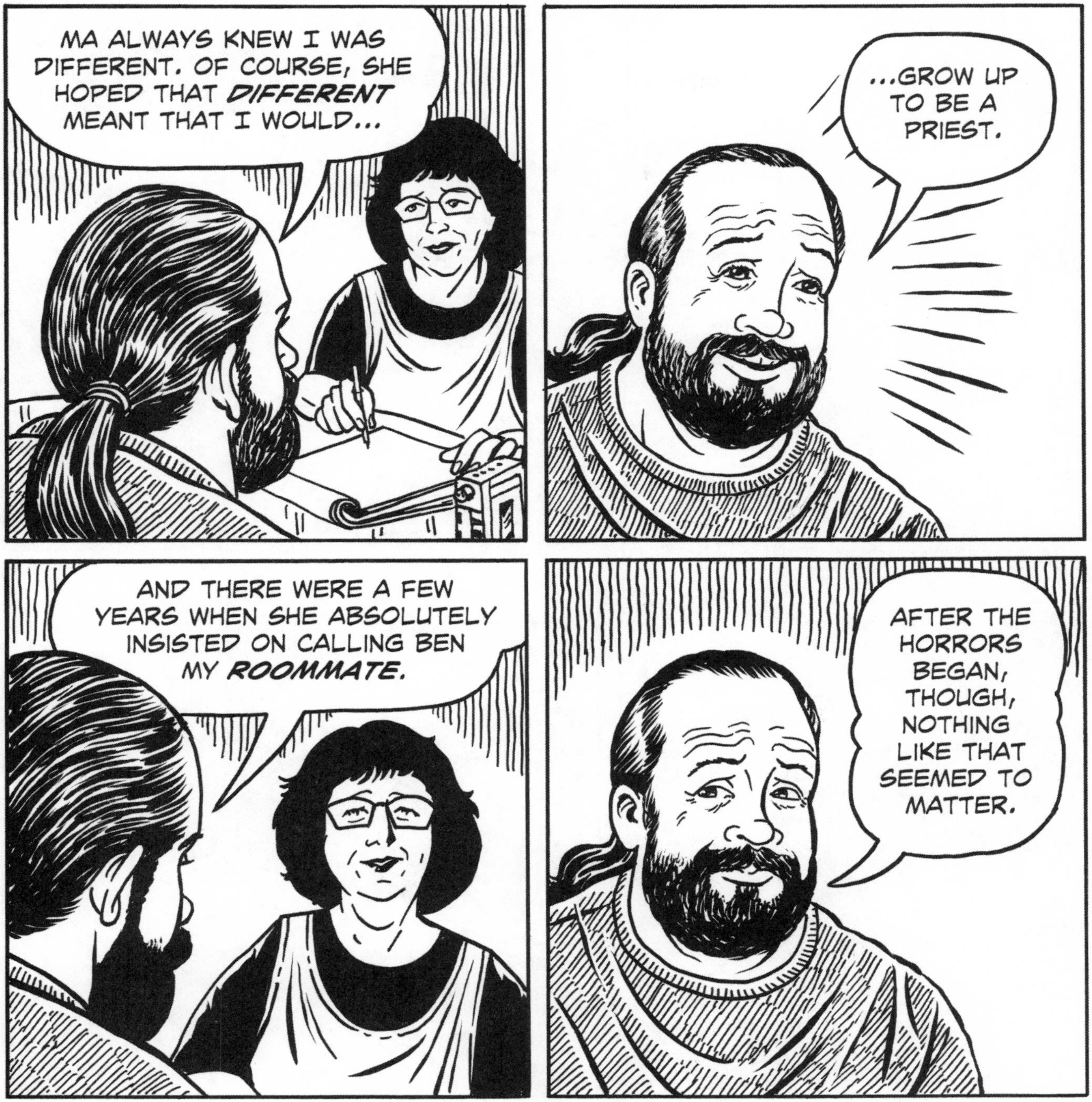
MA ALWAYS KNEW I WAS DIFFERENT. OF COURSE, SHE HOPED THAT *DIFFERENT* MEANT THAT I WOULD...
...GROW UP TO BE A PRIEST.
AND THERE WERE A FEW YEARS WHEN SHE ABSOLUTELY INSISTED ON CALLING BEN MY *ROOMMATE.*
AFTER THE HORRORS BEGAN, THOUGH, NOTHING LIKE THAT SEEMED TO MATTER.

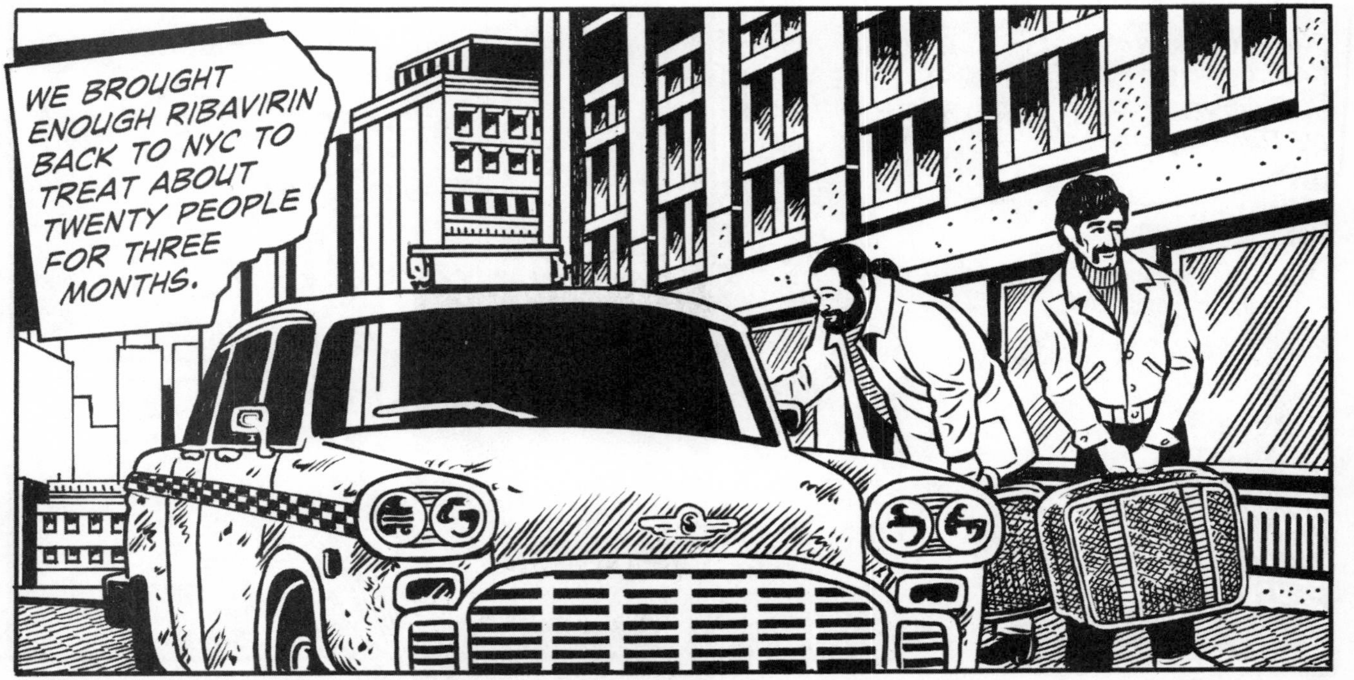
WE BROUGHT ENOUGH RIBAVIRIN BACK TO NYC TO TREAT ABOUT TWENTY PEOPLE FOR THREE MONTHS.

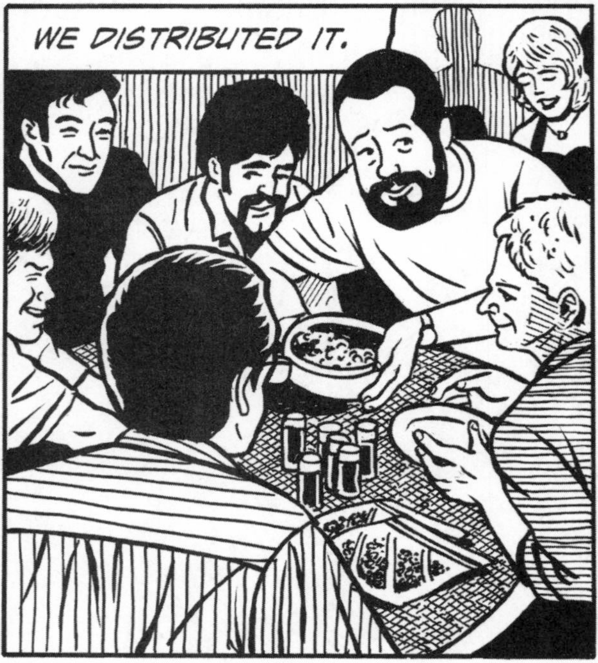
WE DISTRIBUTED IT.

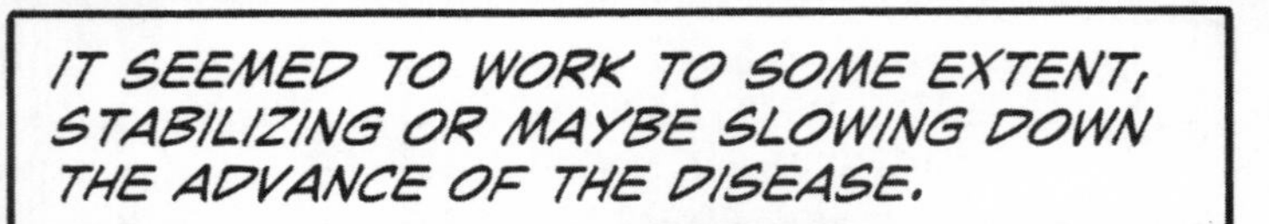
IT SEEMED TO WORK TO SOME EXTENT, STABILIZING OR MAYBE SLOWING DOWN THE ADVANCE OF THE DISEASE.

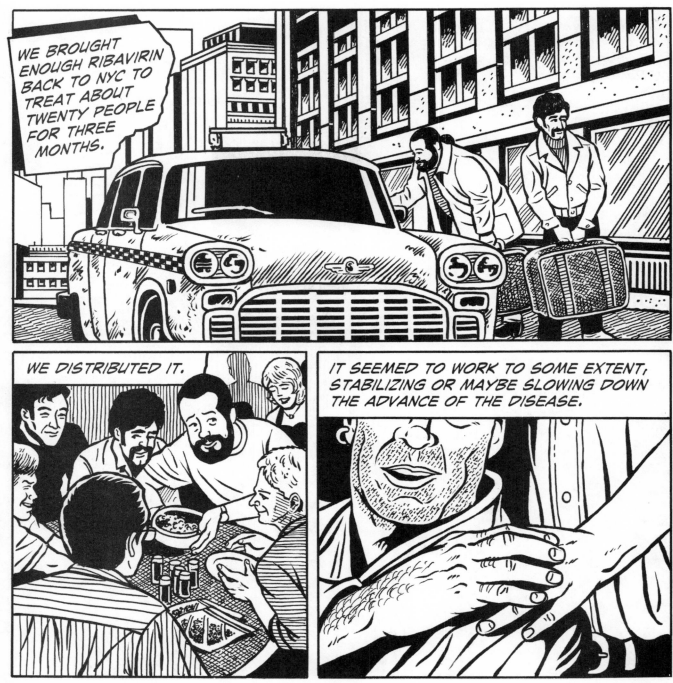

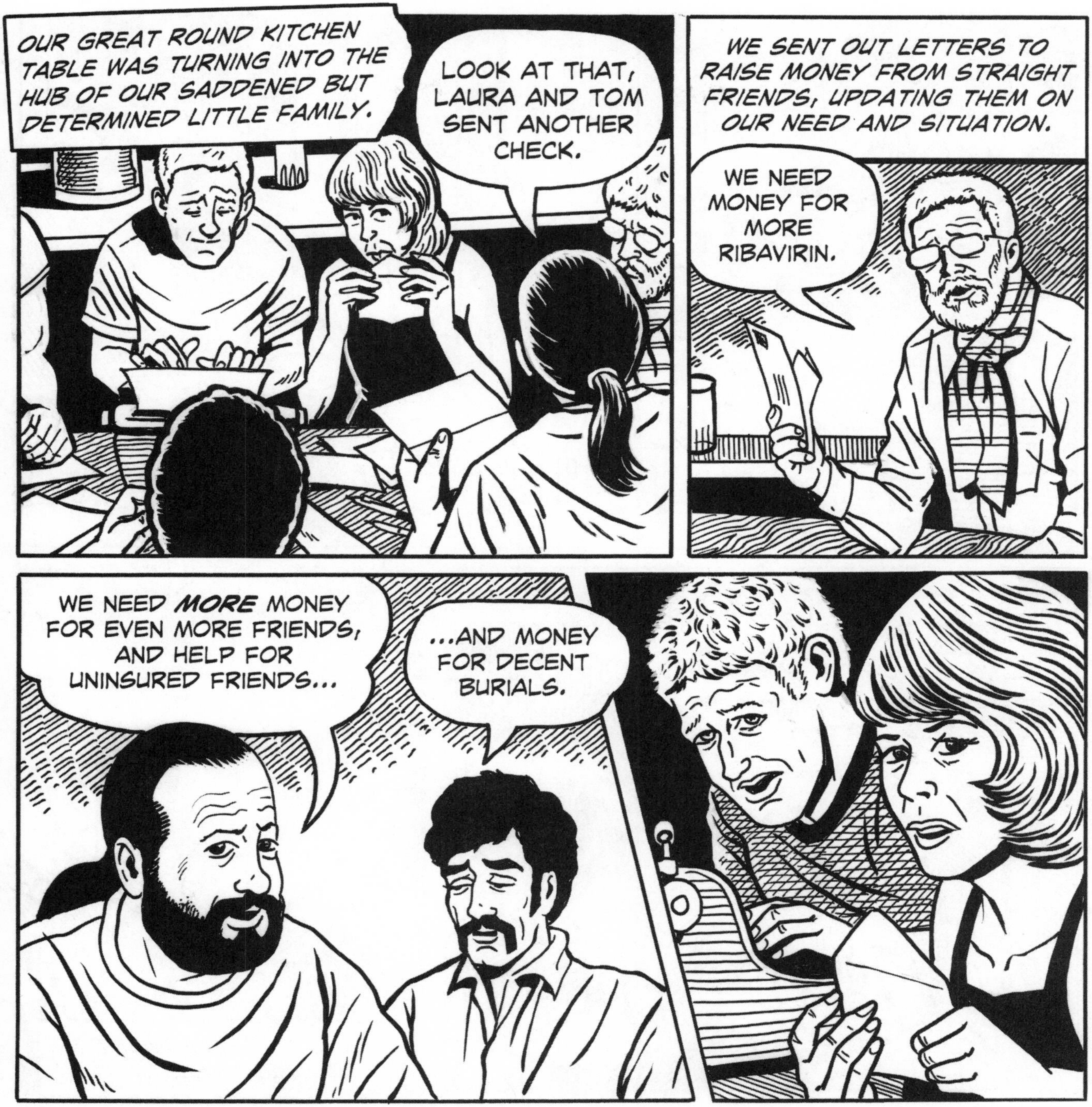
OUR GREAT ROUND KITCHEN TABLE WAS TURNING INTO THE HUB OF OUR SADDENED BUT DETERMINED LITTLE FAMILY.
LOOK AT THAT, LAURA AND TOM SENT ANOTHER CHECK.
WE SENT OUT LETTERS TO RAISE MONEY FROM STRAIGHT FRIENDS, UPDATING THEM ON OUR NEED AND SITUATION.
WE NEED MONEY FOR MORE RIBAVIRIN.
WE NEED *MORE* MONEY FOR EVEN MORE FRIENDS, AND HELP FOR UNINSURED FRIENDS...
...AND MONEY FOR DECENT BURIALS.

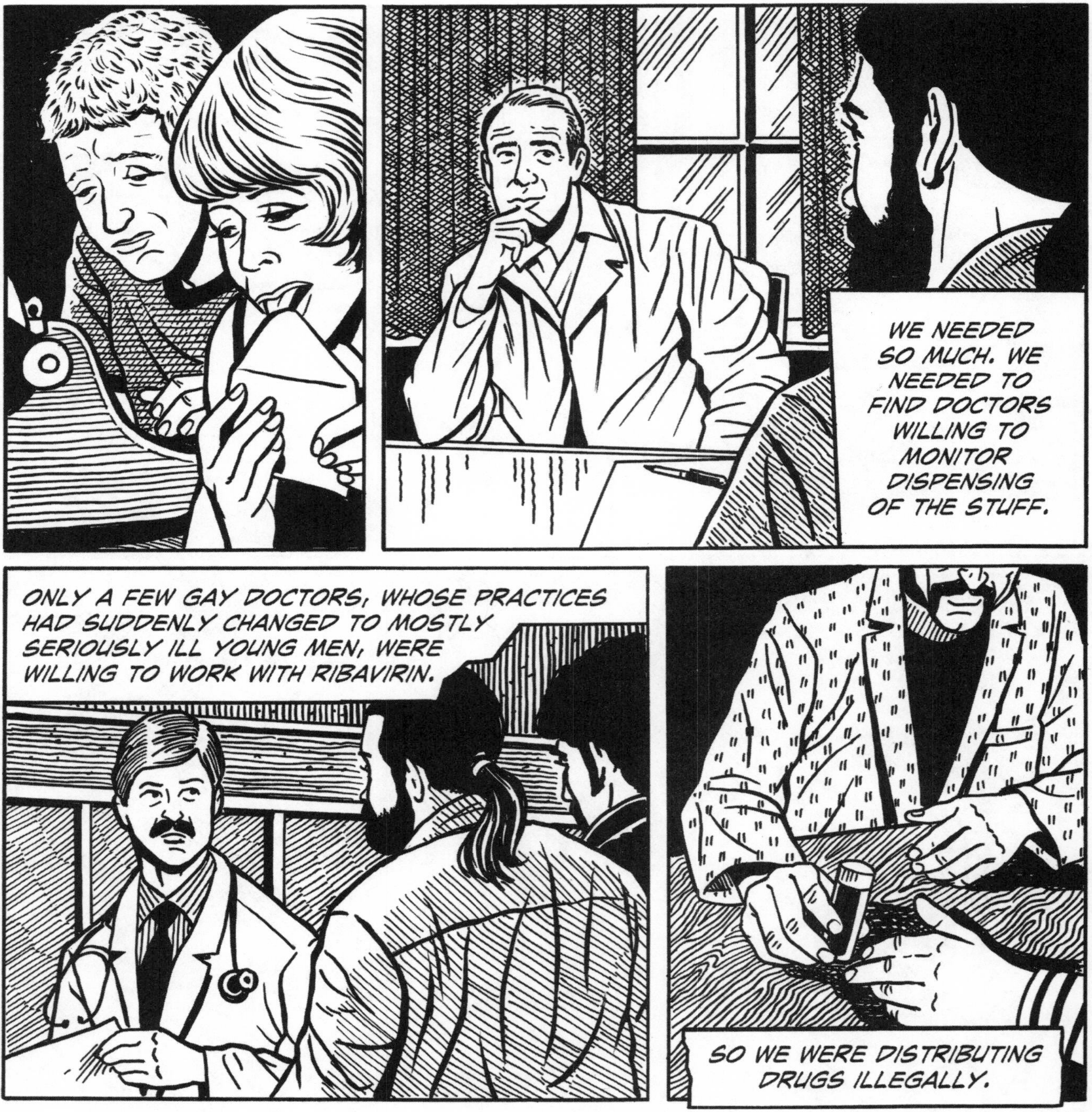
WE NEEDED SO MUCH. WE NEEDED TO FIND DOCTORS WILLING TO MONITOR DISPENSING OF THE STUFF.
ONLY A FEW GAY DOCTORS, WHOSE PRACTICES HAD SUDDENLY CHANGED TO MOSTLY SERIOUSLY ILL YOUNG MEN, WERE WILLING TO WORK WITH RIBAVIRIN.
SO WE WERE DISTRIBUTING DRUGS ILLEGALLY.

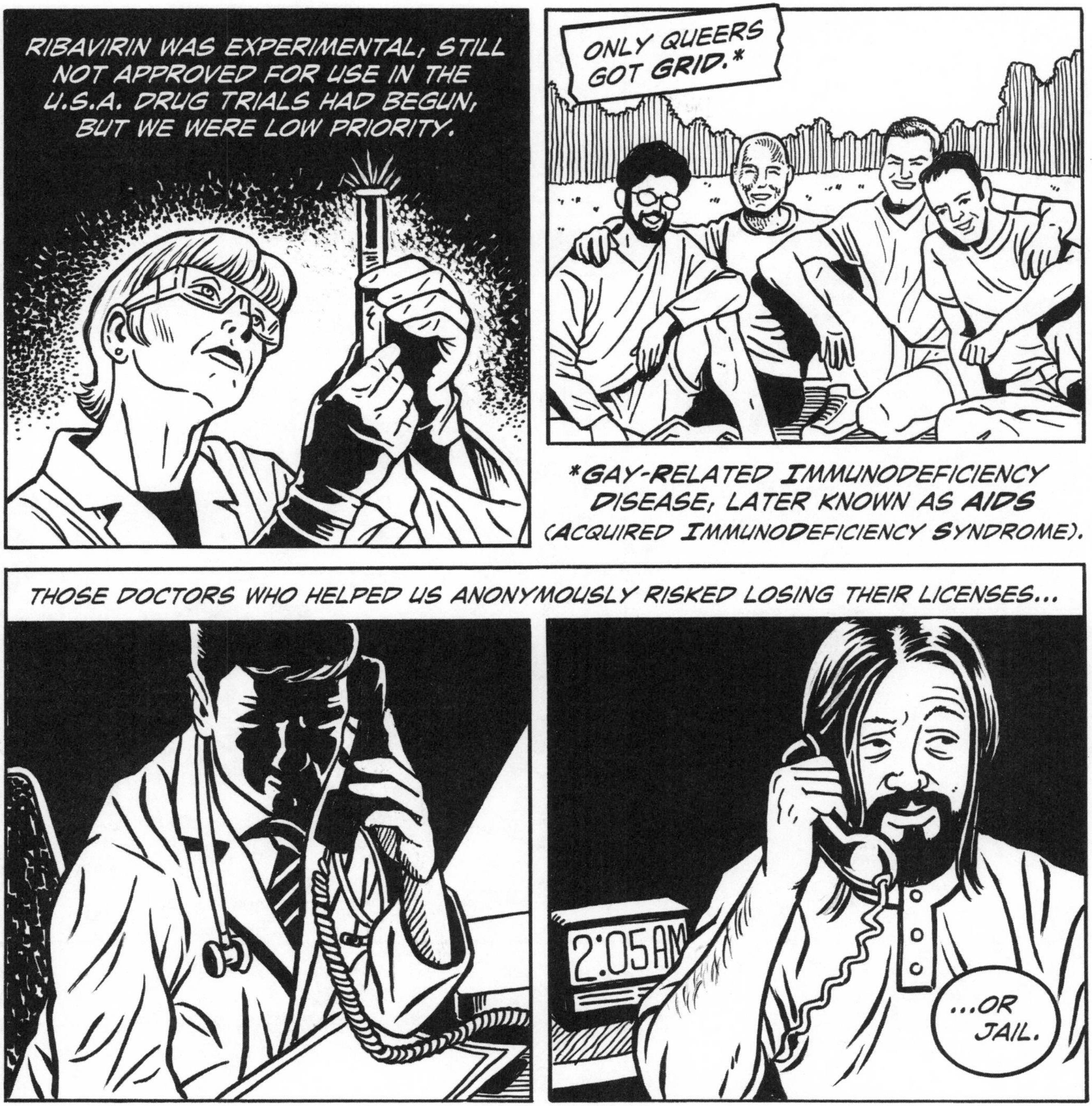
RIBAVIRIN WAS EXPERIMENTAL, STILL NOT APPROVED FOR USE IN THE U.S.A. DRUG TRIALS HAD BEGUN, BUT WE WERE LOW PRIORITY.
ONLY QUEERS GOT GRID.*
*GAY-RELATED IMMUNODEFICIENCY DISEASE, LATER KNOWN AS AIDS (ACQUIRED IMMUNODEFICIENCY SYNDROME).
THOSE DOCTORS WHO HELPED US ANONYMOUSLY RISKED LOSING THEIR LICENSES...
2:05AM
...OR JAIL.

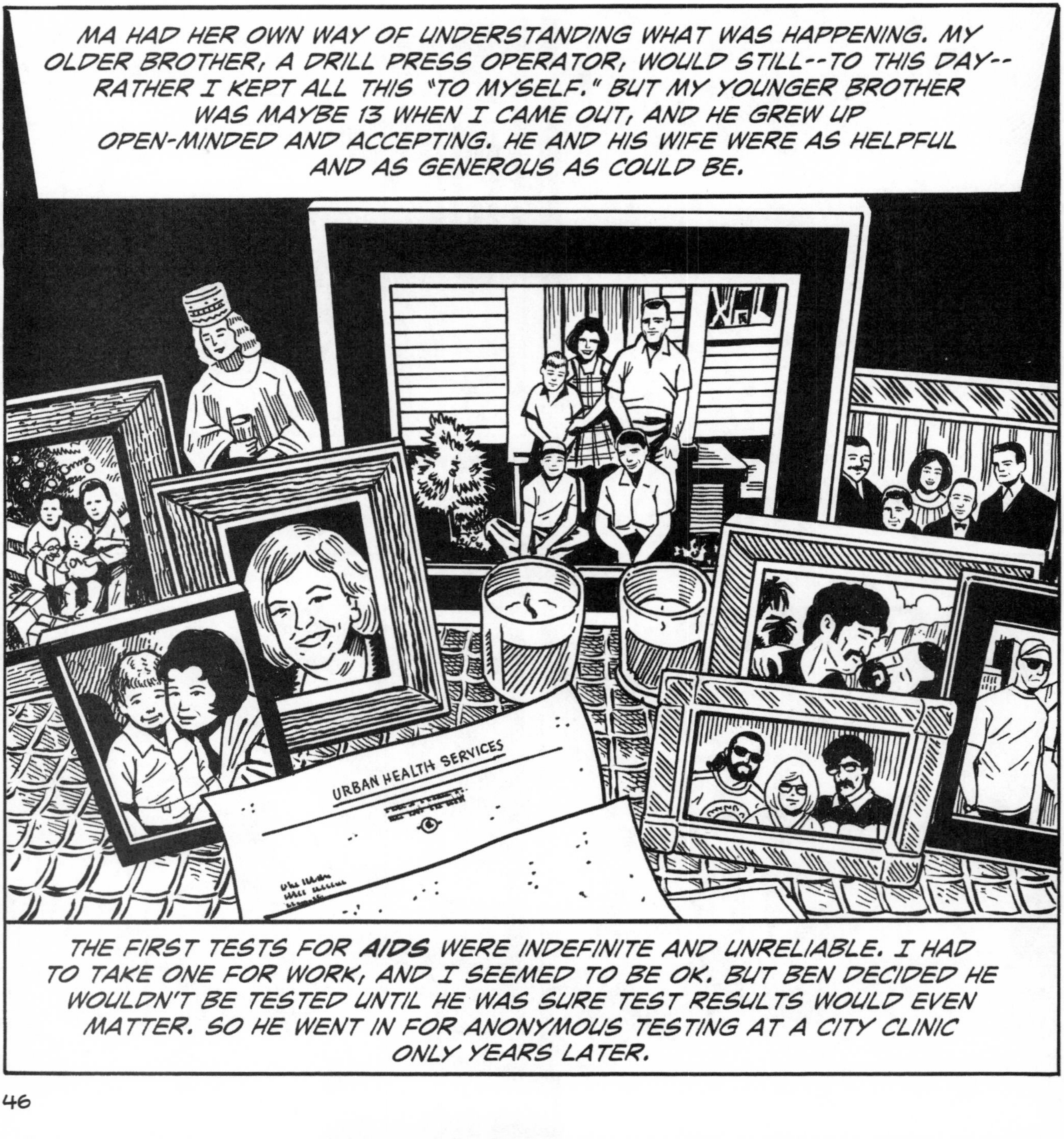
MA HAD HER OWN WAY OF UNDERSTANDING WHAT WAS HAPPENING. MY OLDER BROTHER, A DRILL PRESS OPERATOR, WOULD STILL--TO THIS DAY--RATHER I KEPT ALL THIS "TO MYSELF." BUT MY YOUNGER BROTHER WAS MAYBE 13 WHEN I CAME OUT, AND HE GREW UP OPEN-MINDED AND ACCEPTING. HE AND HIS WIFE WERE AS HELPFUL AND AS GENEROUS AS COULD BE.
URBAN HEALTH SERVICES
THE FIRST TESTS FOR **AIDS** WERE INDEFINITE AND UNRELIABLE. I HAD TO TAKE ONE FOR WORK, AND I SEEMED TO BE OK. BUT BEN DECIDED HE WOULDN'T BE TESTED UNTIL HE WAS SURE TEST RESULTS WOULD EVEN MATTER. SO HE WENT IN FOR ANONYMOUS TESTING AT A CITY CLINIC ONLY YEARS LATER.

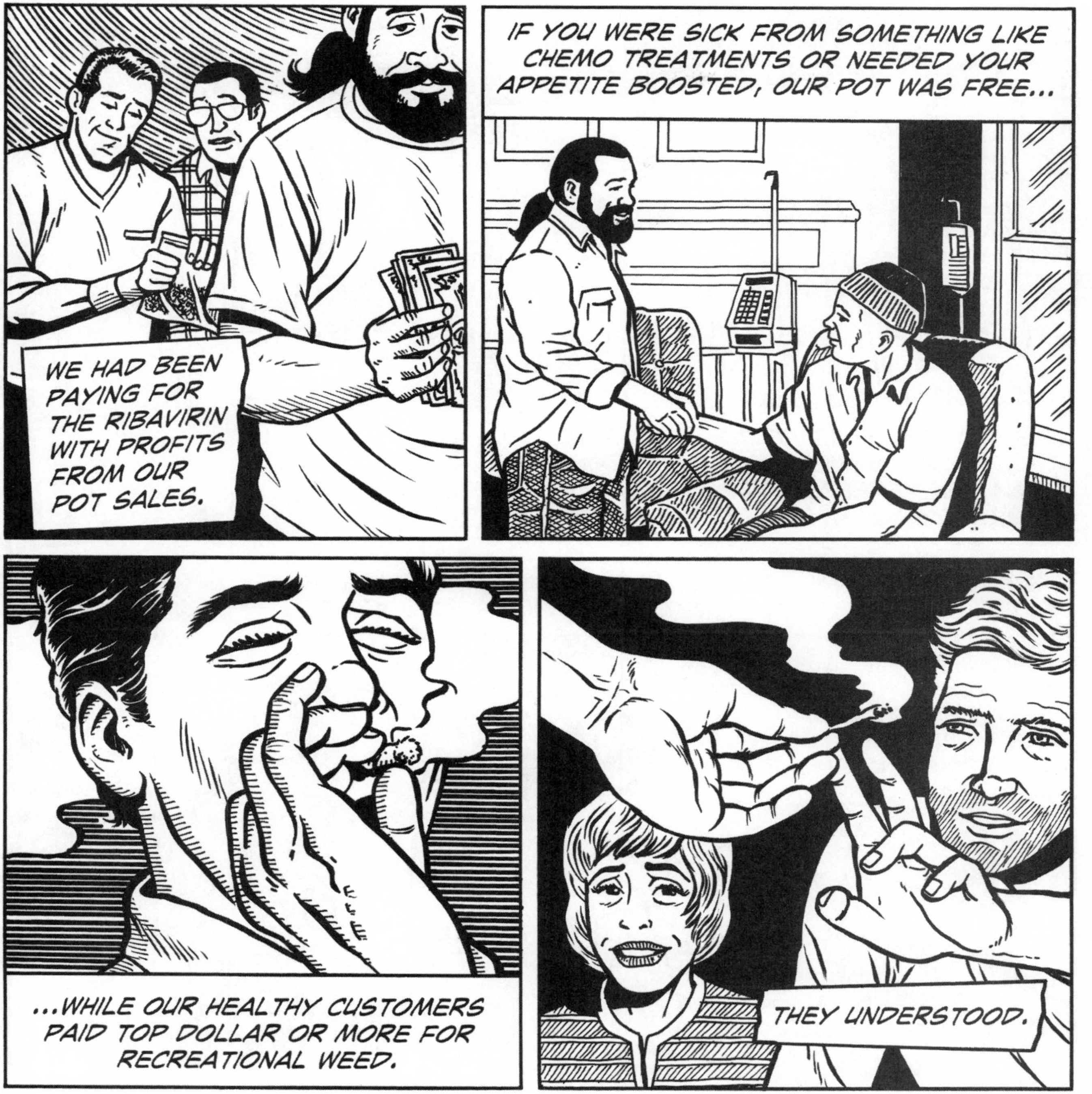
WE HAD BEEN PAYING FOR THE RIBAVIRIN WITH PROFITS FROM OUR POT SALES.
IF YOU WERE SICK FROM SOMETHING LIKE CHEMO TREATMENTS OR NEEDED YOUR APPETITE BOOSTED, OUR POT WAS FREE...
...WHILE OUR HEALTHY CUSTOMERS PAID TOP DOLLAR OR MORE FOR RECREATIONAL WEED.
THEY UNDERSTOOD.

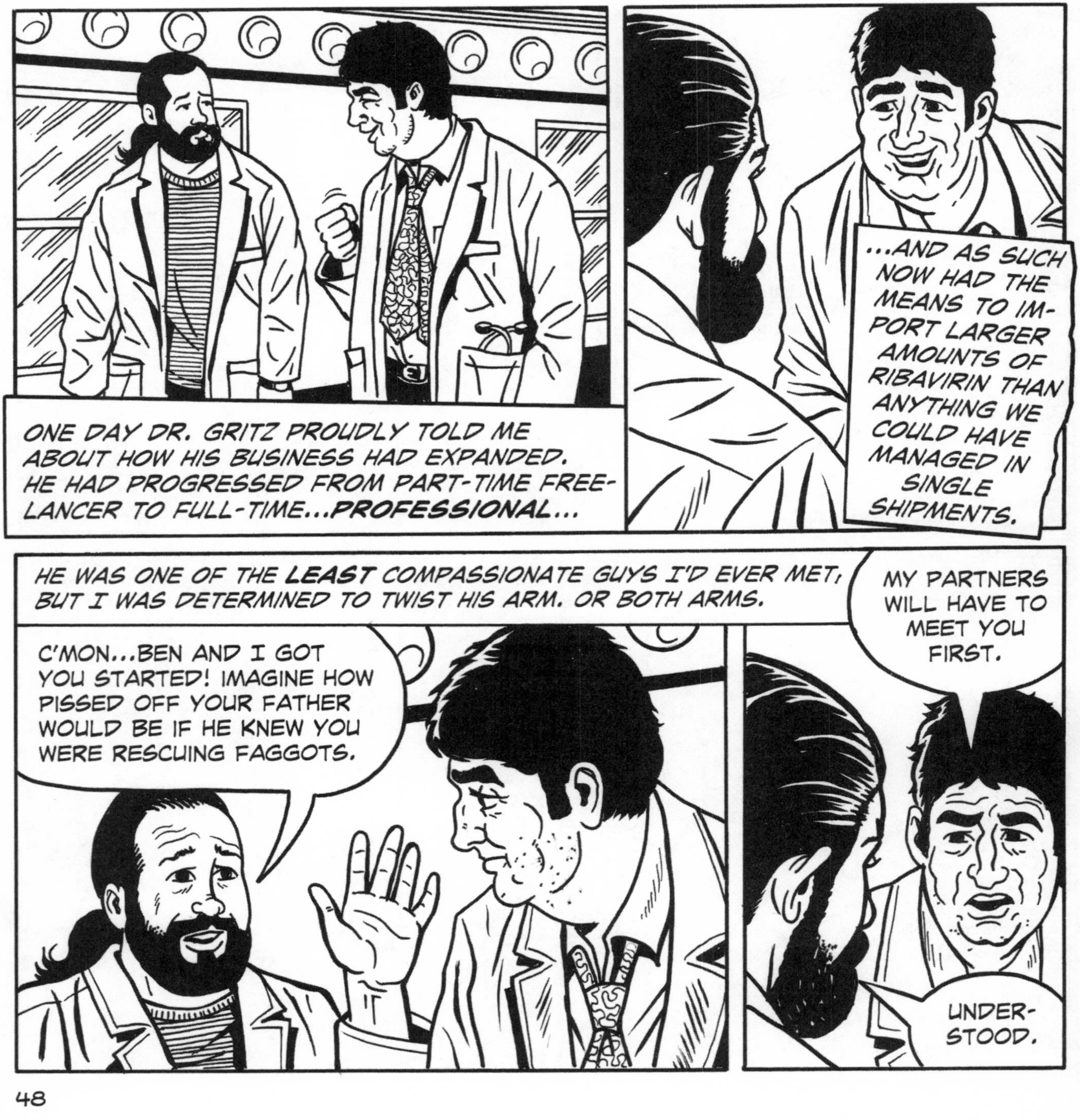
ONE DAY DR. GRITZ PROUDLY TOLD ME ABOUT HOW HIS BUSINESS HAD EXPANDED. HE HAD PROGRESSED FROM PART-TIME FREE-LANCER TO FULL-TIME...PROFESSIONAL...
...AND AS SUCH NOW HAD THE MEANS TO IMPORT LARGER AMOUNTS OF RIBAVIRIN THAN ANYTHING WE COULD HAVE MANAGED IN SINGLE SHIPMENTS.
HE WAS ONE OF THE LEAST COMPASSIONATE GUYS I'D EVER MET, BUT I WAS DETERMINED TO TWIST HIS ARM. OR BOTH ARMS.
C'MON...BEN AND I GOT YOU STARTED! IMAGINE HOW PISSED OFF YOUR FATHER WOULD BE IF HE KNEW YOU WERE RESCUING FAGGOTS.
MY PARTNERS WILL HAVE TO MEET YOU FIRST.
UNDER-STOOD.

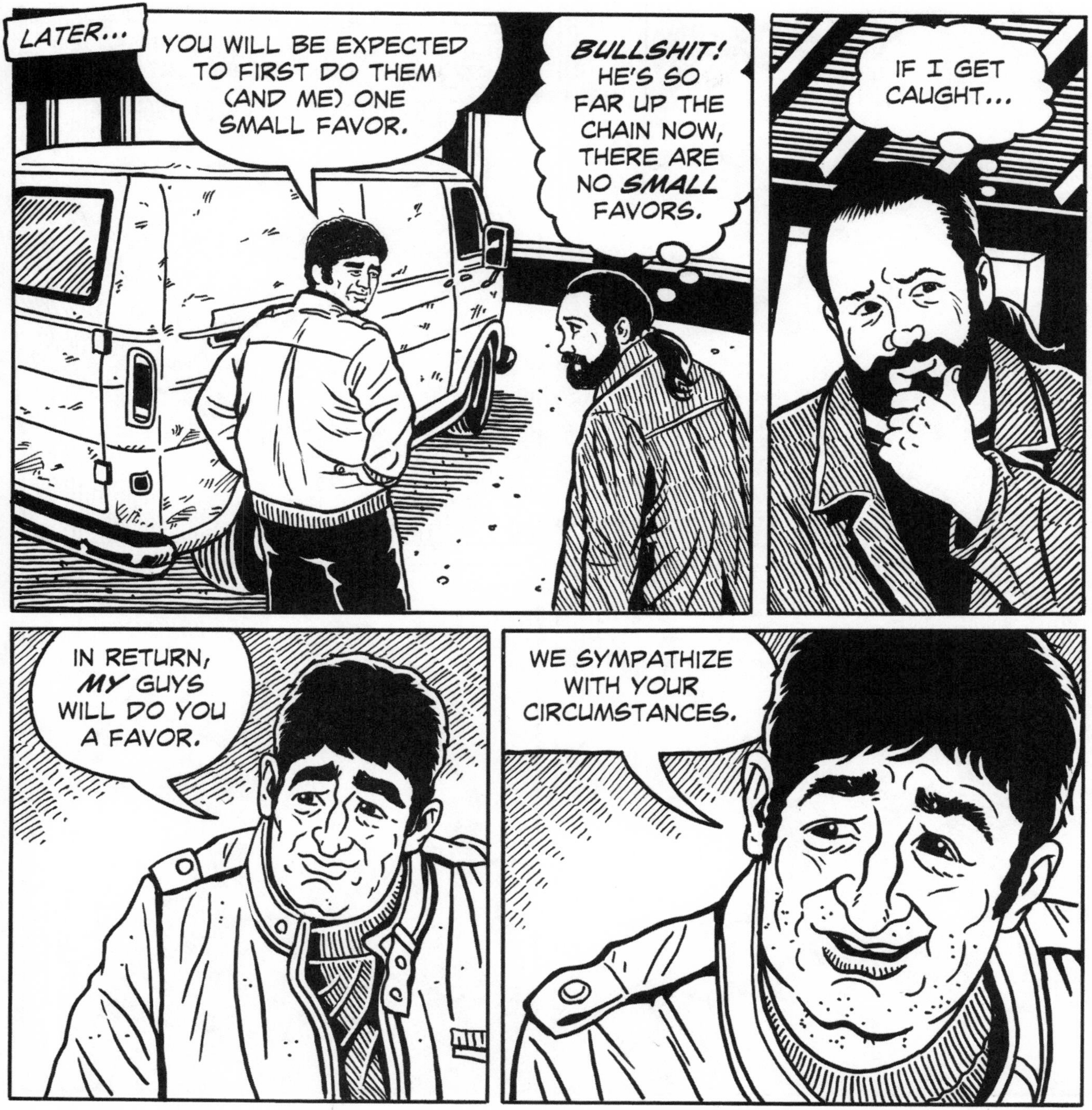
LATER...
YOU WILL BE EXPECTED TO FIRST DO THEM (AND ME) ONE SMALL FAVOR.
BULLSHIT! HE'S SO FAR UP THE CHAIN NOW, THERE ARE NO SMALL FAVORS.
IF I GET CAUGHT...
IN RETURN, MY GUYS WILL DO YOU A FAVOR.
WE SYMPATHIZE WITH YOUR CIRCUMSTANCES.

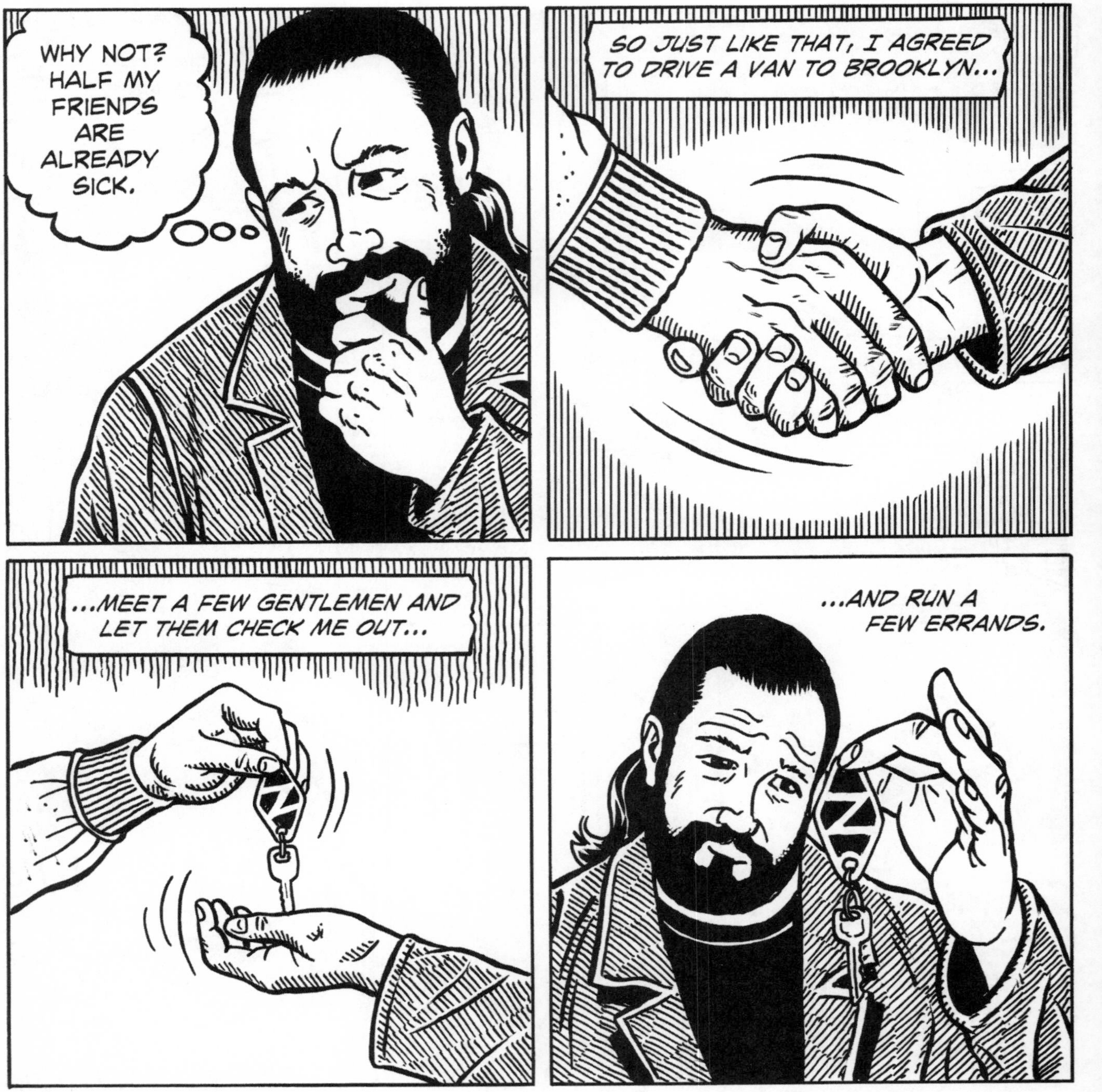
WHY NOT? HALF MY FRIENDS ARE ALREADY SICK.
SO JUST LIKE THAT, I AGREED TO DRIVE A VAN TO BROOKLYN...
...MEET A FEW GENTLEMEN AND LET THEM CHECK ME OUT...
...AND RUN A FEW ERRANDS.

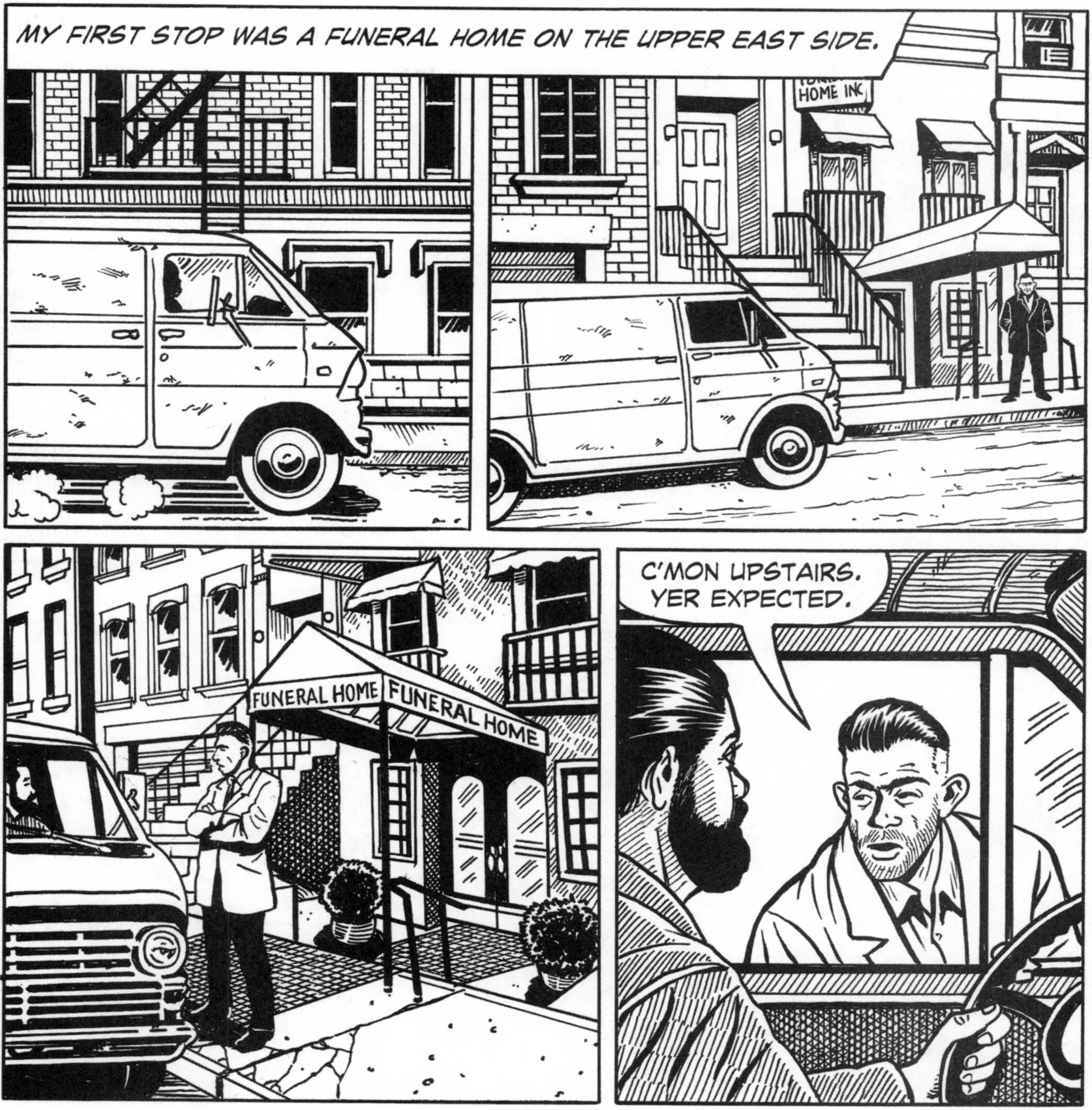
MY FIRST STOP WAS A FUNERAL HOME ON THE UPPER EAST SIDE.
HOME INC
FUNERAL HOME
FUNERAL HOME
C'MON UPSTAIRS. YER EXPECTED.

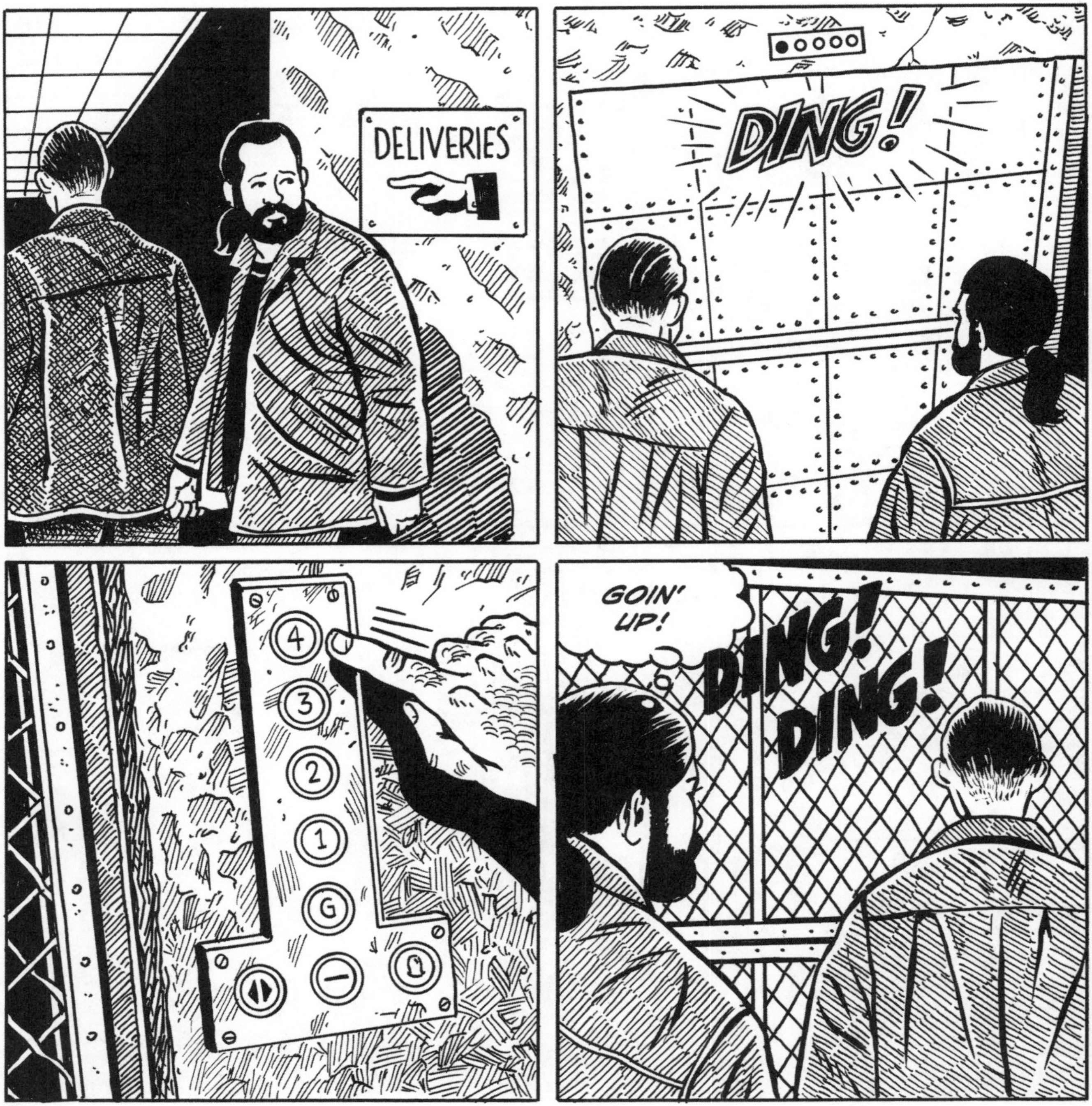
DELIVERIES
DING!
4
3
2
1
G
GOIN' UP!
DING!
DING!

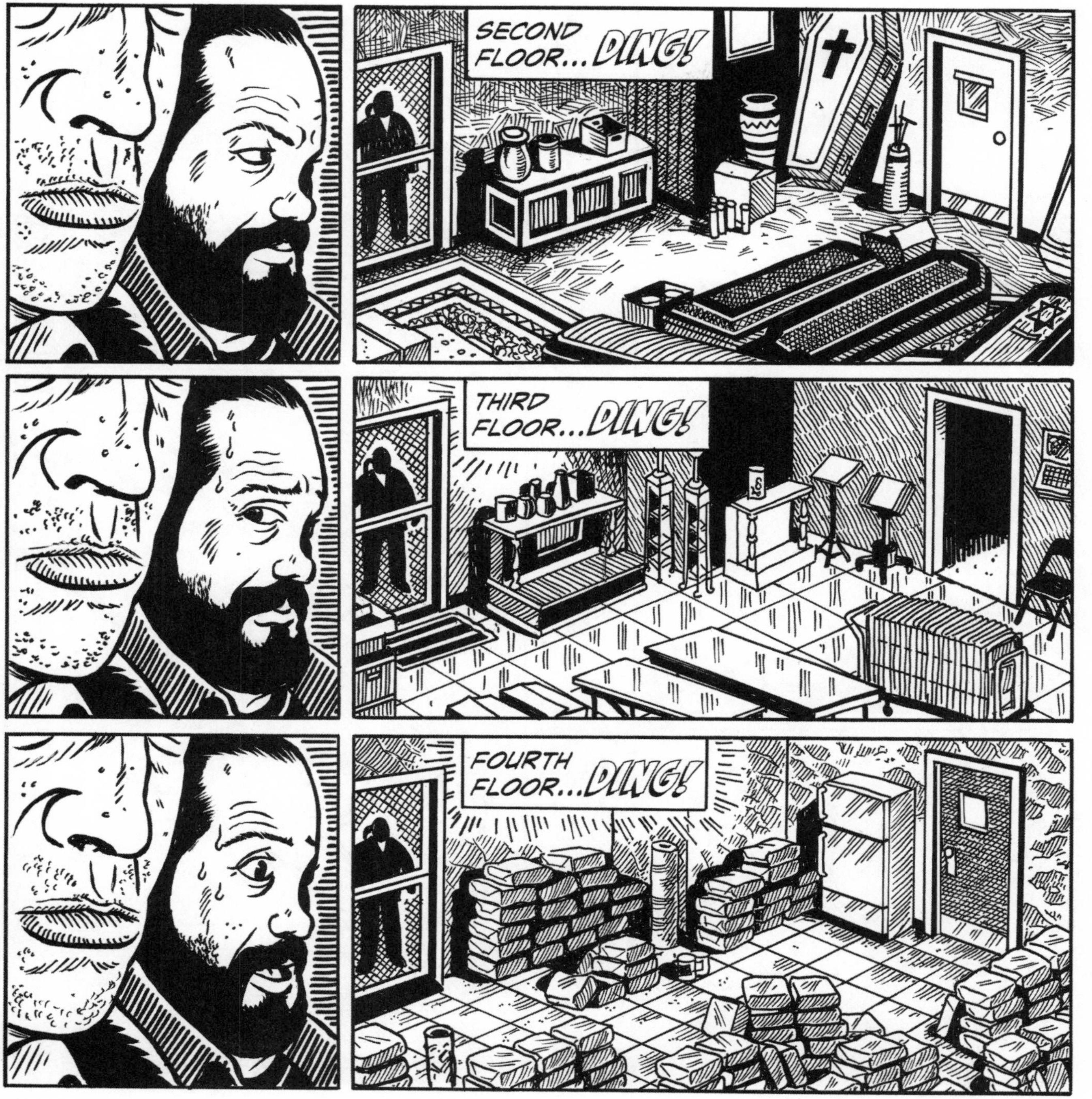
SECOND FLOOR...DING!
THIRD FLOOR...DING!
FOURTH FLOOR...DING!

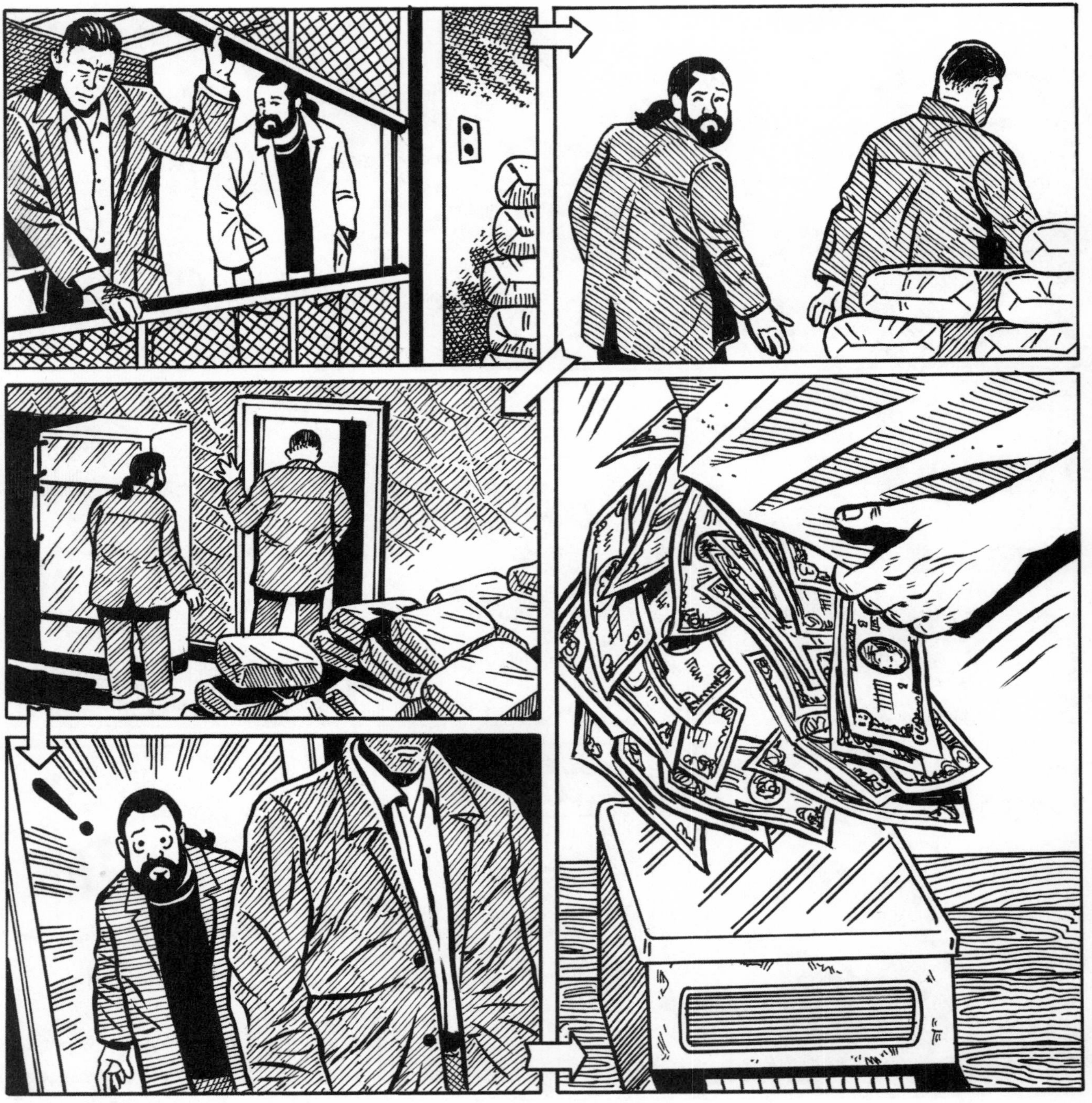
!

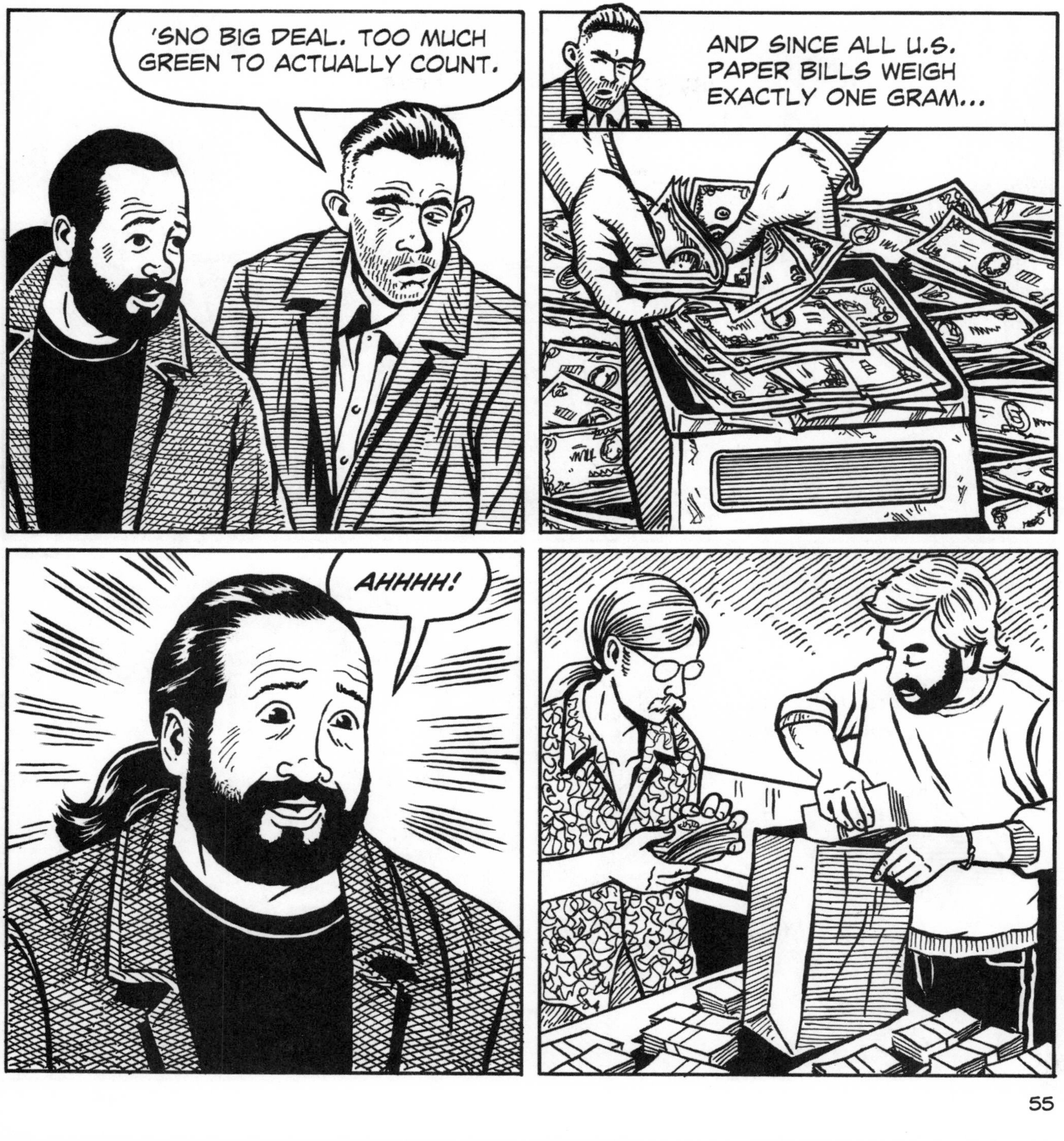
'SNO BIG DEAL. TOO MUCH GREEN TO ACTUALLY COUNT.
AND SINCE ALL U.S. PAPER BILLS WEIGH EXACTLY ONE GRAM...
AHHHH!

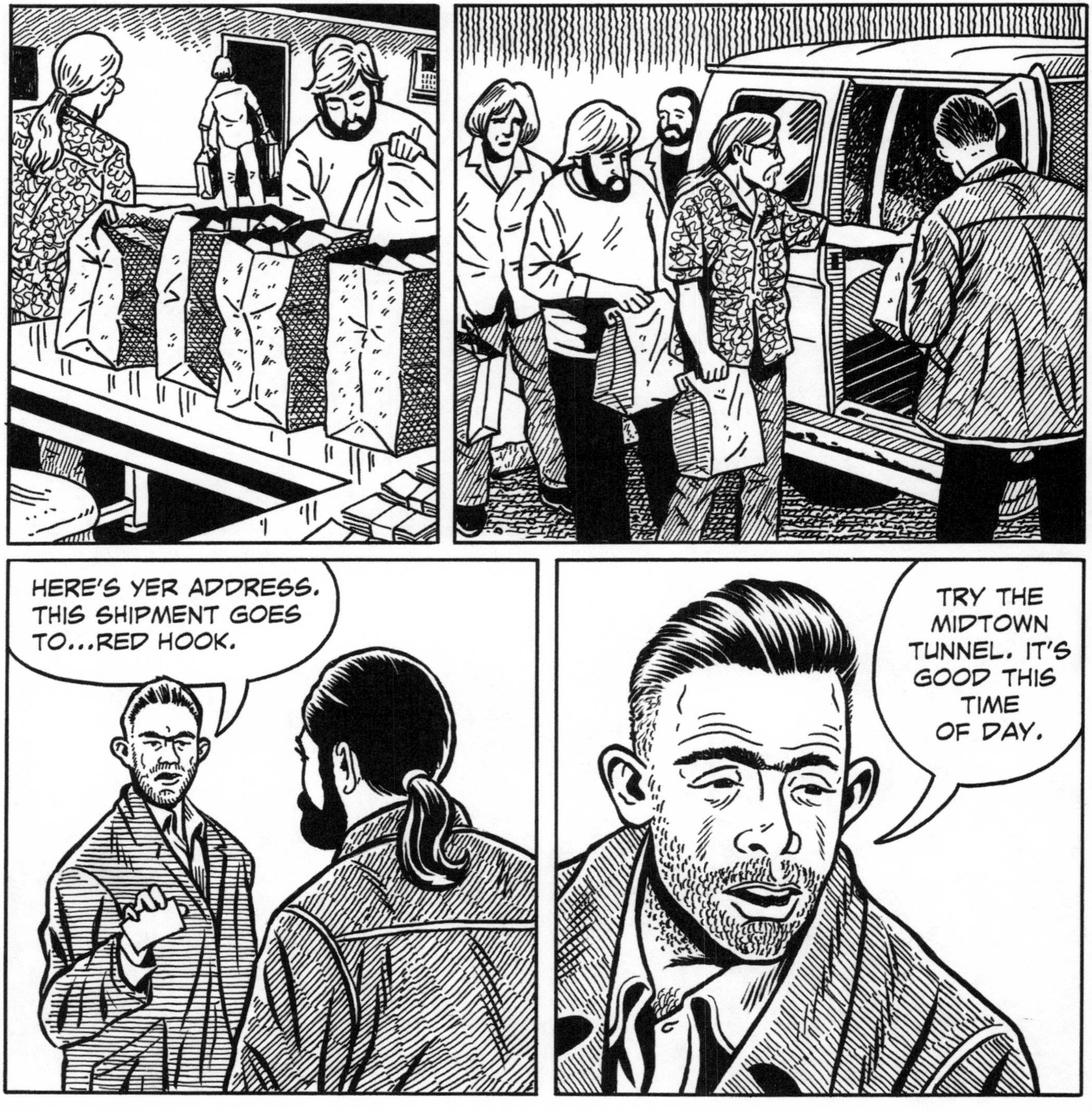
HERE'S YER ADDRESS. THIS SHIPMENT GOES TO...RED HOOK.
TRY THE MIDTOWN TUNNEL. IT'S GOOD THIS TIME OF DAY.

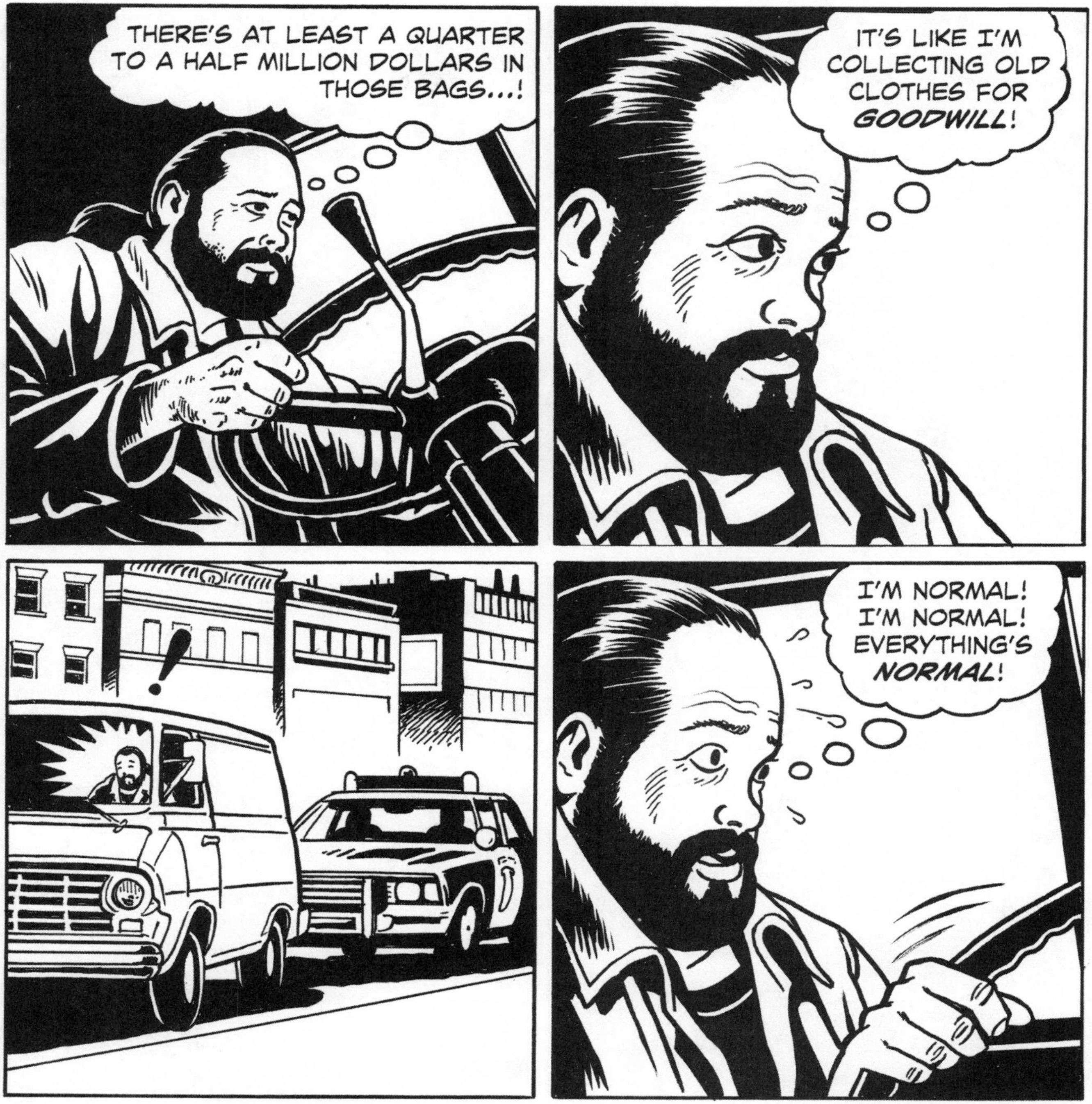
THERE'S AT LEAST A QUARTER TO A HALF MILLION DOLLARS IN THOSE BAGS...!
IT'S LIKE I'M COLLECTING OLD CLOTHES FOR GOODWILL!
!
I'M NORMAL! I'M NORMAL! EVERYTHING'S NORMAL!

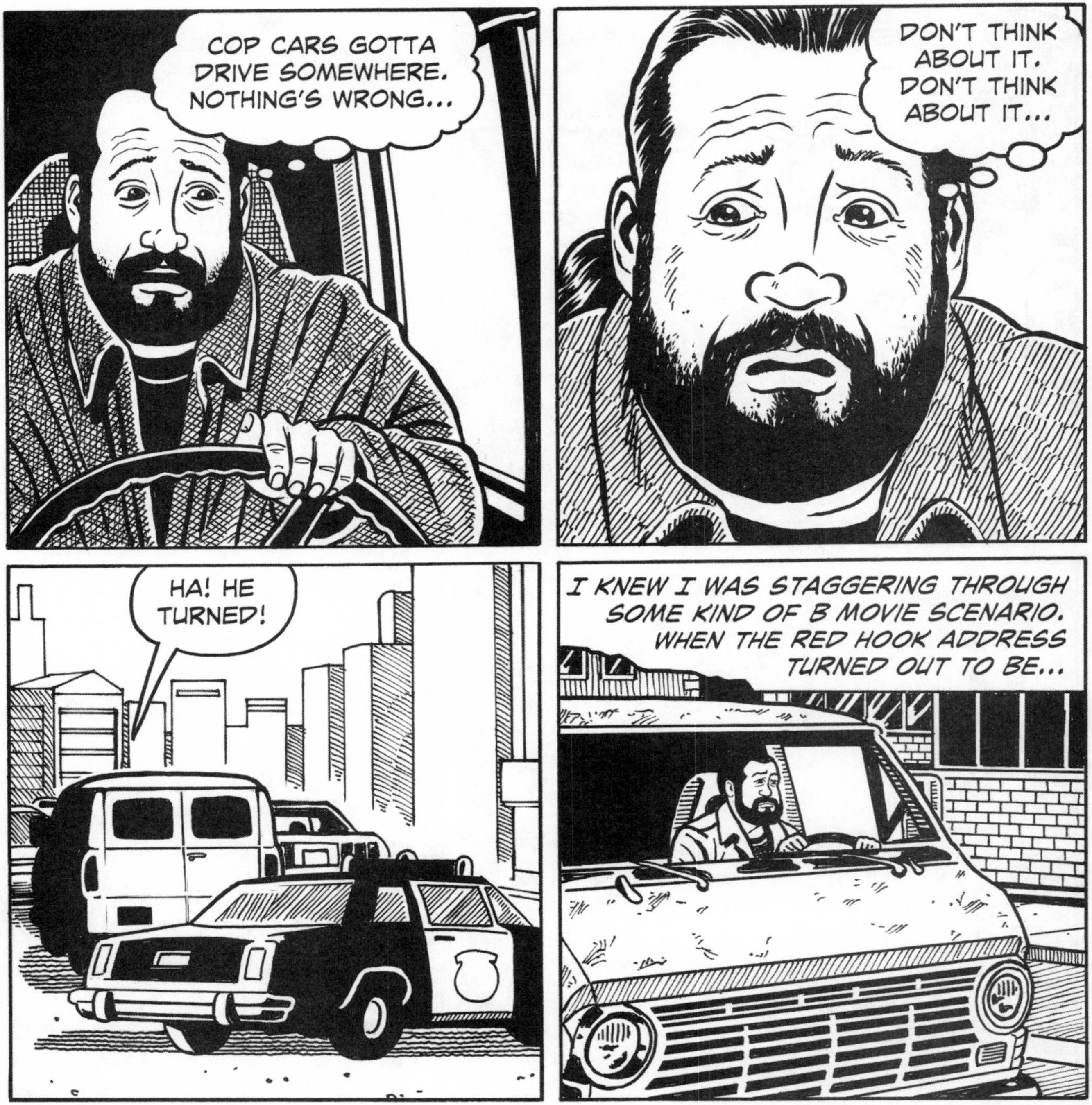
COP CARS GOTTA DRIVE SOMEWHERE. NOTHING'S WRONG...
DON'T THINK ABOUT IT. DON'T THINK ABOUT IT...
HA! HE TURNED!
I KNEW I WAS STAGGERING THROUGH SOME KIND OF B MOVIE SCENARIO. WHEN THE RED HOOK ADDRESS TURNED OUT TO BE...

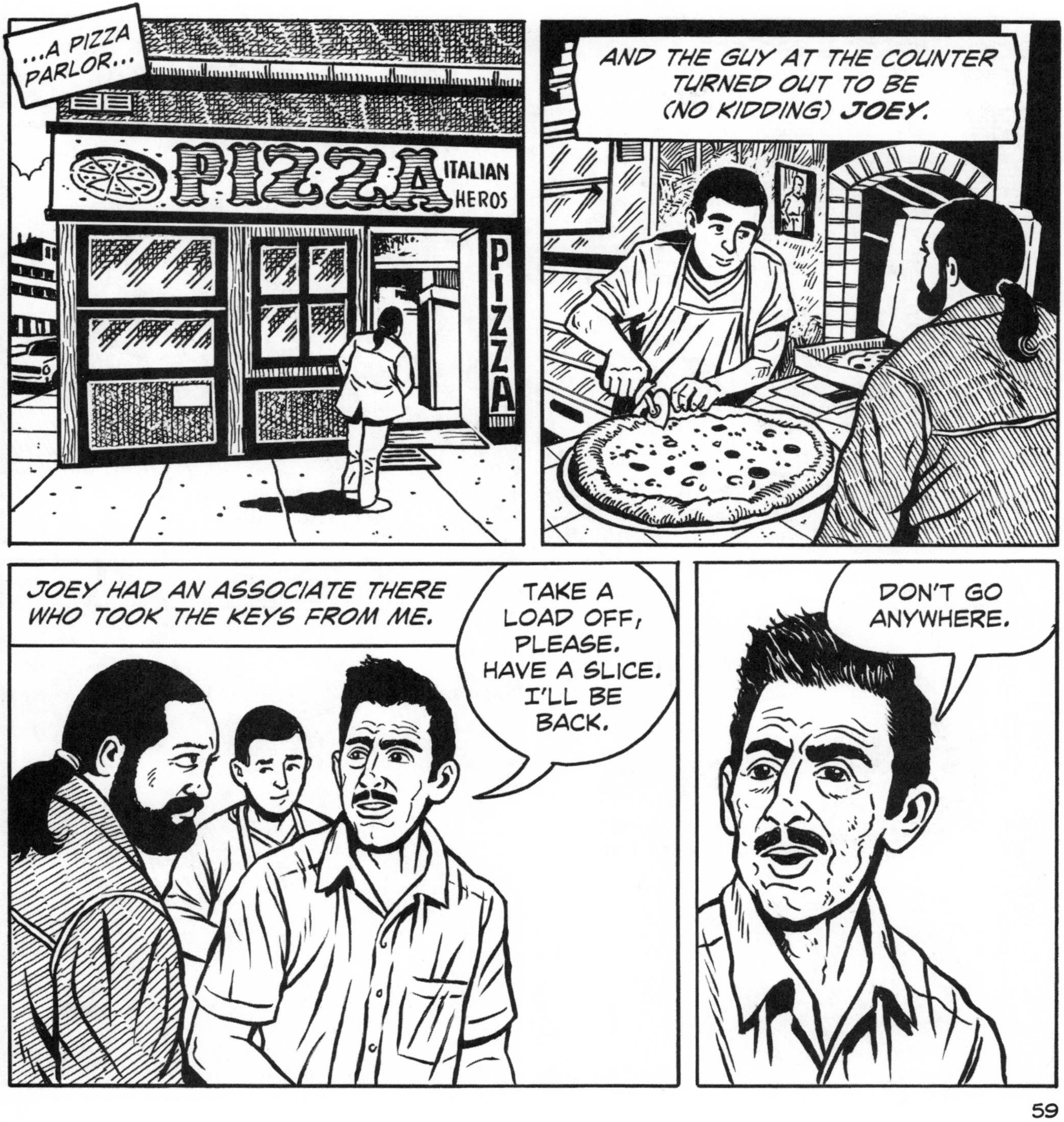
...A PIZZA PARLOR...
PIZZA
ITALIAN HEROS
PIZZA
AND THE GUY AT THE COUNTER TURNED OUT TO BE (NO KIDDING) JOEY.
JOEY HAD AN ASSOCIATE THERE WHO TOOK THE KEYS FROM ME.
TAKE A LOAD OFF, PLEASE. HAVE A SLICE. I'LL BE BACK.
DON'T GO ANYWHERE.

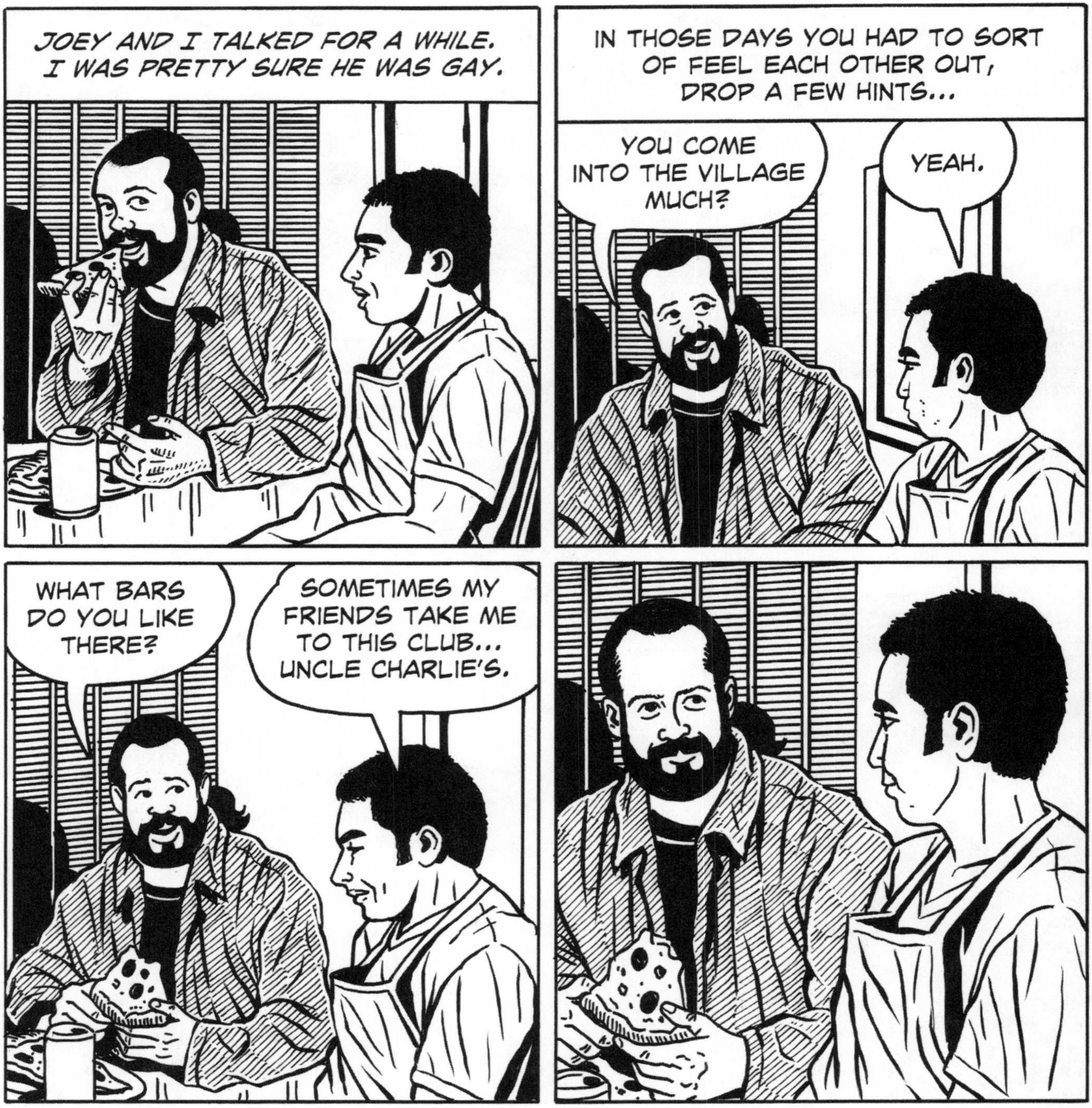
JOEY AND I TALKED FOR A WHILE. I WAS PRETTY SURE HE WAS GAY.
IN THOSE DAYS YOU HAD TO SORT OF FEEL EACH OTHER OUT, DROP A FEW HINTS...
YOU COME INTO THE VILLAGE MUCH?
YEAH.
WHAT BARS DO YOU LIKE THERE?
SOMETIMES MY FRIENDS TAKE ME TO THIS CLUB... UNCLE CHARLIE'S.

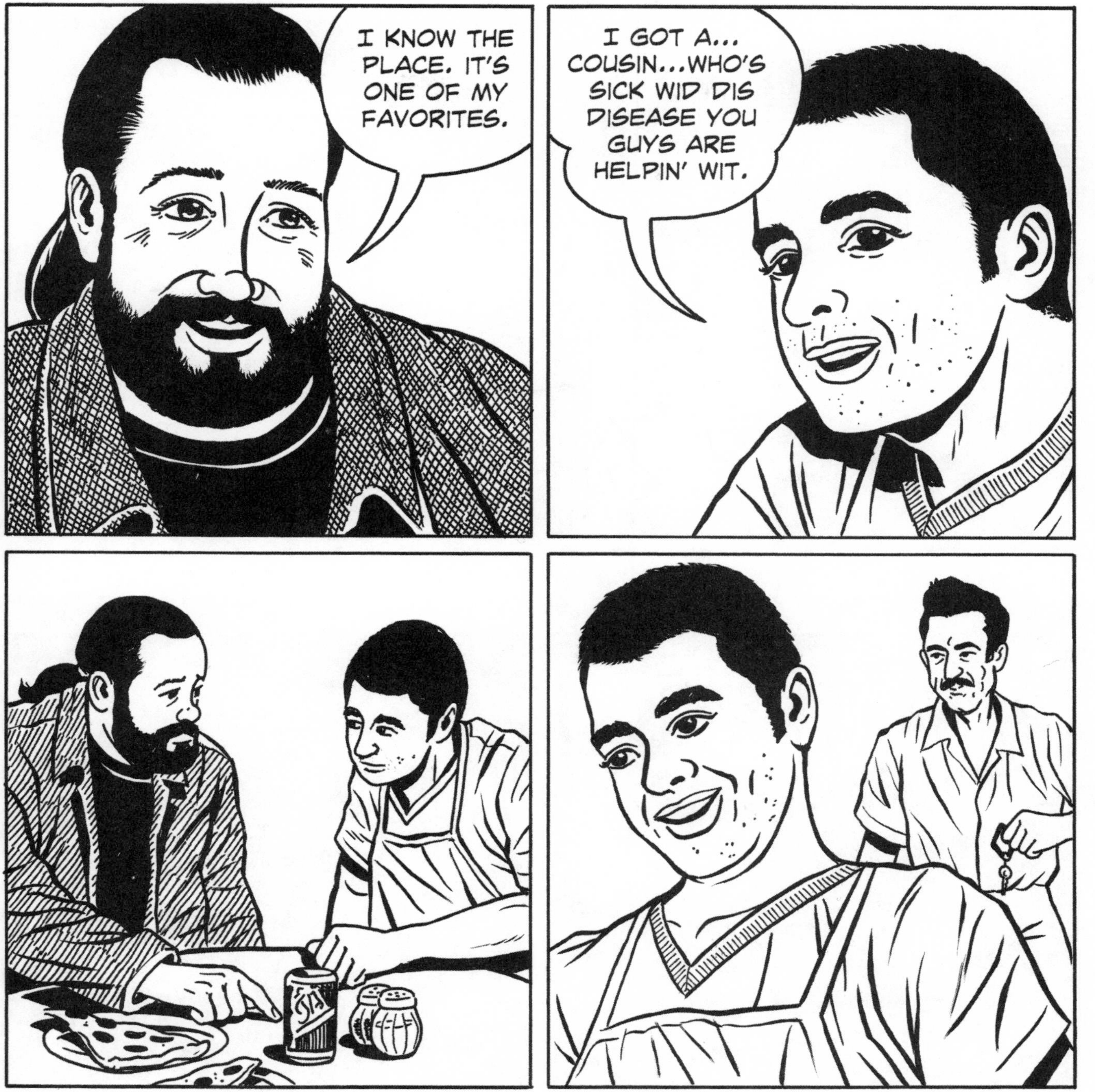
I KNOW THE PLACE. IT'S ONE OF MY FAVORITES.
I GOT A... COUSIN...WHO'S SICK WID DIS DISEASE YOU GUYS ARE HELPIN' WIT.

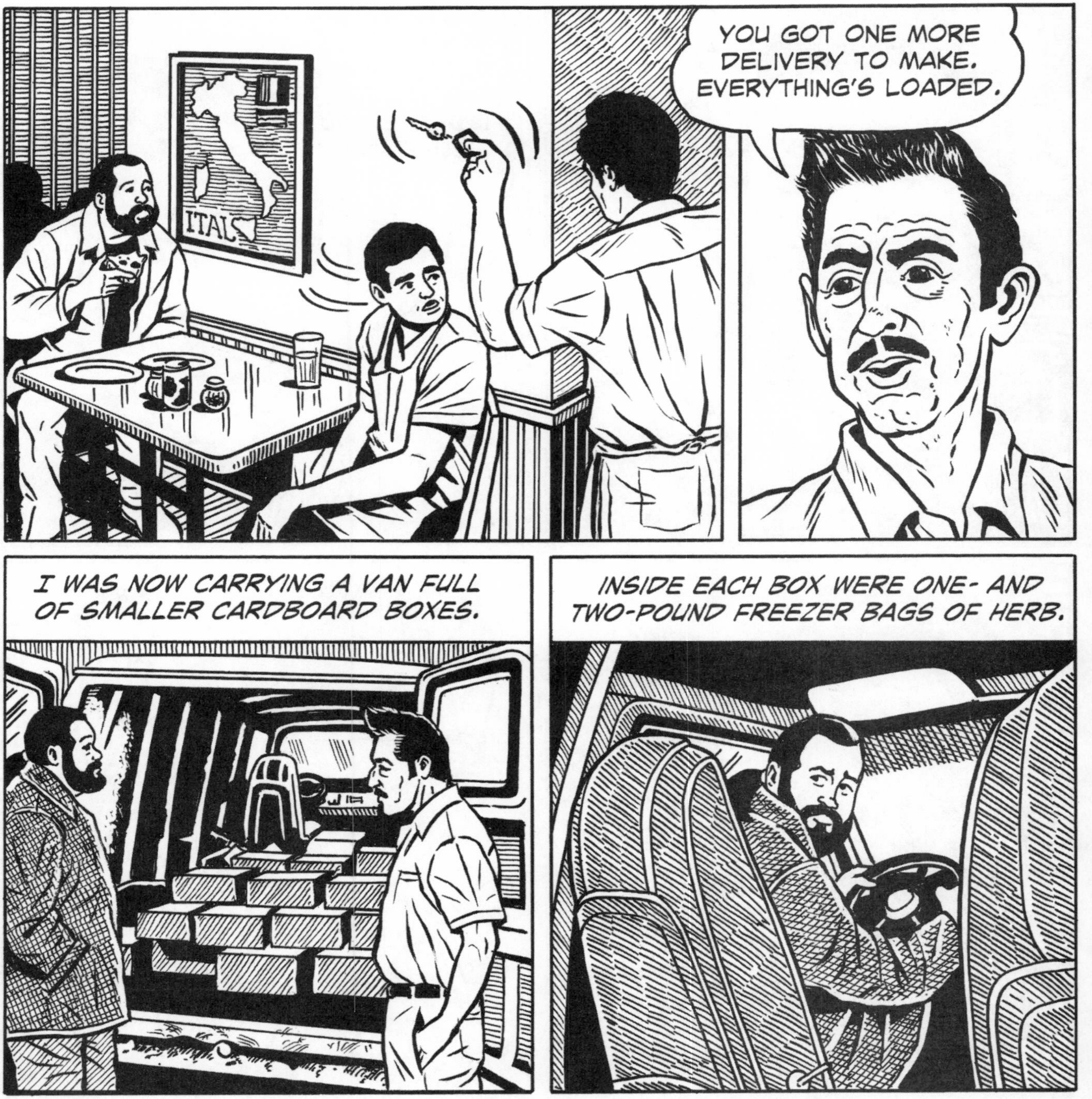
YOU GOT ONE MORE DELIVERY TO MAKE. EVERYTHING'S LOADED.
ITAL
I WAS NOW CARRYING A VAN FULL OF SMALLER CARDBOARD BOXES.
INSIDE EACH BOX WERE ONE- AND TWO-POUND FREEZER BAGS OF HERB.

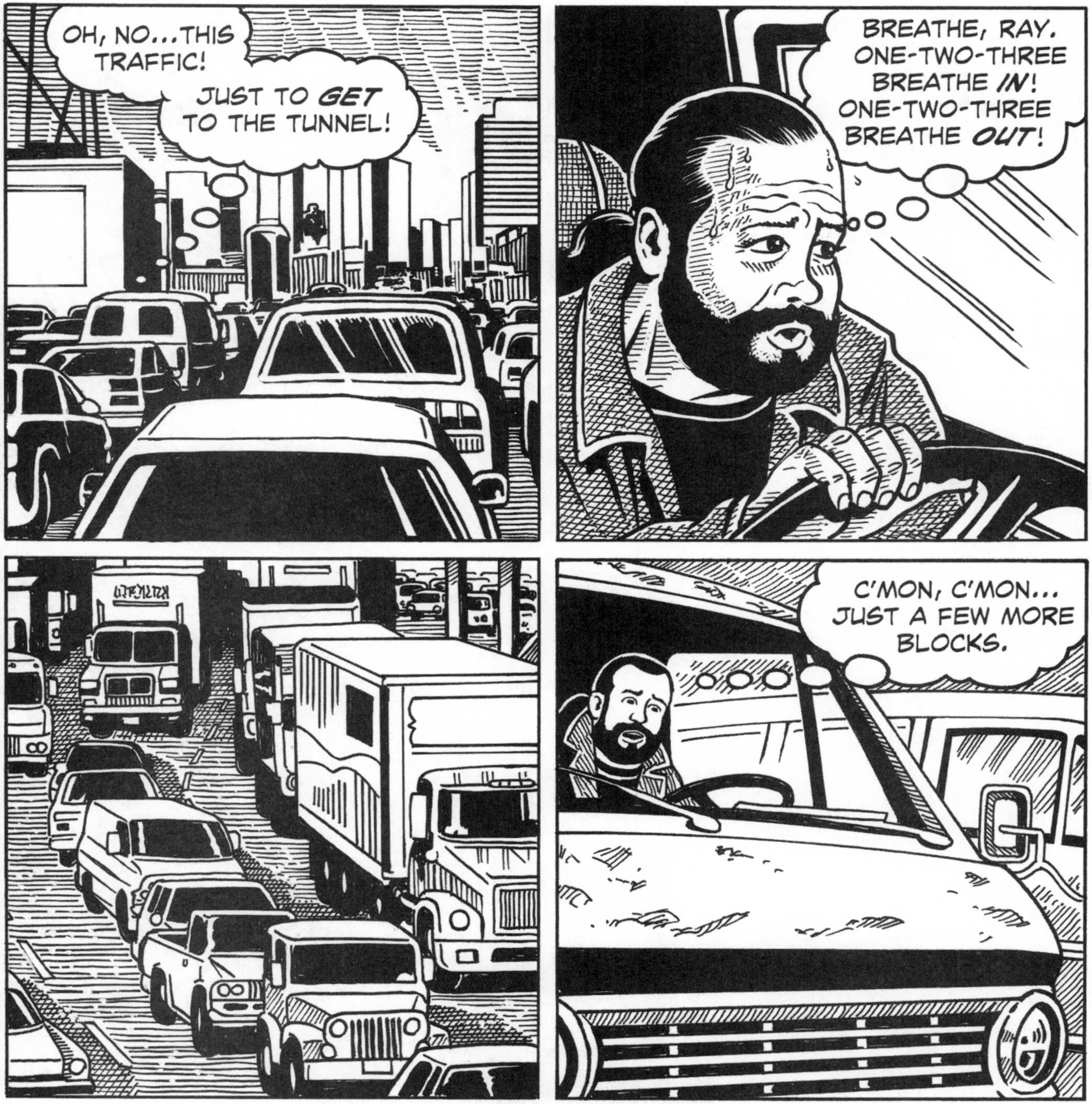
OH, NO...THIS TRAFFIC!
JUST TO **GET** TO THE TUNNEL!
BREATHE, RAY. ONE-TWO-THREE BREATHE **IN**! ONE-TWO-THREE BREATHE **OUT**!
C'MON, C'MON... JUST A FEW MORE BLOCKS.

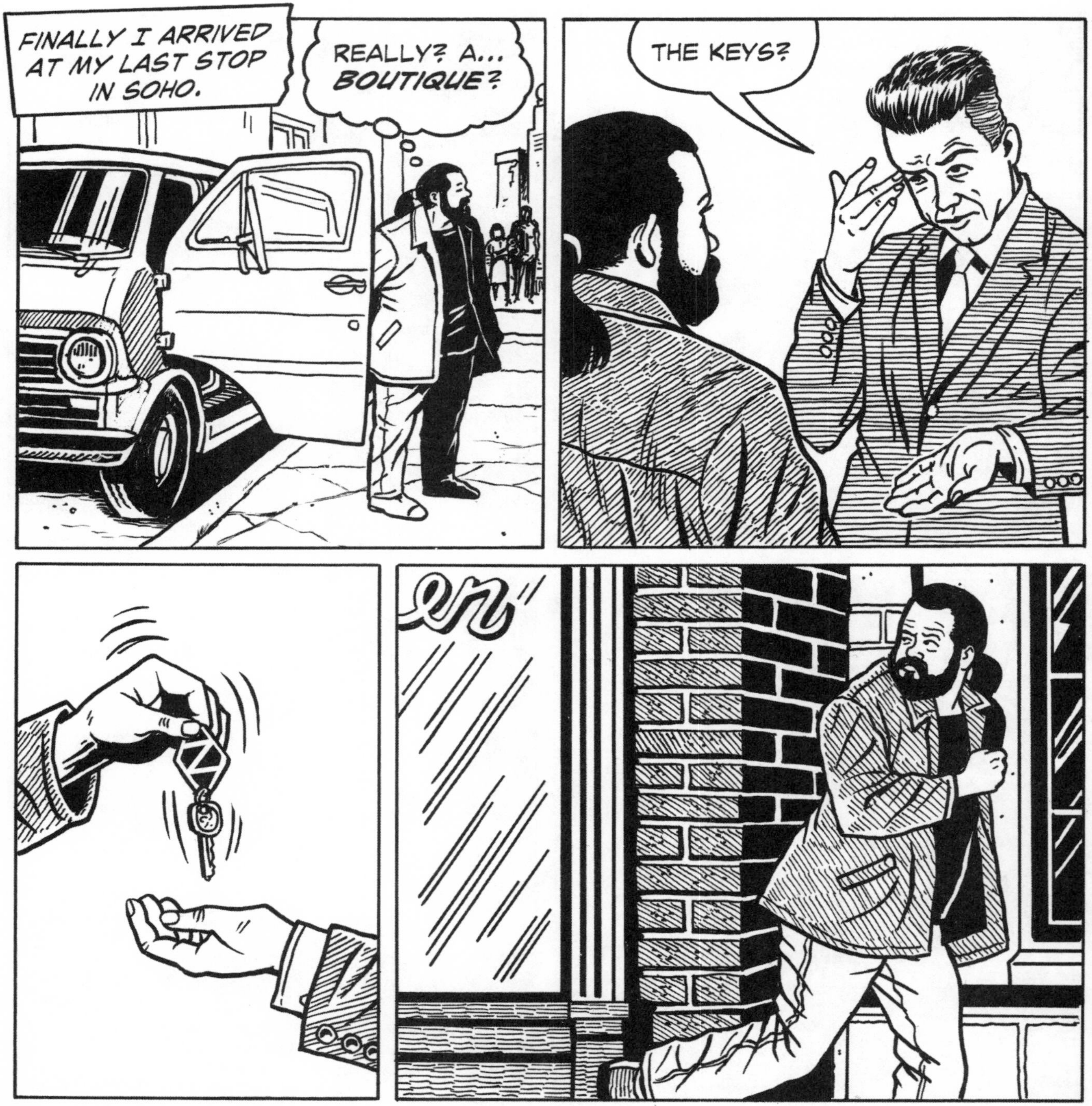
FINALLY I ARRIVED AT MY LAST STOP IN SOHO.
REALLY? A... *BOUTIQUE*?
THE KEYS?
en

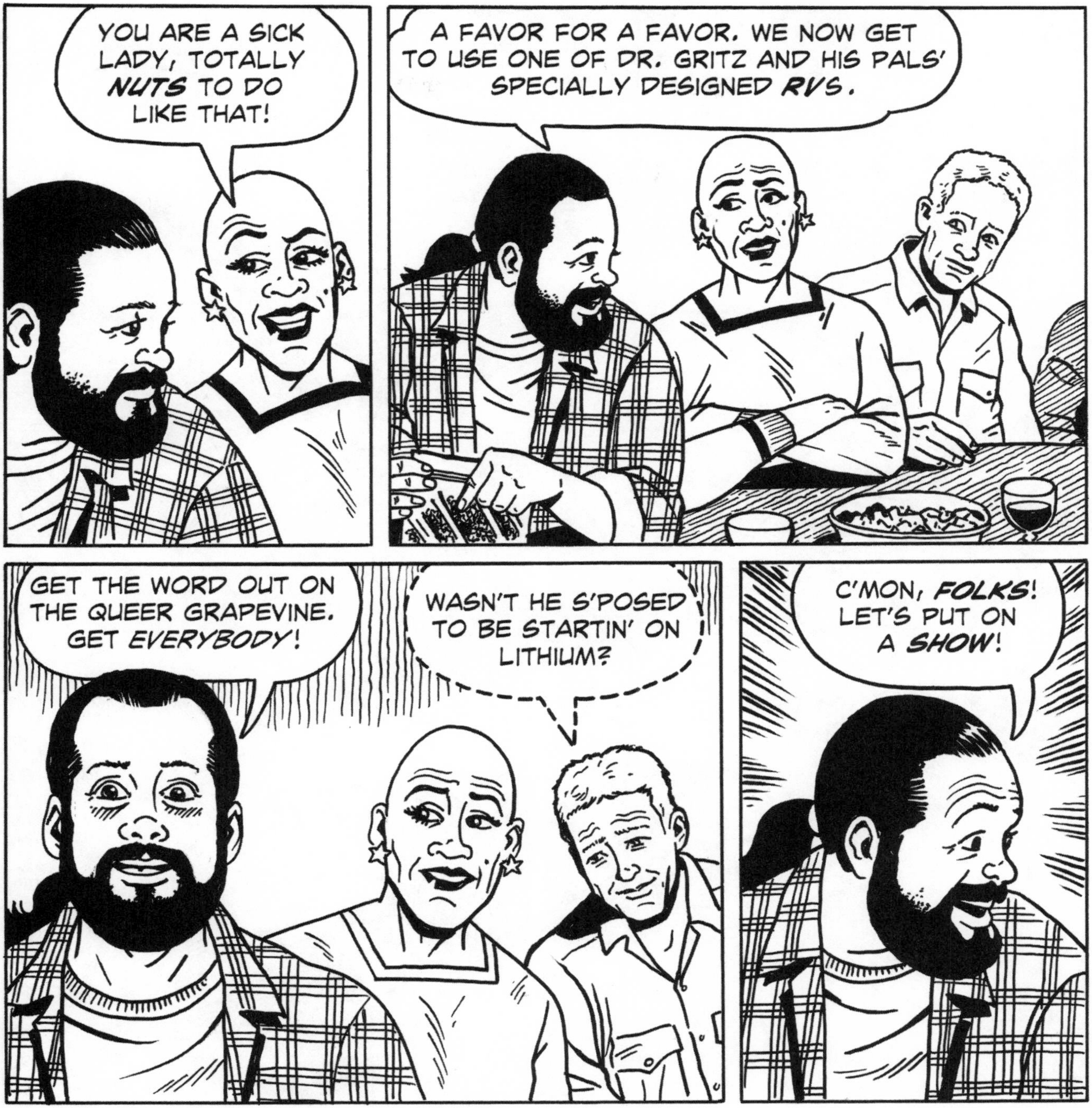
YOU ARE A SICK LADY, TOTALLY NUTS TO DO LIKE THAT!
A FAVOR FOR A FAVOR. WE NOW GET TO USE ONE OF DR. GRITZ AND HIS PALS' SPECIALLY DESIGNED RVS.
GET THE WORD OUT ON THE QUEER GRAPEVINE. GET EVERYBODY!
WASN'T HE S'POSED TO BE STARTIN' ON LITHIUM?
C'MON, FOLKS! LET'S PUT ON A SHOW!

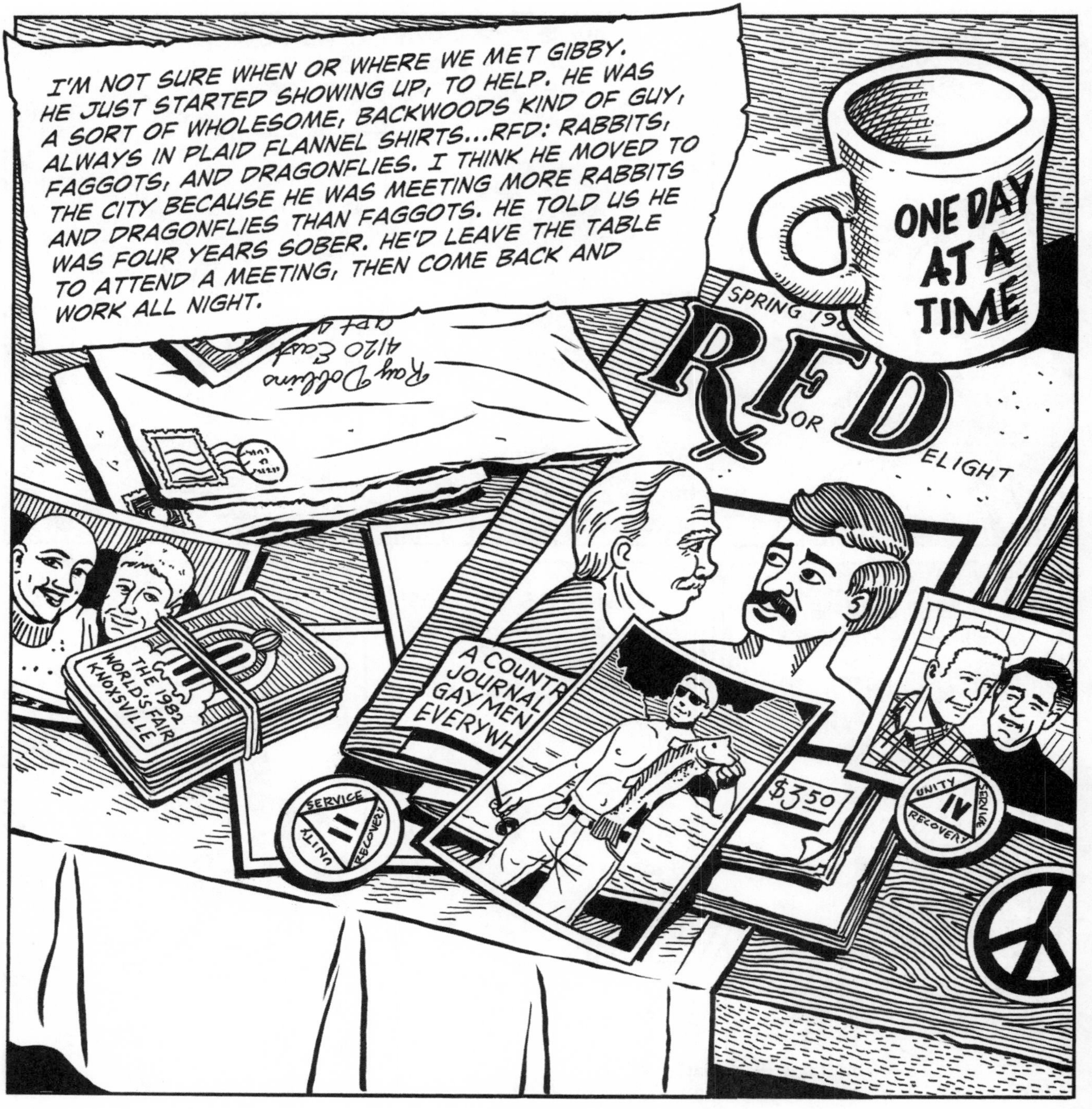
I'M NOT SURE WHEN OR WHERE WE MET GIBBY. HE JUST STARTED SHOWING UP, TO HELP. HE WAS A SORT OF WHOLESOME, BACKWOODS KIND OF GUY, ALWAYS IN PLAID FLANNEL SHIRTS...RFD: RABBITS, FAGGOTS, AND DRAGONFLIES. I THINK HE MOVED TO THE CITY BECAUSE HE WAS MEETING MORE RABBITS AND DRAGONFLIES THAN FAGGOTS. HE TOLD US HE WAS FOUR YEARS SOBER. HE'D LEAVE THE TABLE TO ATTEND A MEETING, THEN COME BACK AND WORK ALL NIGHT.
ONE DAY AT A TIME
RFD
THE 1982 WORLD'S FAIR KNOXSVILLE
$3.50
SERVICE UNITY RECOVERY
UNITY SERVICE RECOVERY IV

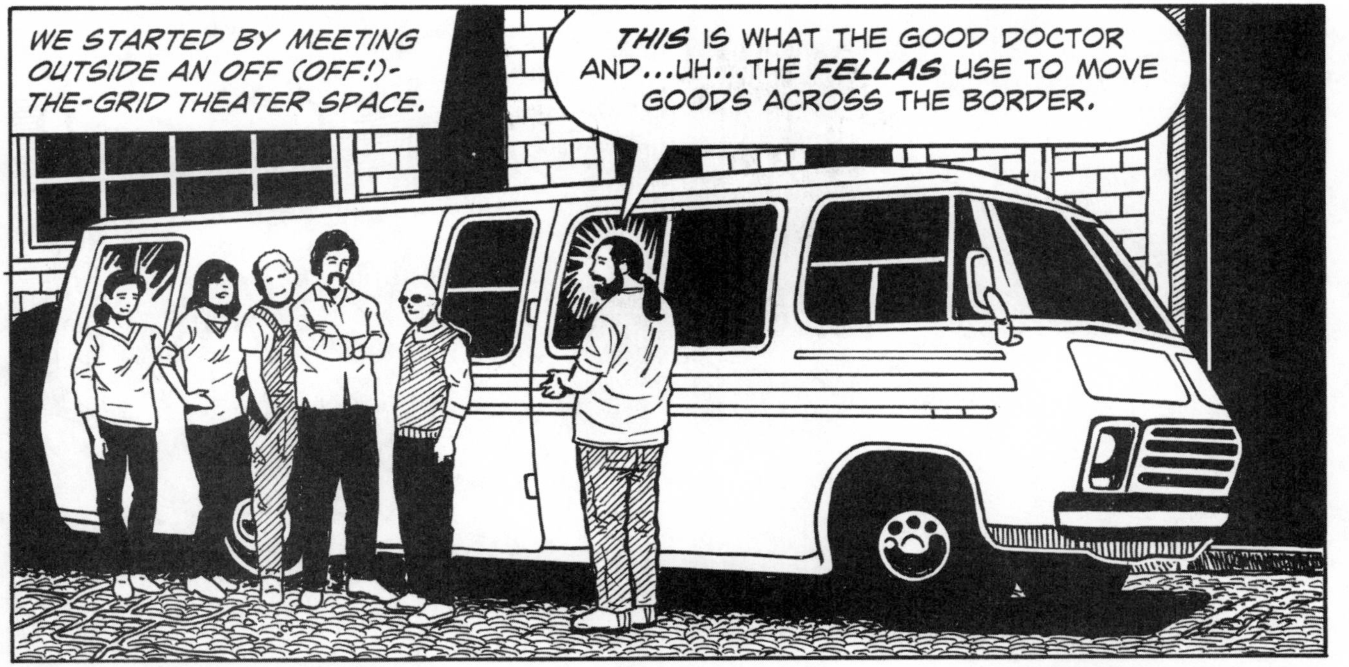
WE STARTED BY MEETING OUTSIDE AN OFF (OFF!)-THE-GRID THEATER SPACE.
THIS IS WHAT THE GOOD DOCTOR AND...UH...THE FELLAS USE TO MOVE GOODS ACROSS THE BORDER.

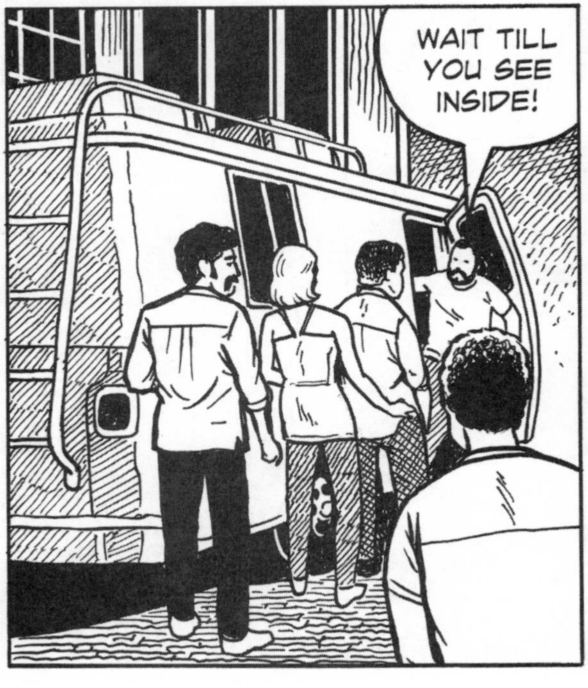
WAIT TILL YOU SEE INSIDE!

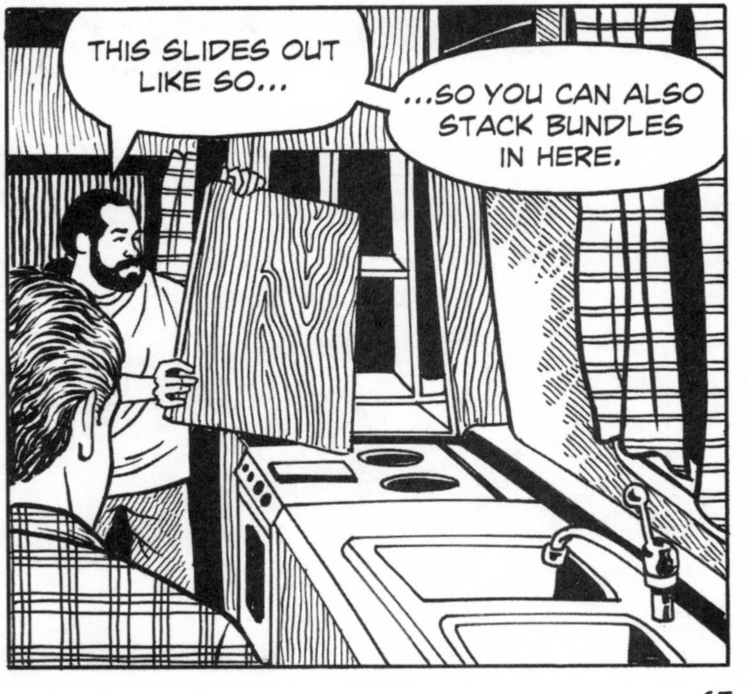
THIS SLIDES OUT LIKE SO...
...SO YOU CAN ALSO STACK BUNDLES IN HERE.

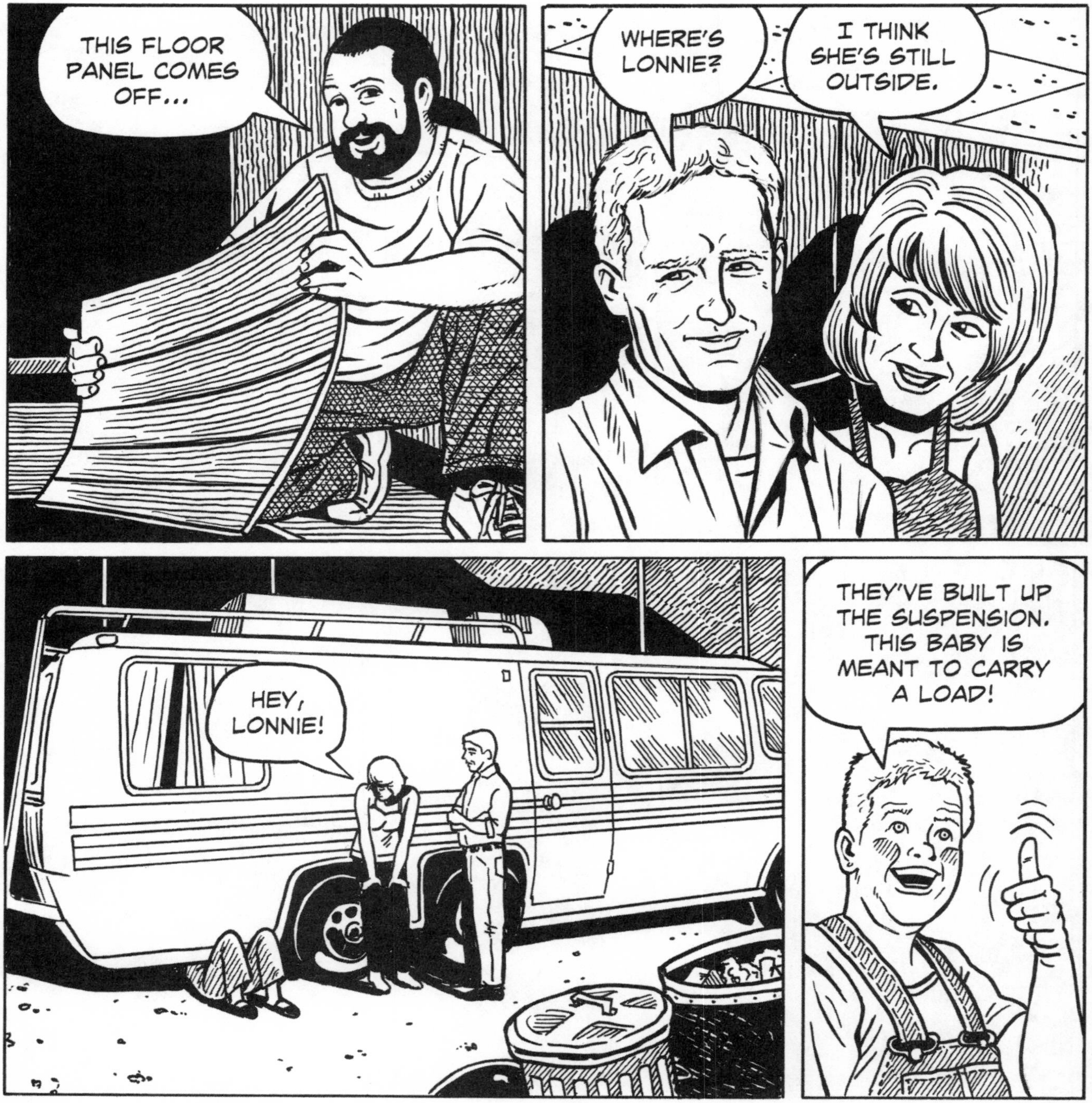
THIS FLOOR PANEL COMES OFF...
WHERE'S LONNIE?
I THINK SHE'S STILL OUTSIDE.
HEY, LONNIE!
THEY'VE BUILT UP THE SUSPENSION. THIS BABY IS MEANT TO CARRY A LOAD!

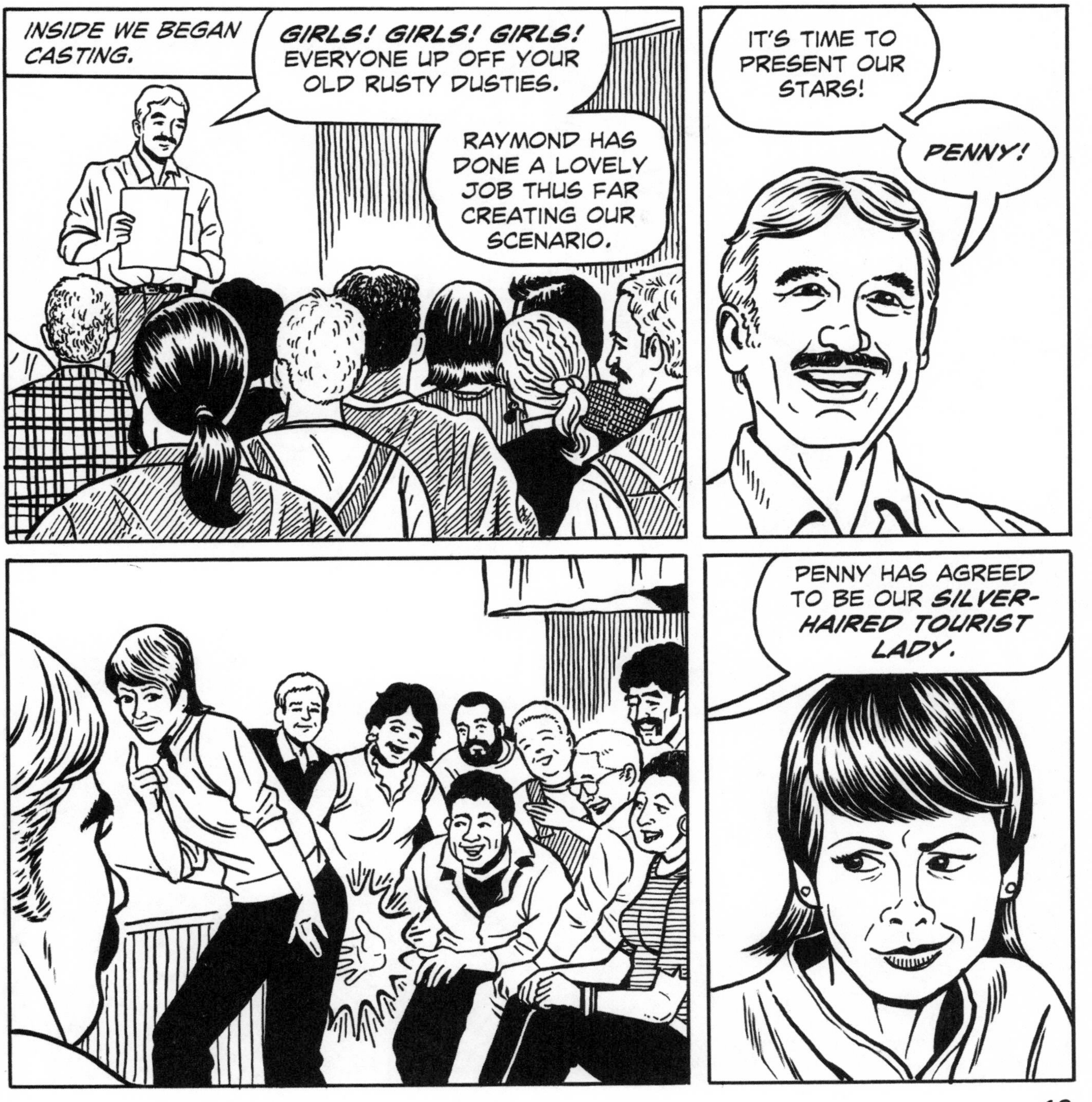
INSIDE WE BEGAN CASTING.
GIRLS! GIRLS! GIRLS! EVERYONE UP OFF YOUR OLD RUSTY DUSTIES.
RAYMOND HAS DONE A LOVELY JOB THUS FAR CREATING OUR SCENARIO.
IT'S TIME TO PRESENT OUR STARS!
PENNY!
PENNY HAS AGREED TO BE OUR SILVER-HAIRED TOURIST LADY.

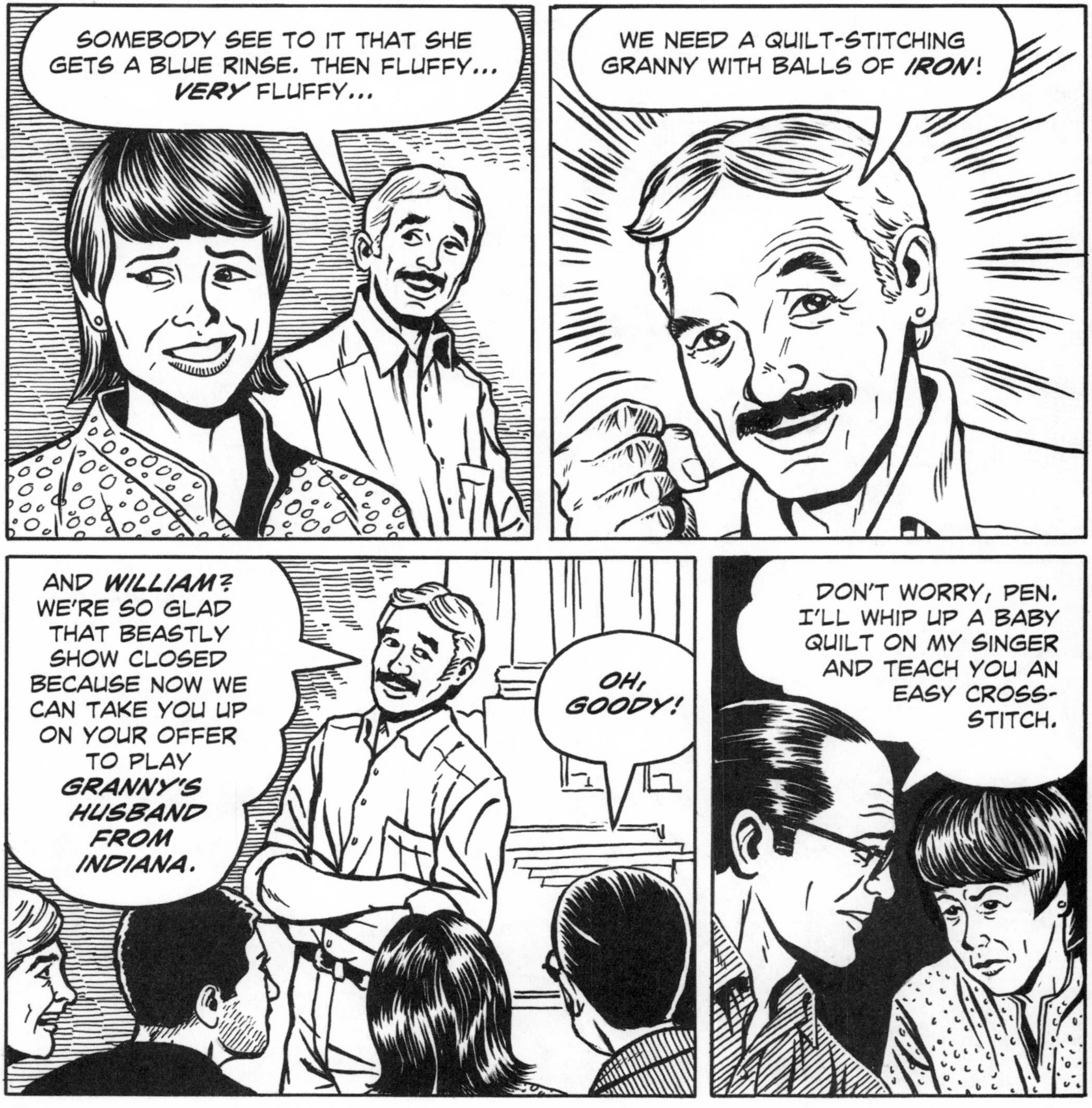
SOMEBODY SEE TO IT THAT SHE GETS A BLUE RINSE. THEN FLUFFY... *VERY* FLUFFY...
WE NEED A QUILT-STITCHING GRANNY WITH BALLS OF *IRON*!
AND *WILLIAM*? WE'RE SO GLAD THAT BEASTLY SHOW CLOSED BECAUSE NOW WE CAN TAKE YOU UP ON YOUR OFFER TO PLAY *GRANNY'S HUSBAND FROM INDIANA*.
OH, GOODY!
DON'T WORRY, PEN. I'LL WHIP UP A BABY QUILT ON MY SINGER AND TEACH YOU AN EASY CROSS-STITCH.

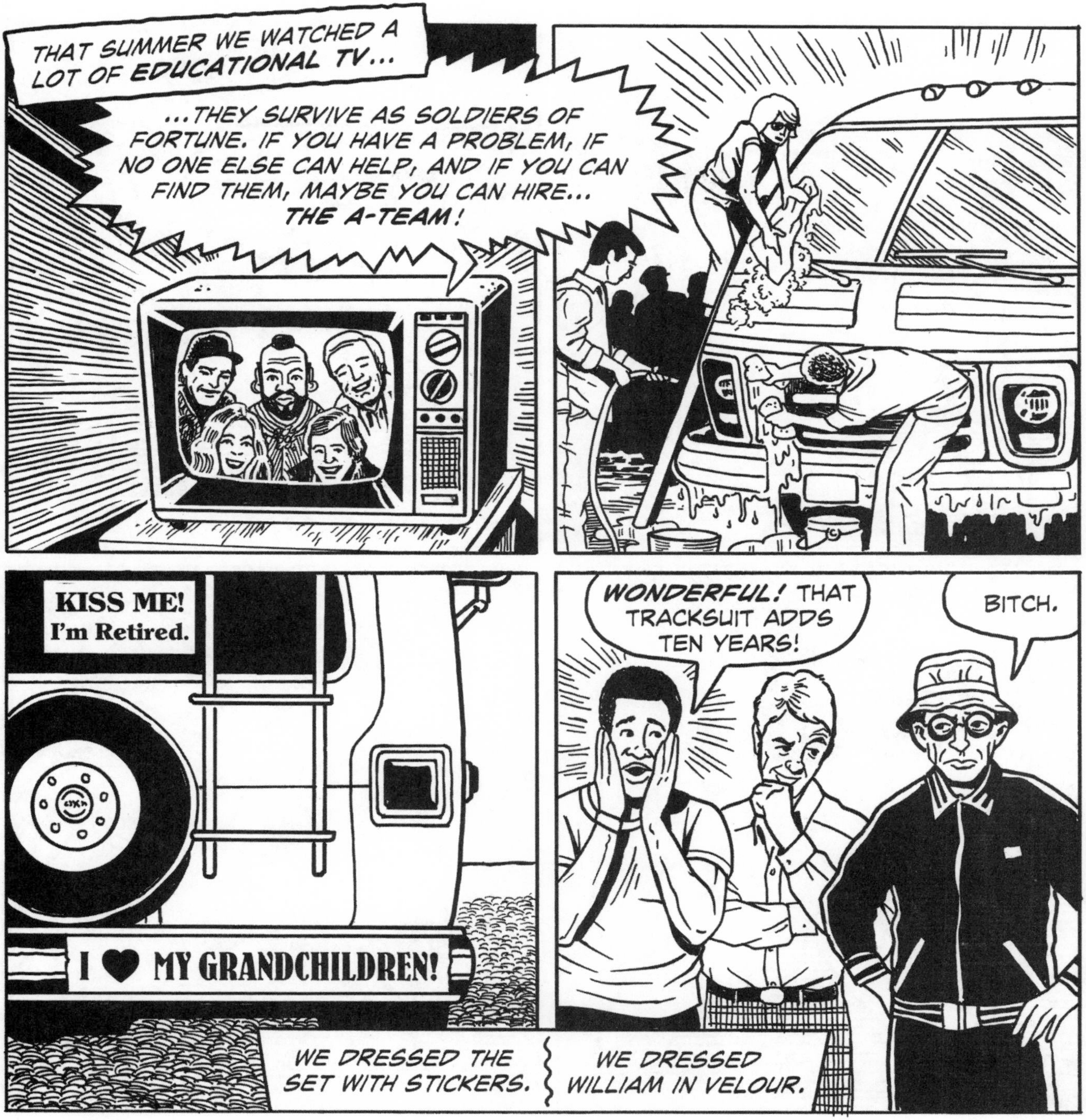

THAT SUMMER WE WATCHED A LOT OF EDUCATIONAL TV...
...THEY SURVIVE AS SOLDIERS OF FORTUNE. IF YOU HAVE A PROBLEM, IF NO ONE ELSE CAN HELP, AND IF YOU CAN FIND THEM, MAYBE YOU CAN HIRE... THE A-TEAM!
KISS ME! I'm Retired.
I ♥ MY GRANDCHILDREN!
WONDERFUL! THAT TRACKSUIT ADDS TEN YEARS!
BITCH.
WE DRESSED THE SET WITH STICKERS.
WE DRESSED WILLIAM IN VELOUR.

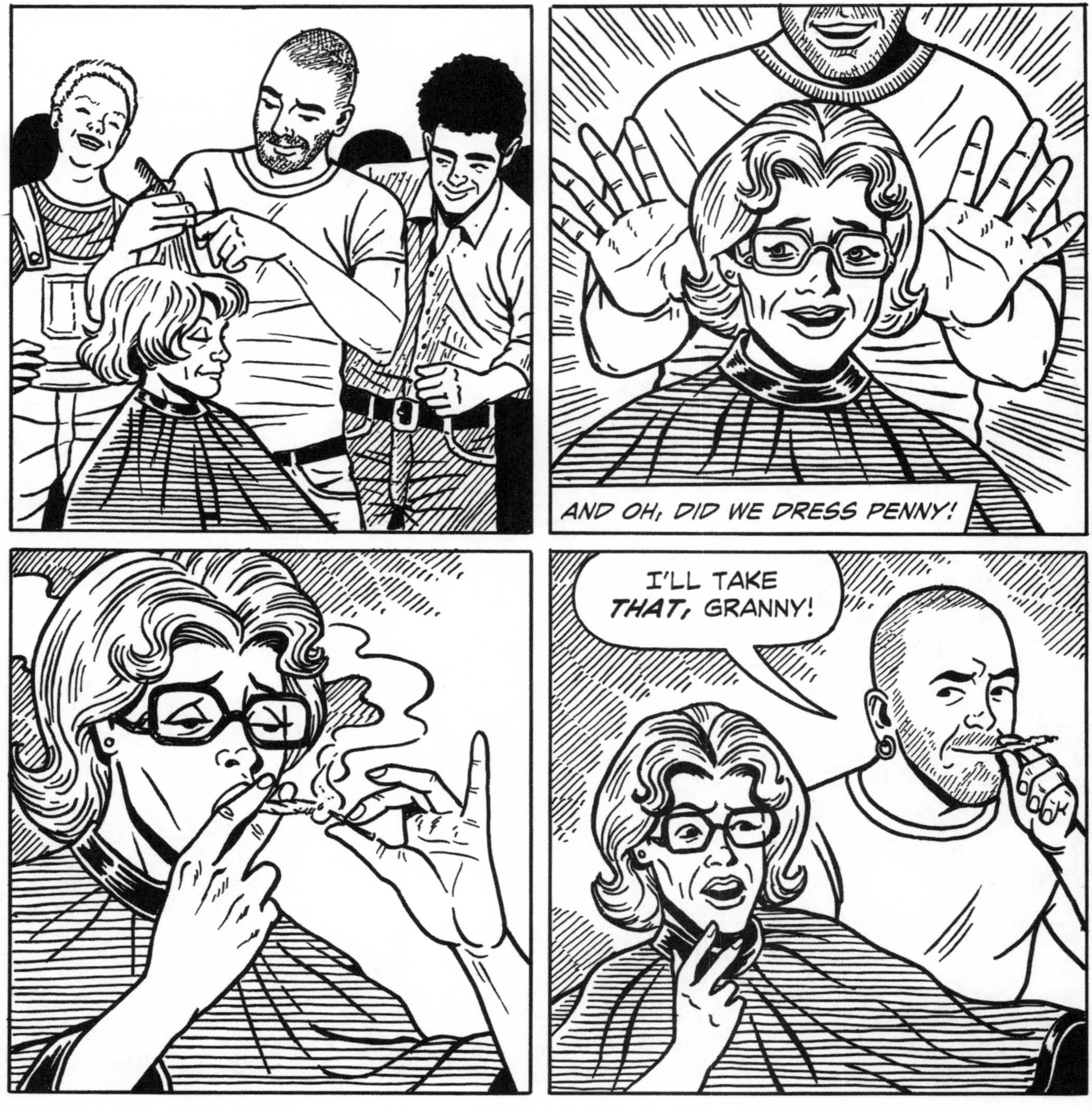
AND OH, DID WE DRESS PENNY!
I'LL TAKE *THAT,* GRANNY!

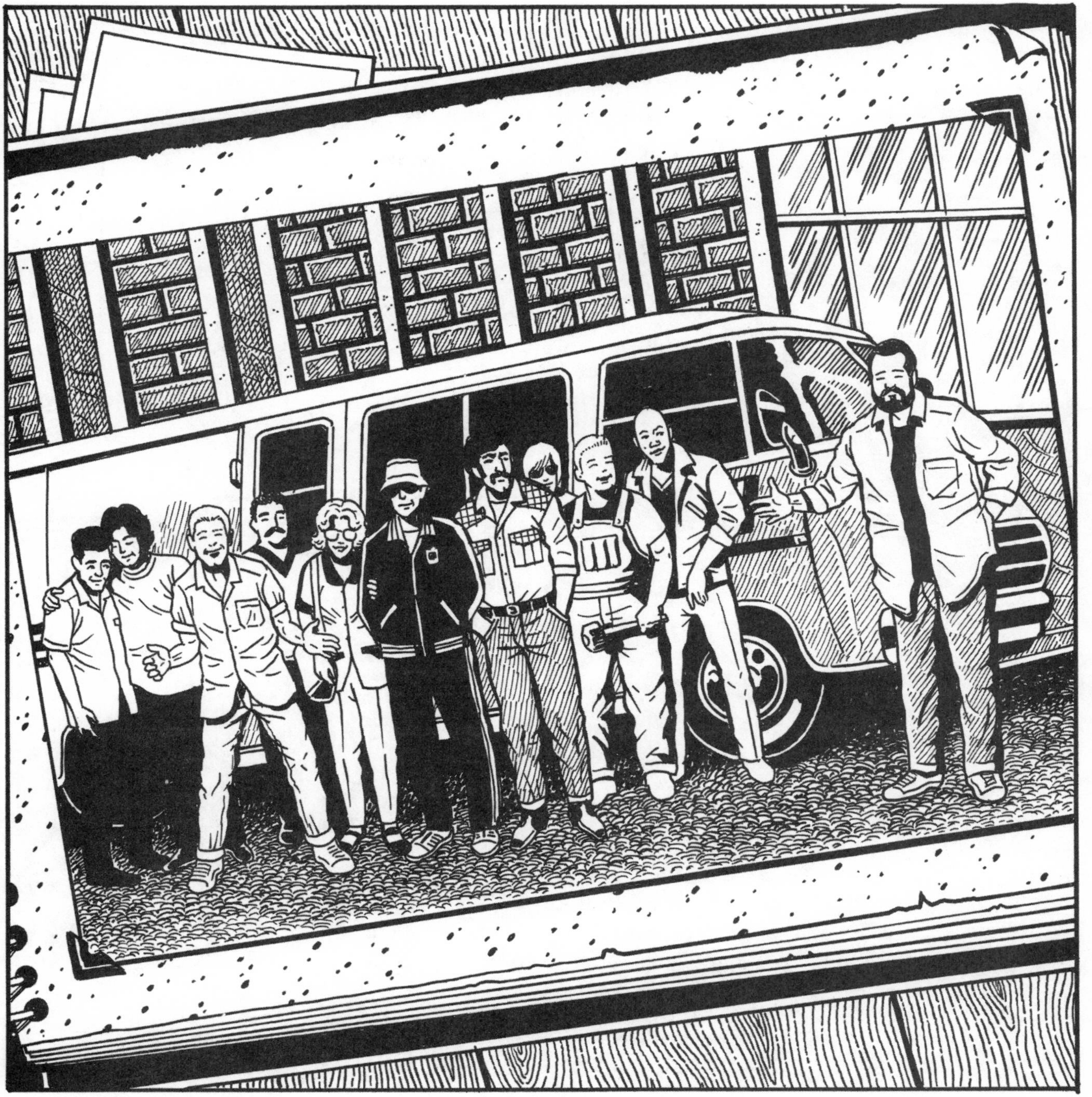

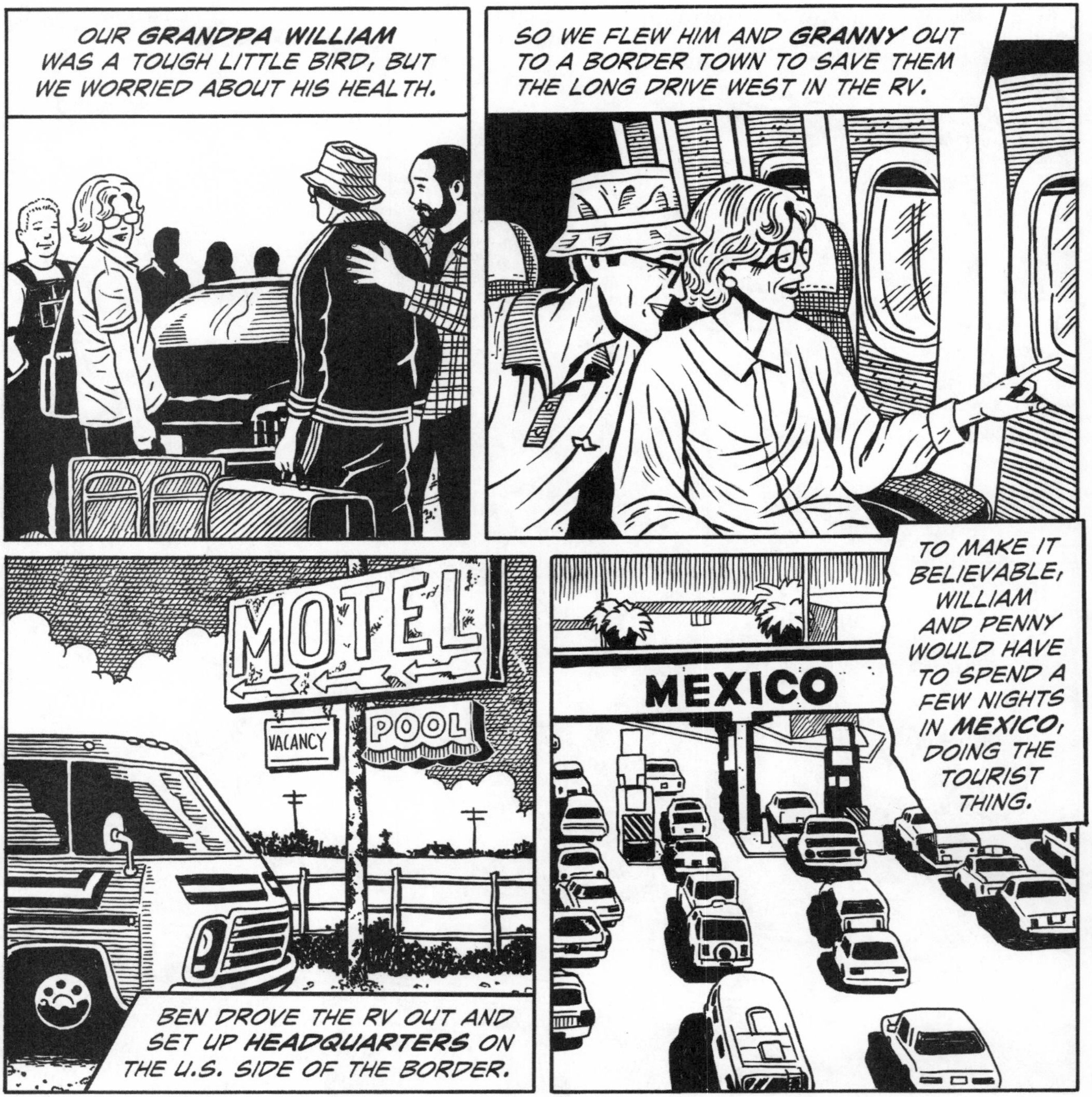
OUR GRANDPA WILLIAM WAS A TOUGH LITTLE BIRD, BUT WE WORRIED ABOUT HIS HEALTH.
SO WE FLEW HIM AND GRANNY OUT TO A BORDER TOWN TO SAVE THEM THE LONG DRIVE WEST IN THE RV.
MOTEL
VACANCY
POOL
BEN DROVE THE RV OUT AND SET UP HEADQUARTERS ON THE U.S. SIDE OF THE BORDER.
TO MAKE IT BELIEVABLE, WILLIAM AND PENNY WOULD HAVE TO SPEND A FEW NIGHTS IN MEXICO, DOING THE TOURIST THING.
MEXICO

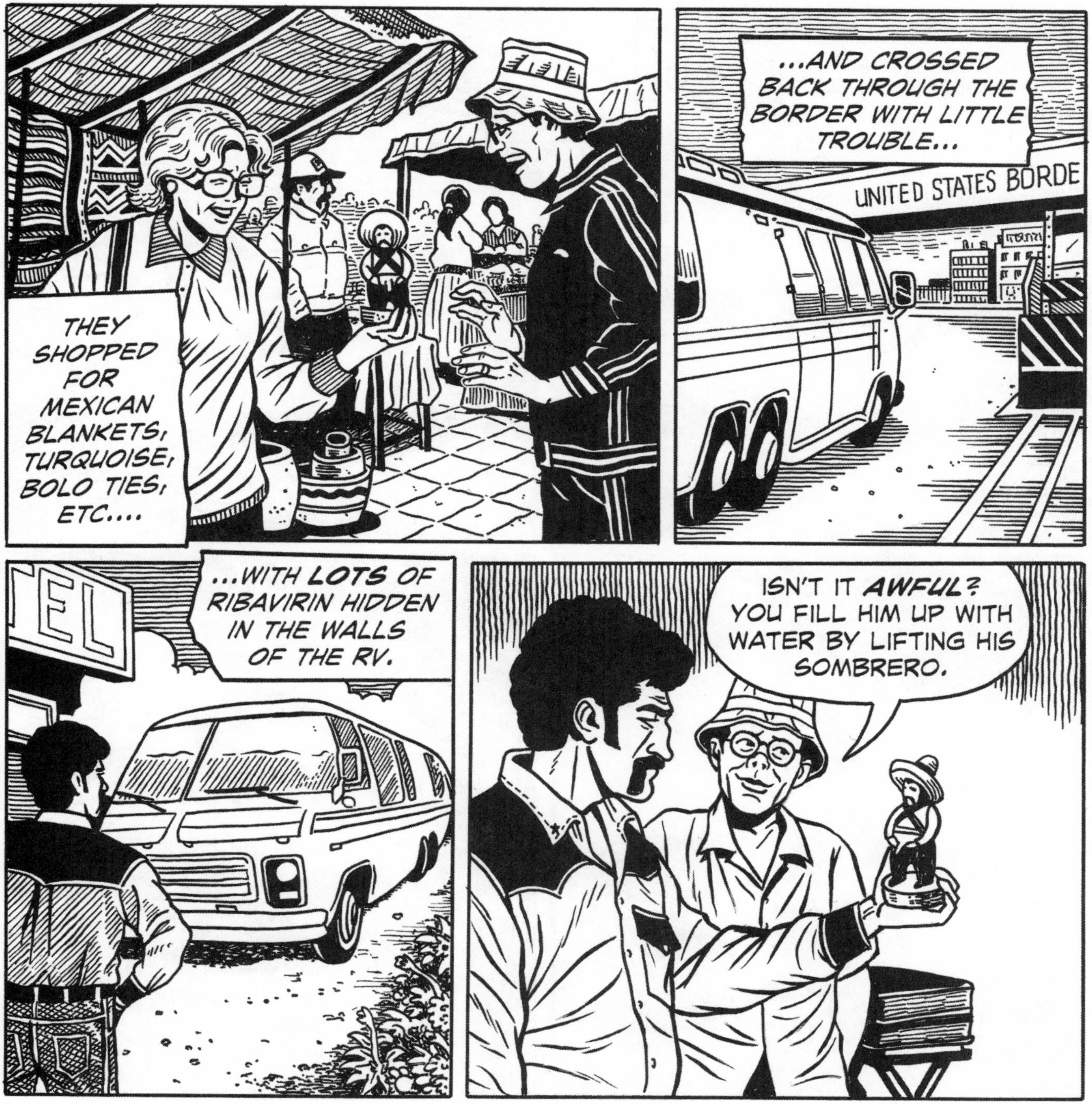
THEY SHOPPED FOR MEXICAN BLANKETS, TURQUOISE, BOLO TIES, ETC....
...AND CROSSED BACK THROUGH THE BORDER WITH LITTLE TROUBLE...
UNITED STATES BORDE
...WITH LOTS OF RIBAVIRIN HIDDEN IN THE WALLS OF THE RV.
TEL
ISN'T IT AWFUL? YOU FILL HIM UP WITH WATER BY LIFTING HIS SOMBRERO.

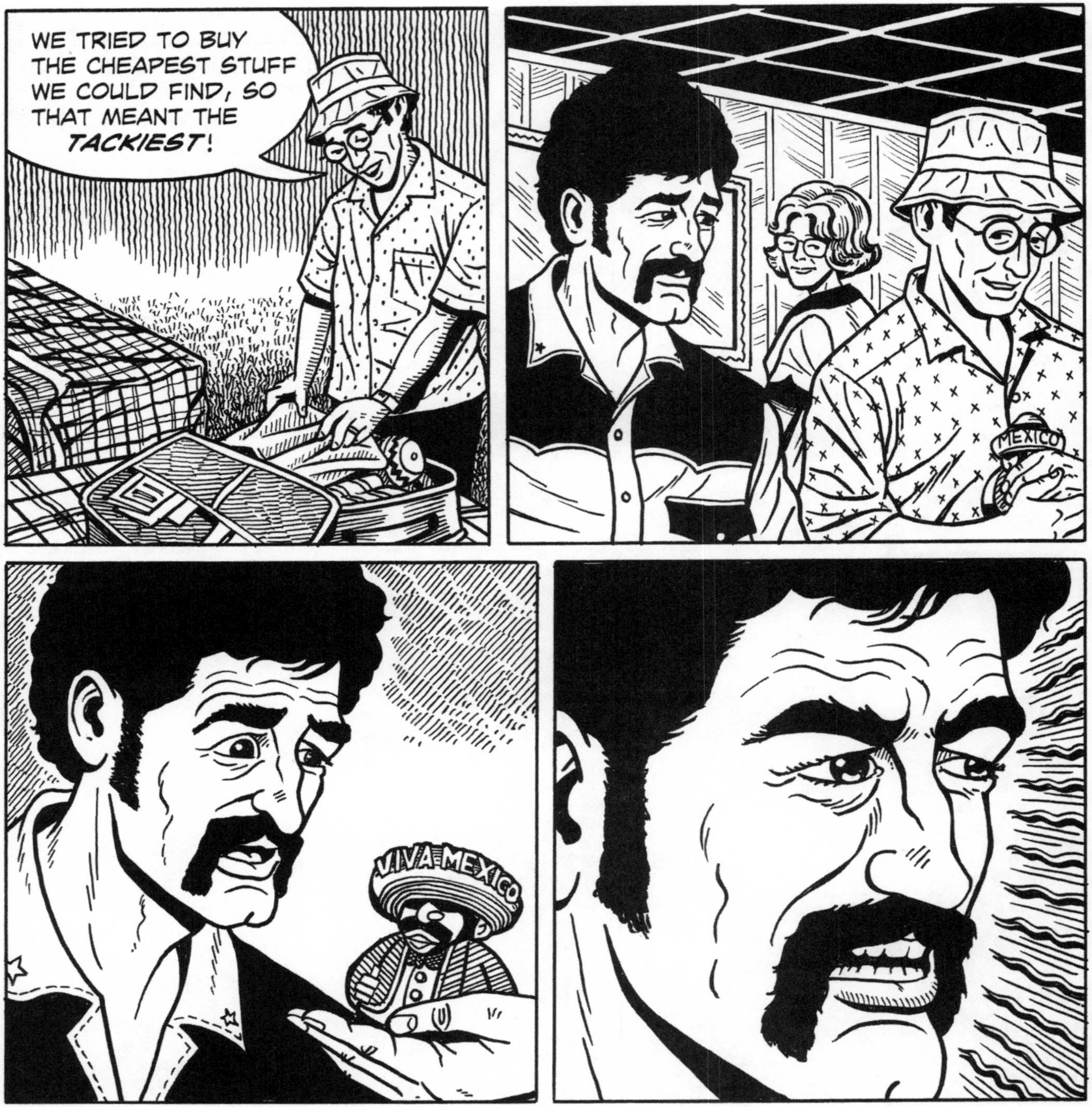
WE TRIED TO BUY THE CHEAPEST STUFF WE COULD FIND, SO THAT MEANT THE *TACKIEST*!
MEXICO
VIVA MEXICO

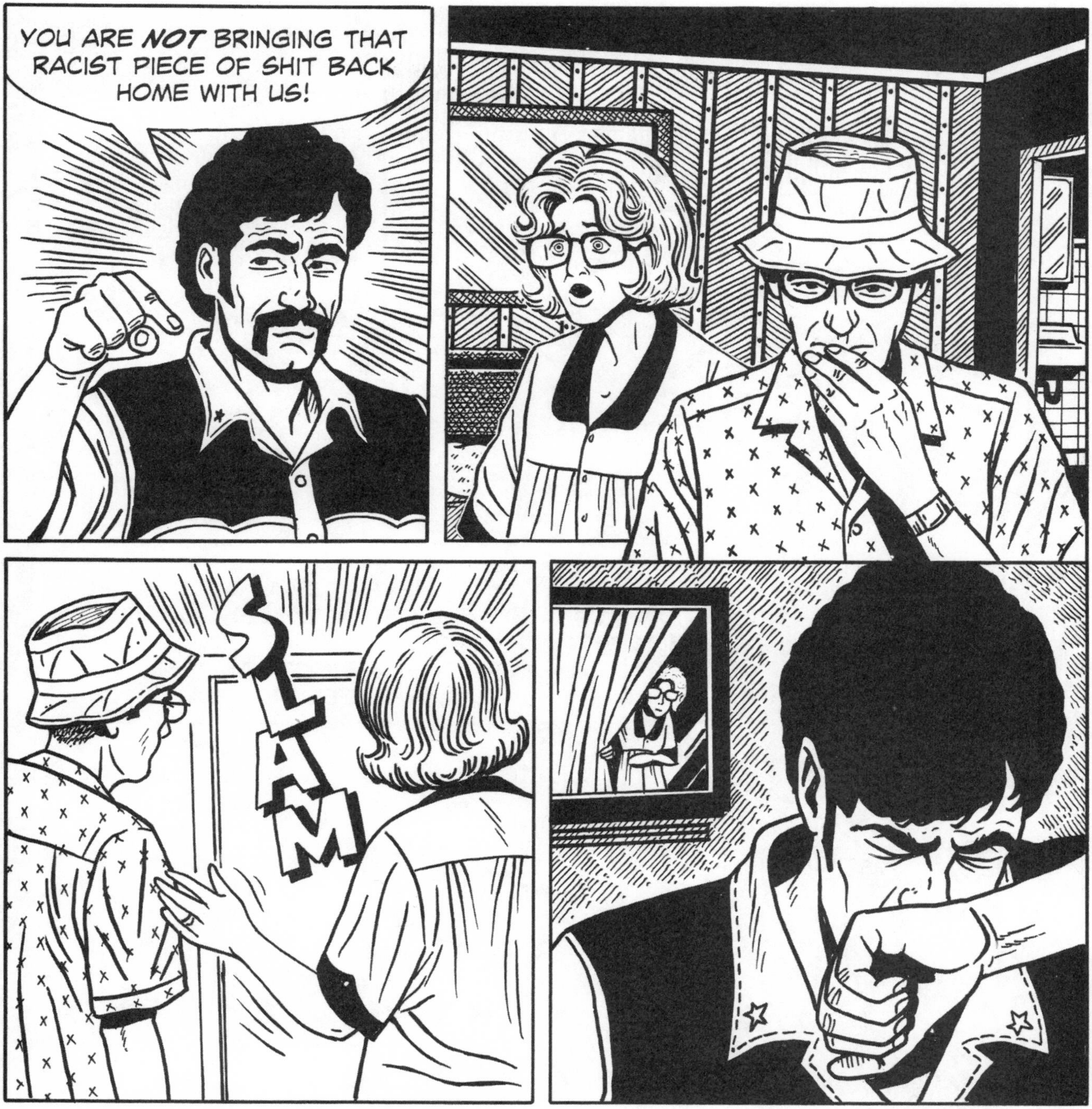
YOU ARE *NOT* BRINGING THAT RACIST PIECE OF SHIT BACK HOME WITH US!
SLAMM

I DIDN'T MEAN... WEREN'T WE SUPPOSED TO...?
LEAVE IT, WILLY. THIS HAS NOTHING TO DO WITH YOU.
JUST AFTER WE LEFT, RAY CALLED BEN ABOUT MICHAEL AND HECTOR.
HECTOR? THAT REALLY YOUNG, SORTA SLOW LITTLE SWEETHEART? HE AND MICHAEL?
MOST OF HECTOR'S FAMILY IS STILL IN THE DOMINICAN REPUBLIC. IT'S A *GREEN CARD* MESS. HE'S GOT NO MONEY, WILLY, NO INSURANCE, AND HIS CASEWORKER IS A BIGOT WHO THINKS HE SHOULD BE DEPORTED.

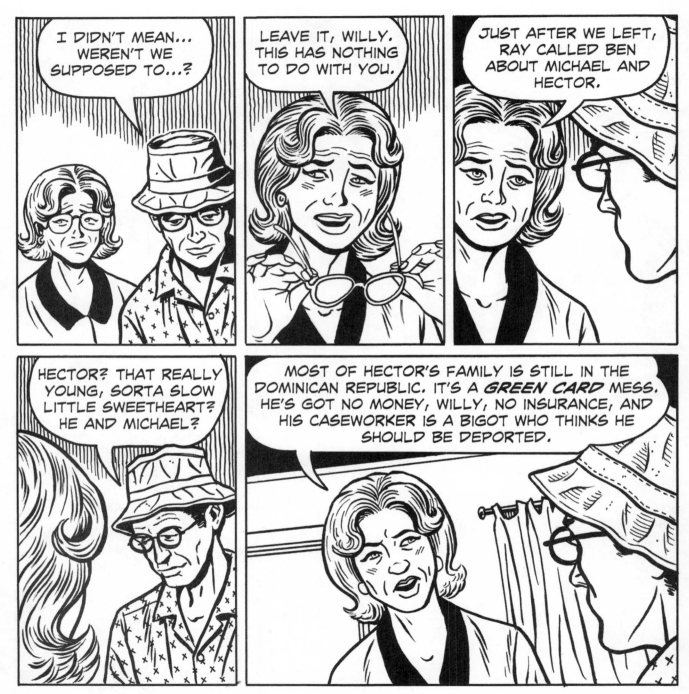

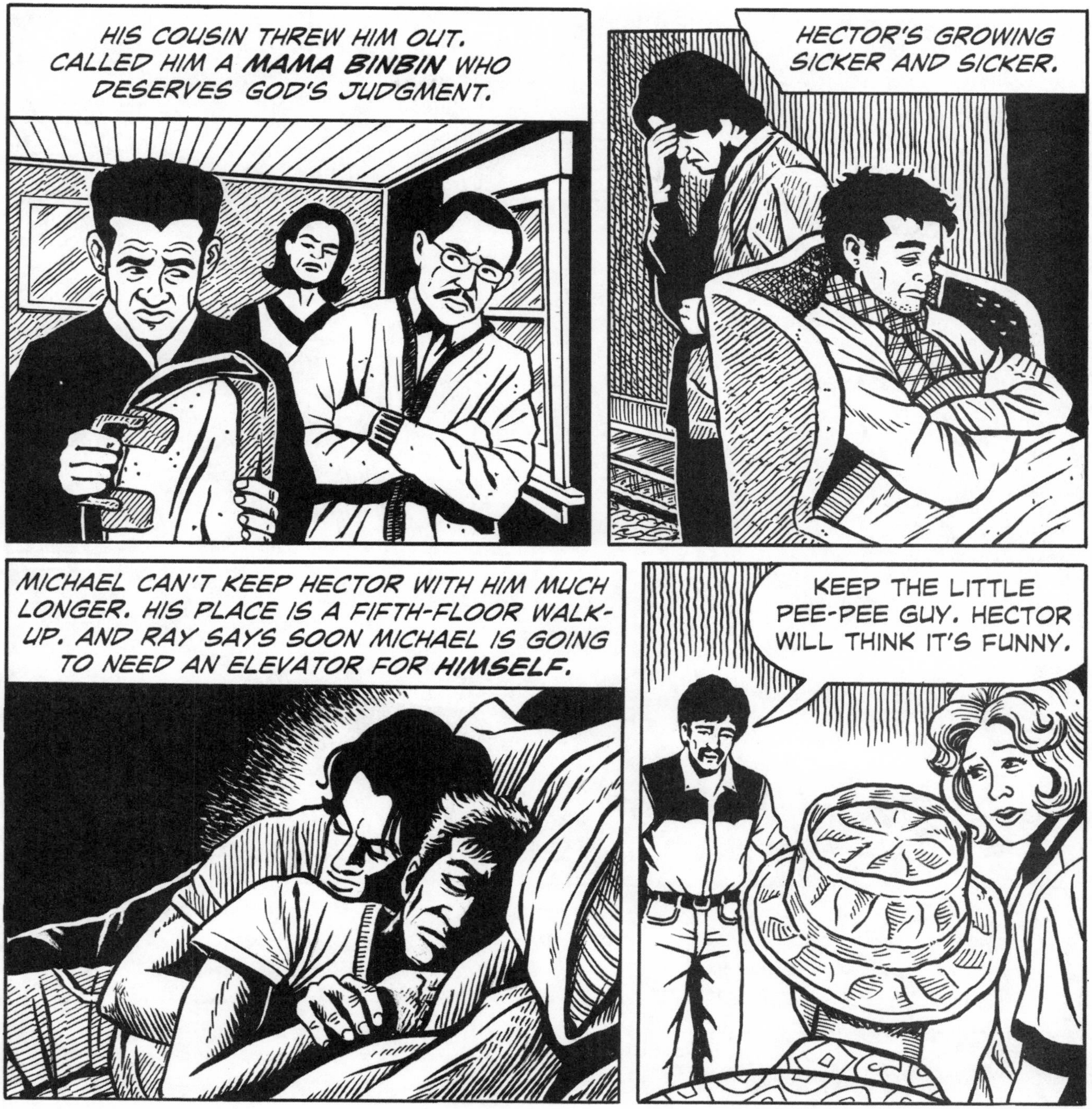
HIS COUSIN THREW HIM OUT. CALLED HIM A **MAMA BINBIN** WHO DESERVES GOD'S JUDGMENT.
HECTOR'S GROWING SICKER AND SICKER.
MICHAEL CAN'T KEEP HECTOR WITH HIM MUCH LONGER. HIS PLACE IS A FIFTH-FLOOR WALK-UP. AND RAY SAYS SOON MICHAEL IS GOING TO NEED AN ELEVATOR FOR **HIMSELF**.
KEEP THE LITTLE PEE-PEE GUY. HECTOR WILL THINK IT'S FUNNY.

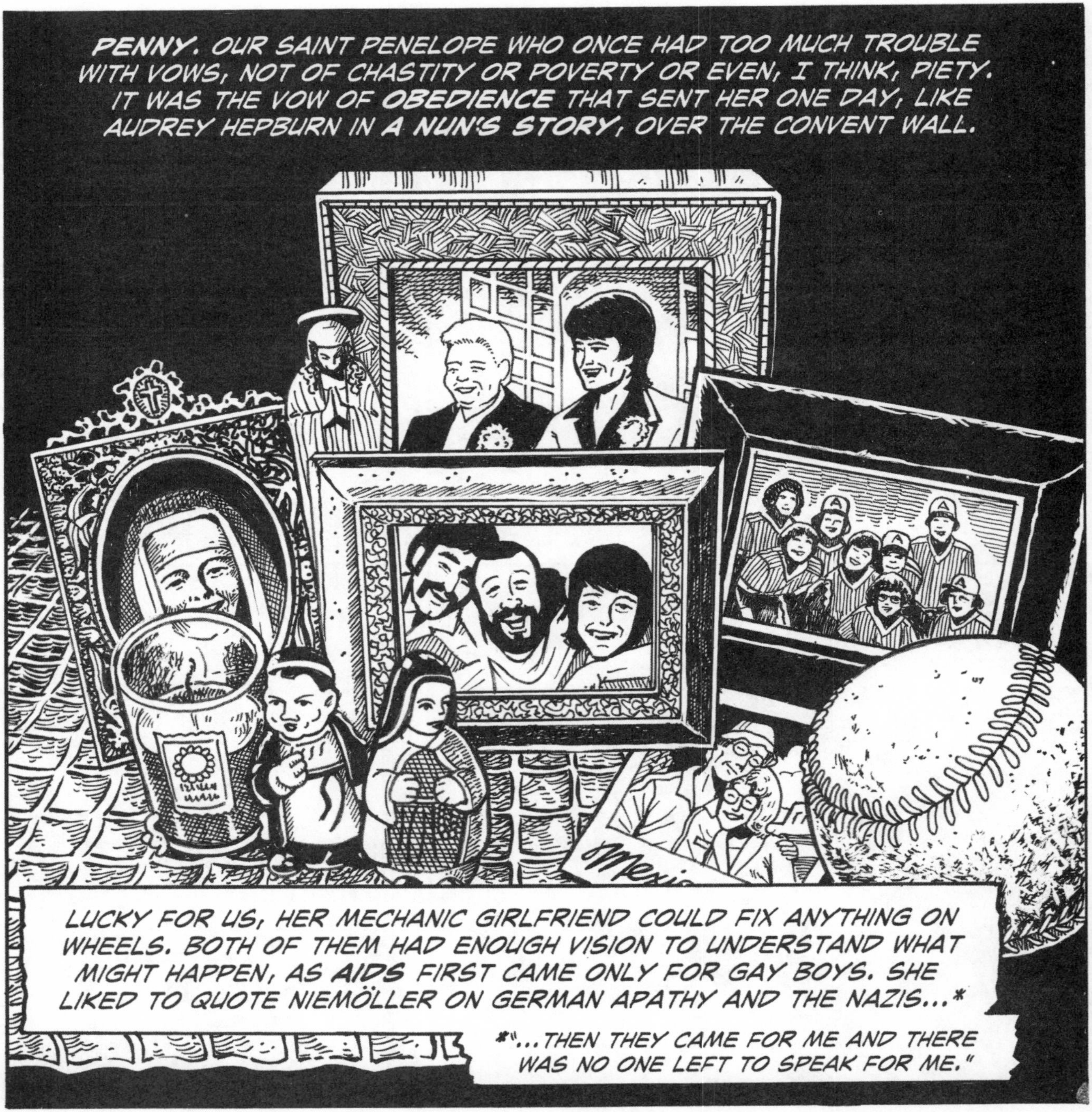
PENNY. OUR SAINT PENELOPE WHO ONCE HAD TOO MUCH TROUBLE WITH VOWS, NOT OF CHASTITY OR POVERTY OR EVEN, I THINK, PIETY. IT WAS THE VOW OF OBEDIENCE THAT SENT HER ONE DAY, LIKE AUDREY HEPBURN IN A NUN'S STORY, OVER THE CONVENT WALL.
LUCKY FOR US, HER MECHANIC GIRLFRIEND COULD FIX ANYTHING ON WHEELS. BOTH OF THEM HAD ENOUGH VISION TO UNDERSTAND WHAT MIGHT HAPPEN, AS AIDS FIRST CAME ONLY FOR GAY BOYS. SHE LIKED TO QUOTE NIEMÖLLER ON GERMAN APATHY AND THE NAZIS...*
*"...THEN THEY CAME FOR ME AND THERE WAS NO ONE LEFT TO SPEAK FOR ME."

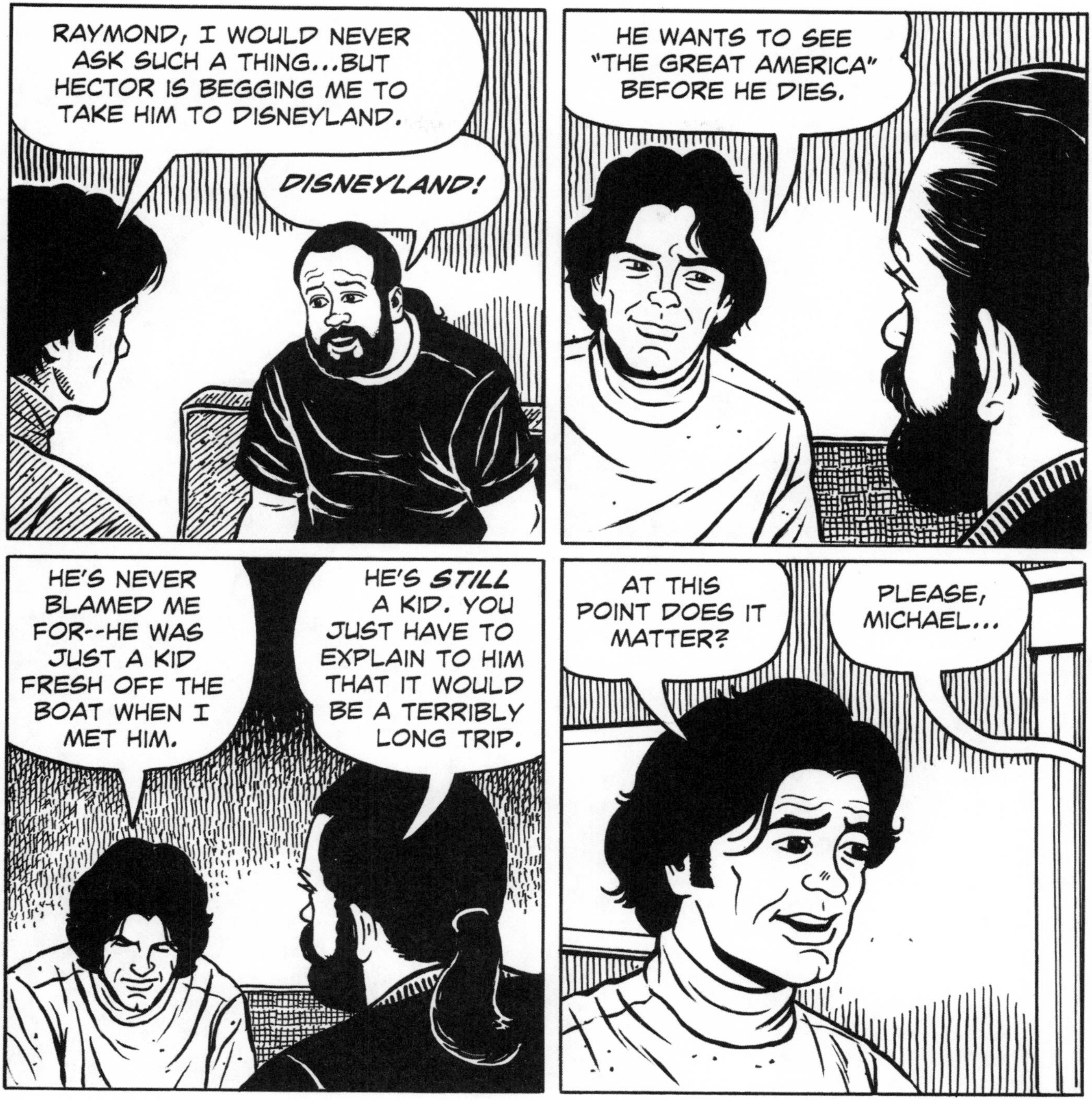
RAYMOND, I WOULD NEVER ASK SUCH A THING...BUT HECTOR IS BEGGING ME TO TAKE HIM TO DISNEYLAND.
DISNEYLAND!
HE WANTS TO SEE "THE GREAT AMERICA" BEFORE HE DIES.
HE'S NEVER BLAMED ME FOR--HE WAS JUST A KID FRESH OFF THE BOAT WHEN I MET HIM.
HE'S STILL A KID. YOU JUST HAVE TO EXPLAIN TO HIM THAT IT WOULD BE A TERRIBLY LONG TRIP.
AT THIS POINT DOES IT MATTER?
PLEASE, MICHAEL...

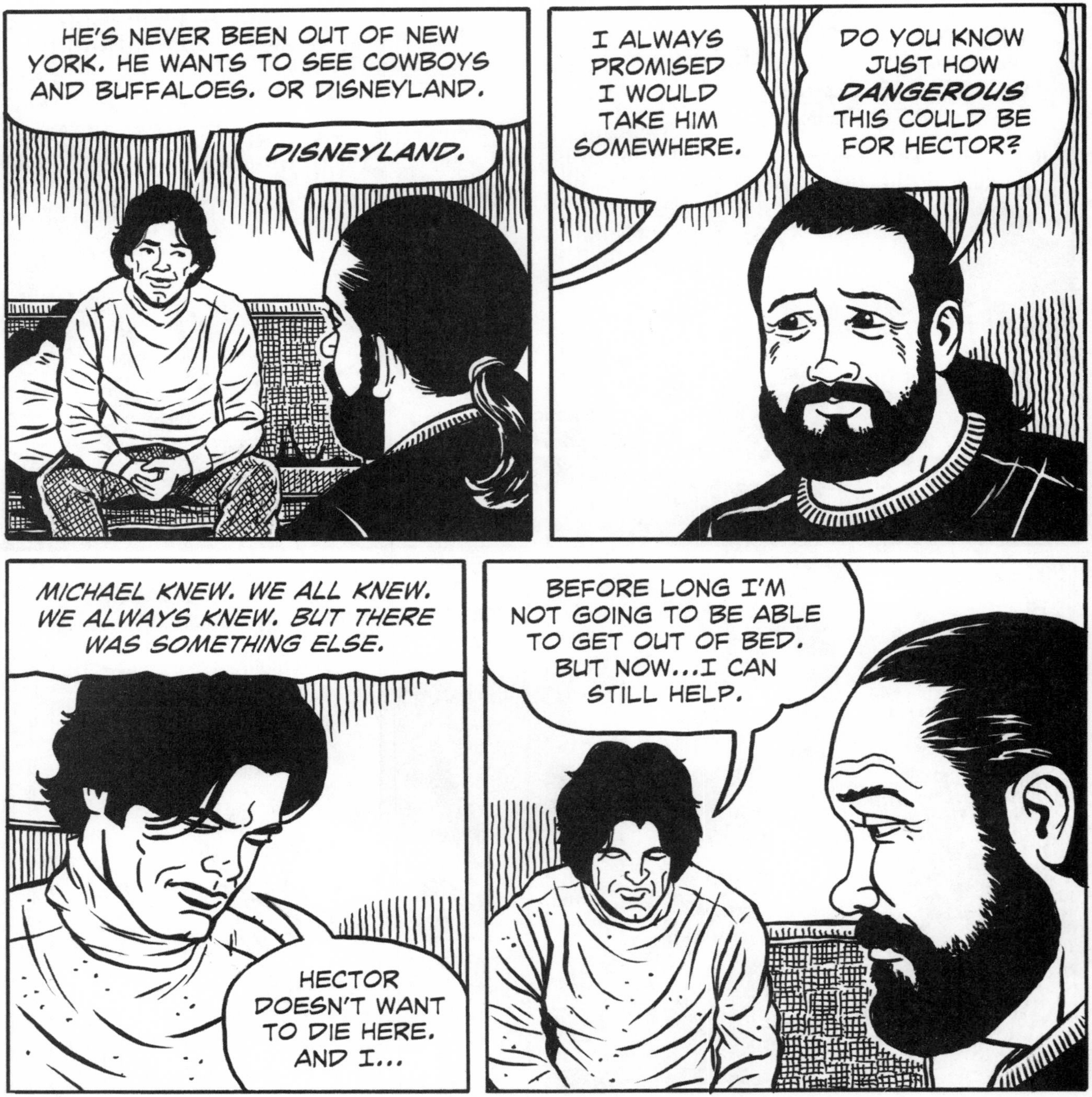
HE'S NEVER BEEN OUT OF NEW YORK. HE WANTS TO SEE COWBOYS AND BUFFALOES. OR DISNEYLAND.
DISNEYLAND.
I ALWAYS PROMISED I WOULD TAKE HIM SOMEWHERE.
DO YOU KNOW JUST HOW ***DANGEROUS*** THIS COULD BE FOR HECTOR?
MICHAEL KNEW. WE ALL KNEW. WE ALWAYS KNEW. BUT THERE WAS SOMETHING ELSE.
HECTOR DOESN'T WANT TO DIE HERE. AND I...
BEFORE LONG I'M NOT GOING TO BE ABLE TO GET OUT OF BED. BUT NOW...I CAN STILL HELP.

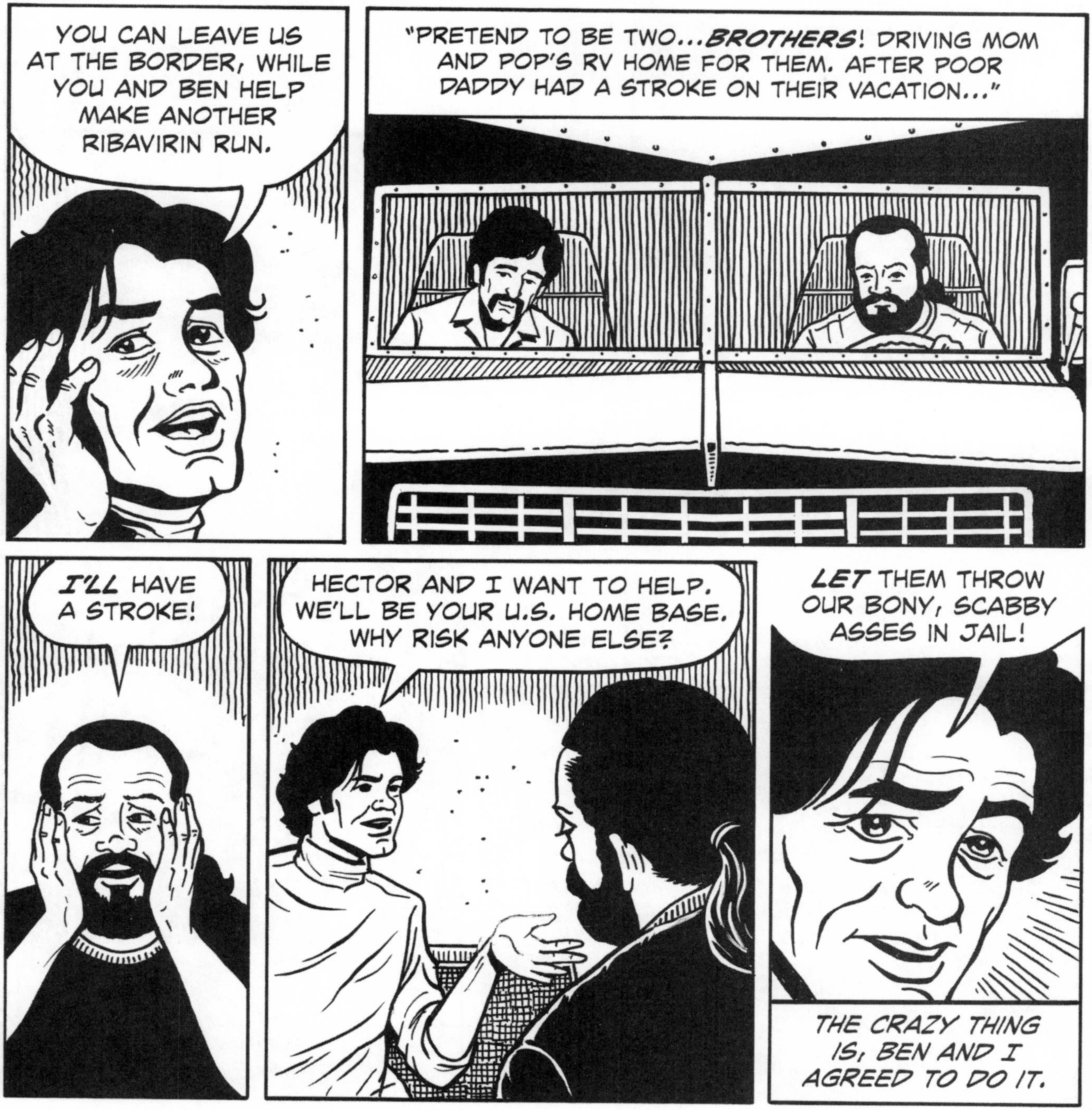
YOU CAN LEAVE US AT THE BORDER, WHILE YOU AND BEN HELP MAKE ANOTHER RIBAVIRIN RUN.
"PRETEND TO BE TWO...BROTHERS! DRIVING MOM AND POP'S RV HOME FOR THEM. AFTER POOR DADDY HAD A STROKE ON THEIR VACATION..."
I'LL HAVE A STROKE!
HECTOR AND I WANT TO HELP. WE'LL BE YOUR U.S. HOME BASE. WHY RISK ANYONE ELSE?
LET THEM THROW OUR BONY, SCABBY ASSES IN JAIL!
THE CRAZY THING IS, BEN AND I AGREED TO DO IT.

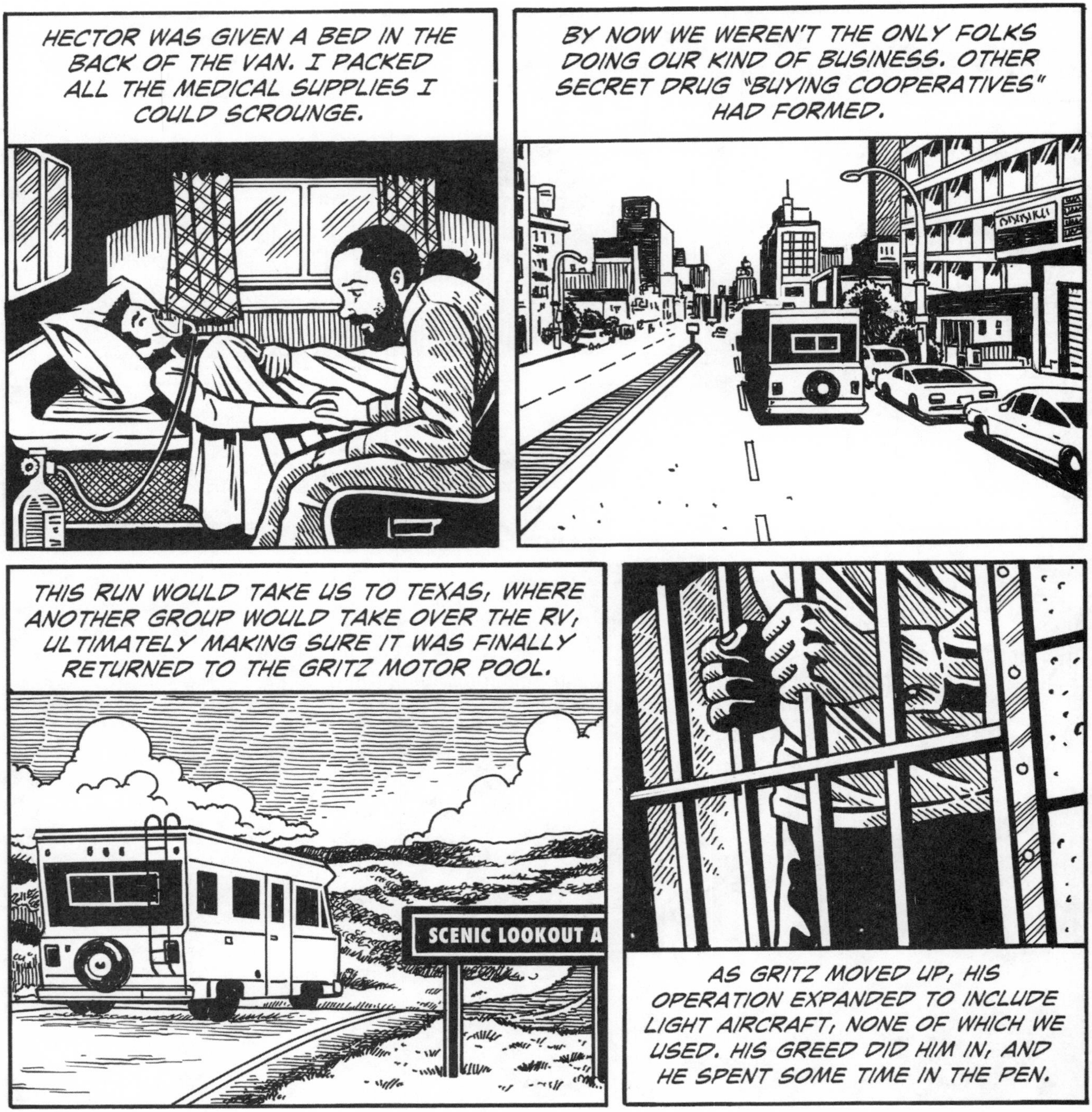
HECTOR WAS GIVEN A BED IN THE BACK OF THE VAN. I PACKED ALL THE MEDICAL SUPPLIES I COULD SCROUNGE.
BY NOW WE WEREN'T THE ONLY FOLKS DOING OUR KIND OF BUSINESS. OTHER SECRET DRUG "BUYING COOPERATIVES" HAD FORMED.
THIS RUN WOULD TAKE US TO TEXAS, WHERE ANOTHER GROUP WOULD TAKE OVER THE RV, ULTIMATELY MAKING SURE IT WAS FINALLY RETURNED TO THE GRITZ MOTOR POOL.
SCENIC LOOKOUT A
AS GRITZ MOVED UP, HIS OPERATION EXPANDED TO INCLUDE LIGHT AIRCRAFT, NONE OF WHICH WE USED. HIS GREED DID HIM IN, AND HE SPENT SOME TIME IN THE PEN.

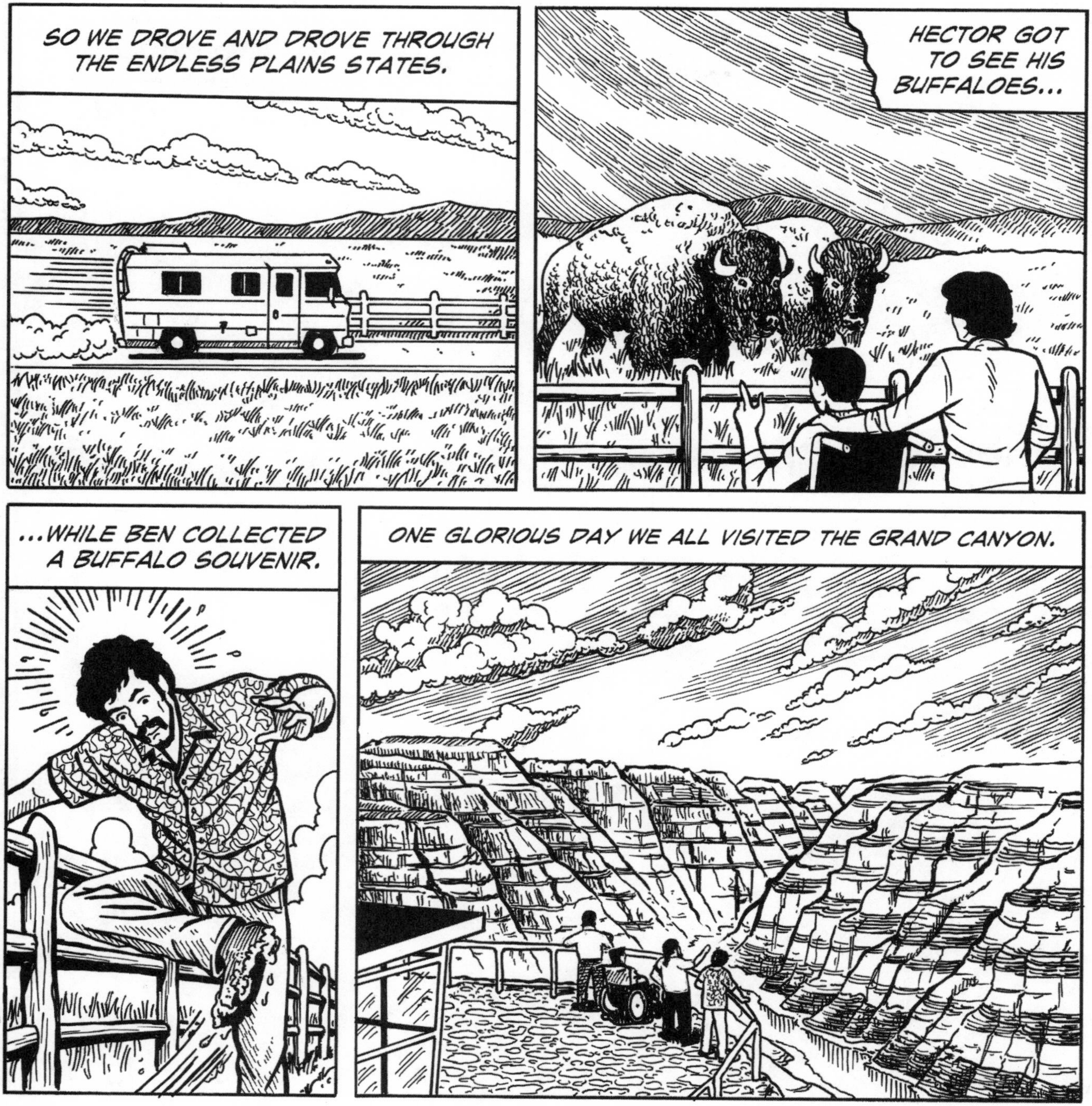
SO WE DROVE AND DROVE THROUGH THE ENDLESS PLAINS STATES.
HECTOR GOT TO SEE HIS BUFFALOES...
...WHILE BEN COLLECTED A BUFFALO SOUVENIR.
ONE GLORIOUS DAY WE ALL VISITED THE GRAND CANYON.

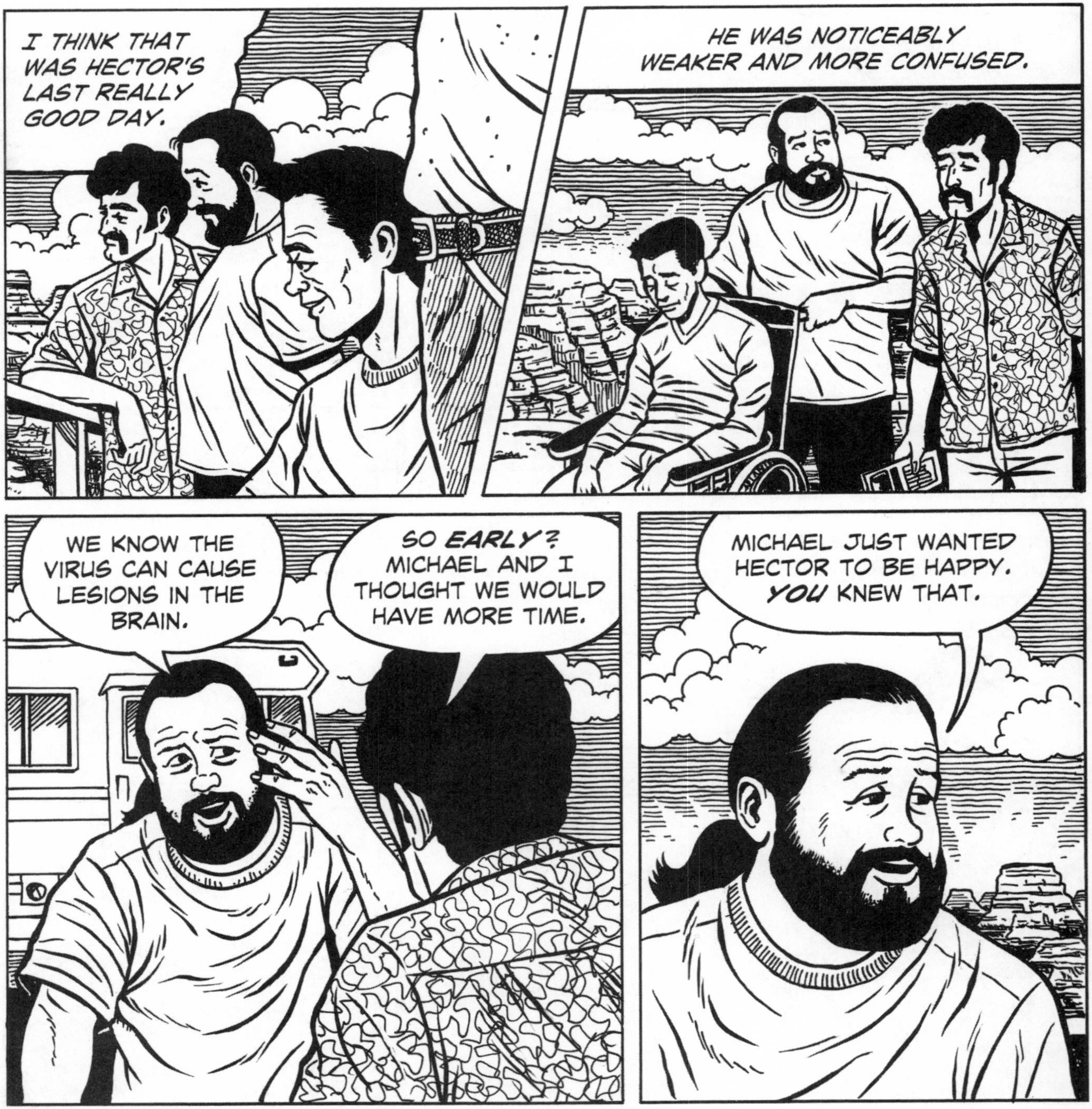
I THINK THAT WAS HECTOR'S LAST REALLY GOOD DAY.
HE WAS NOTICEABLY WEAKER AND MORE CONFUSED.
WE KNOW THE VIRUS CAN CAUSE LESIONS IN THE BRAIN.
SO *EARLY*? MICHAEL AND I THOUGHT WE WOULD HAVE MORE TIME.
MICHAEL JUST WANTED HECTOR TO BE HAPPY. *YOU* KNEW THAT.

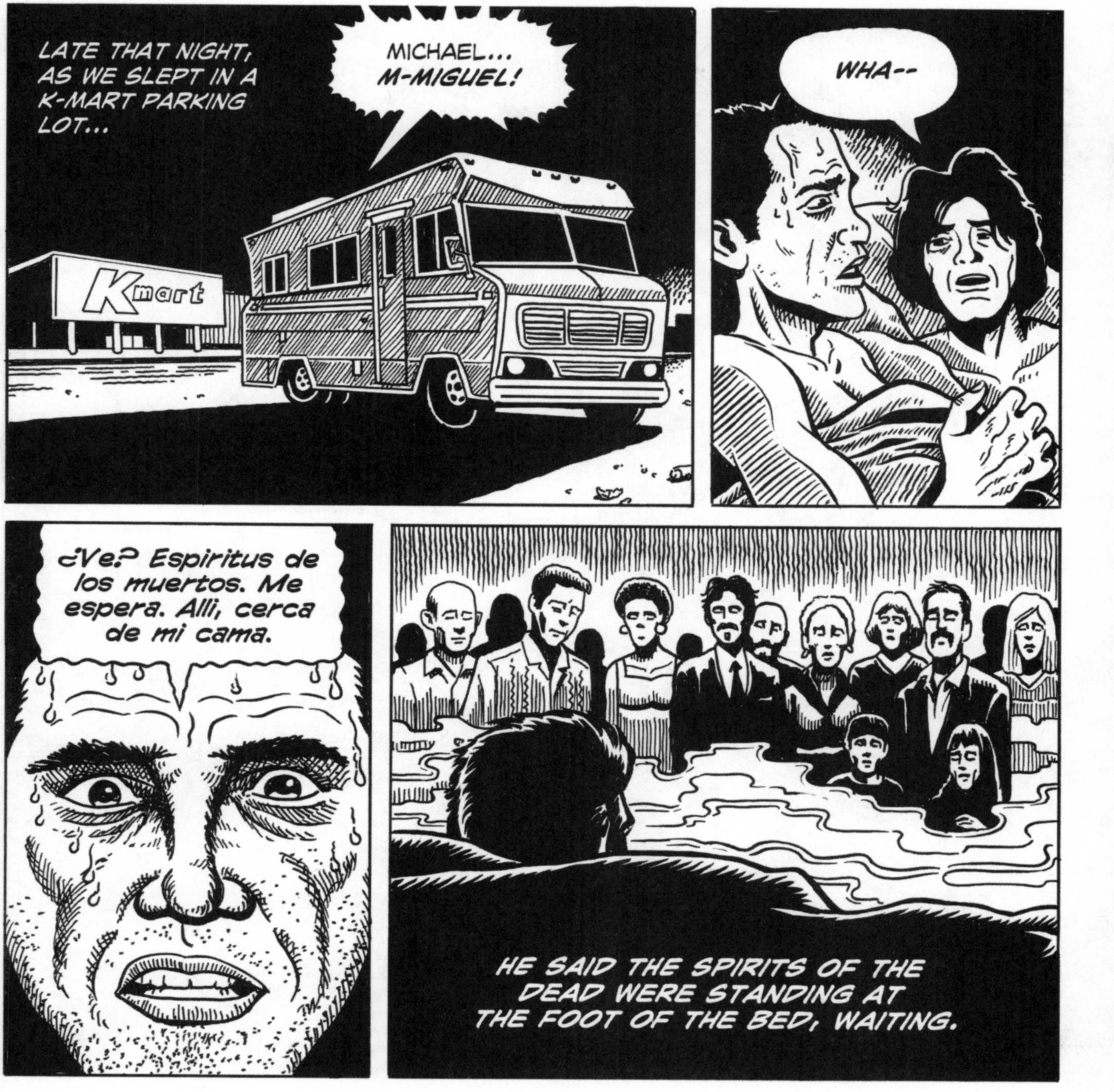

LATE THAT NIGHT, AS WE SLEPT IN A K-MART PARKING LOT...
Kmart
MICHAEL... M-MIGUEL!
WHA--
¿Ve? Espiritus de los muertos. Me espera. Alli, cerca de mi cama.
HE SAID THE SPIRITS OF THE DEAD WERE STANDING AT THE FOOT OF THE BED, WAITING.

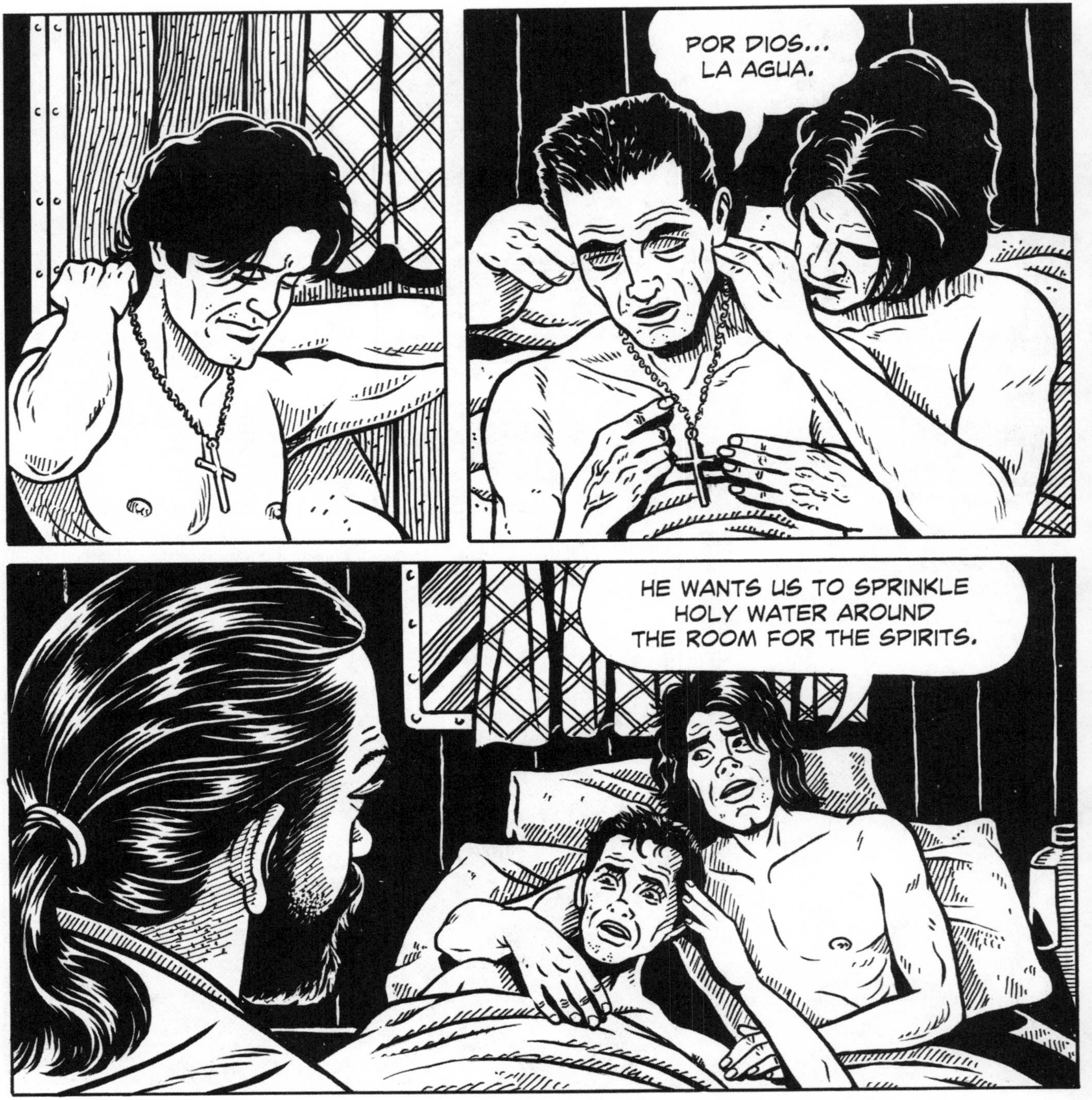
POR DIOS... LA AGUA.
HE WANTS US TO SPRINKLE HOLY WATER AROUND THE ROOM FOR THE SPIRITS.

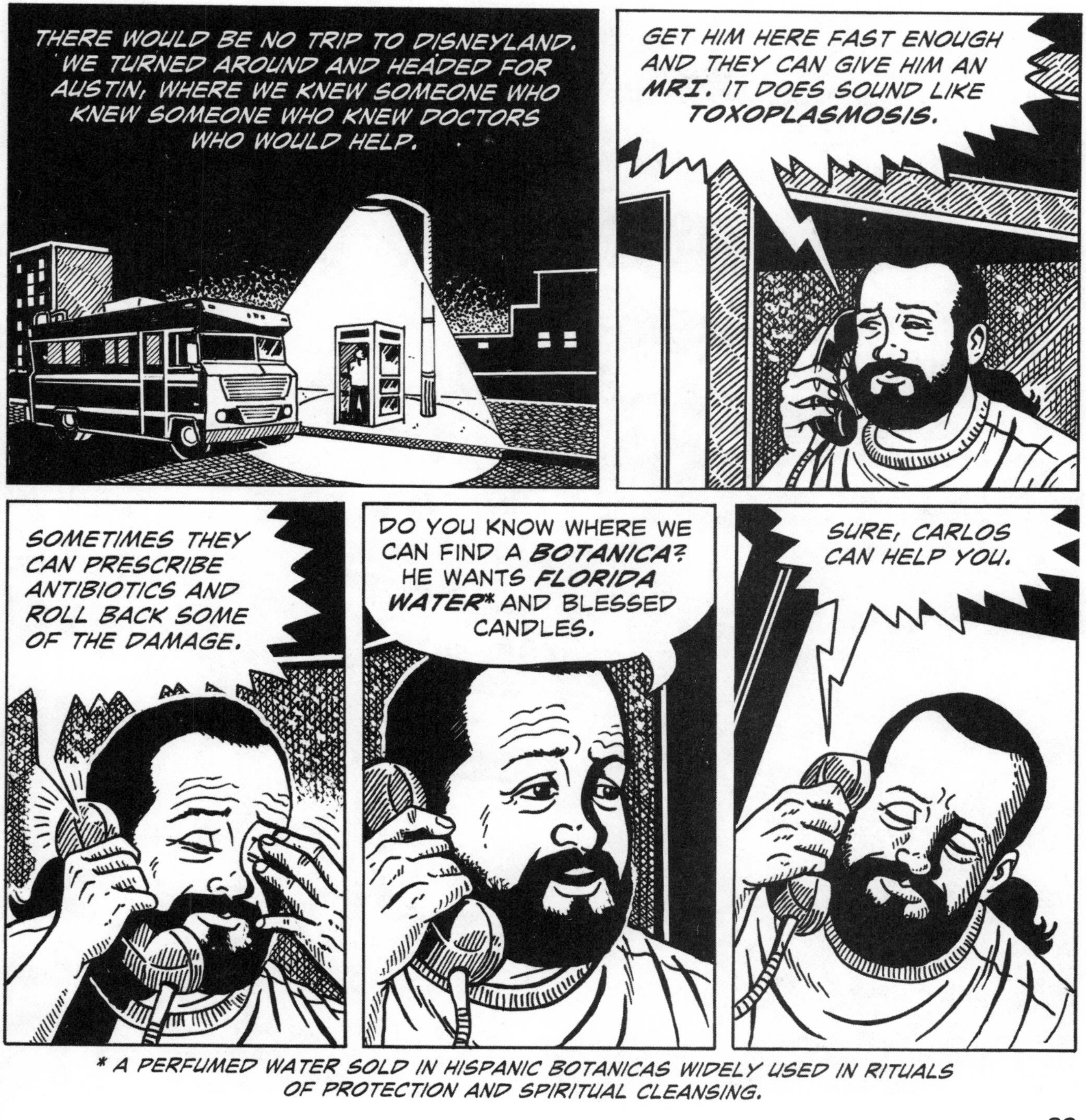
THERE WOULD BE NO TRIP TO DISNEYLAND. WE TURNED AROUND AND HEADED FOR AUSTIN, WHERE WE KNEW SOMEONE WHO KNEW SOMEONE WHO KNEW DOCTORS WHO WOULD HELP.
GET HIM HERE FAST ENOUGH AND THEY CAN GIVE HIM AN ***MRI***. IT DOES SOUND LIKE ***TOXOPLASMOSIS***.
SOMETIMES THEY CAN PRESCRIBE ANTIBIOTICS AND ROLL BACK SOME OF THE DAMAGE.
DO YOU KNOW WHERE WE CAN FIND A ***BOTANICA***? HE WANTS ***FLORIDA WATER**** AND BLESSED CANDLES.
SURE, CARLOS CAN HELP YOU.

* A PERFUMED WATER SOLD IN HISPANIC BOTANICAS WIDELY USED IN RITUALS OF PROTECTION AND SPIRITUAL CLEANSING.

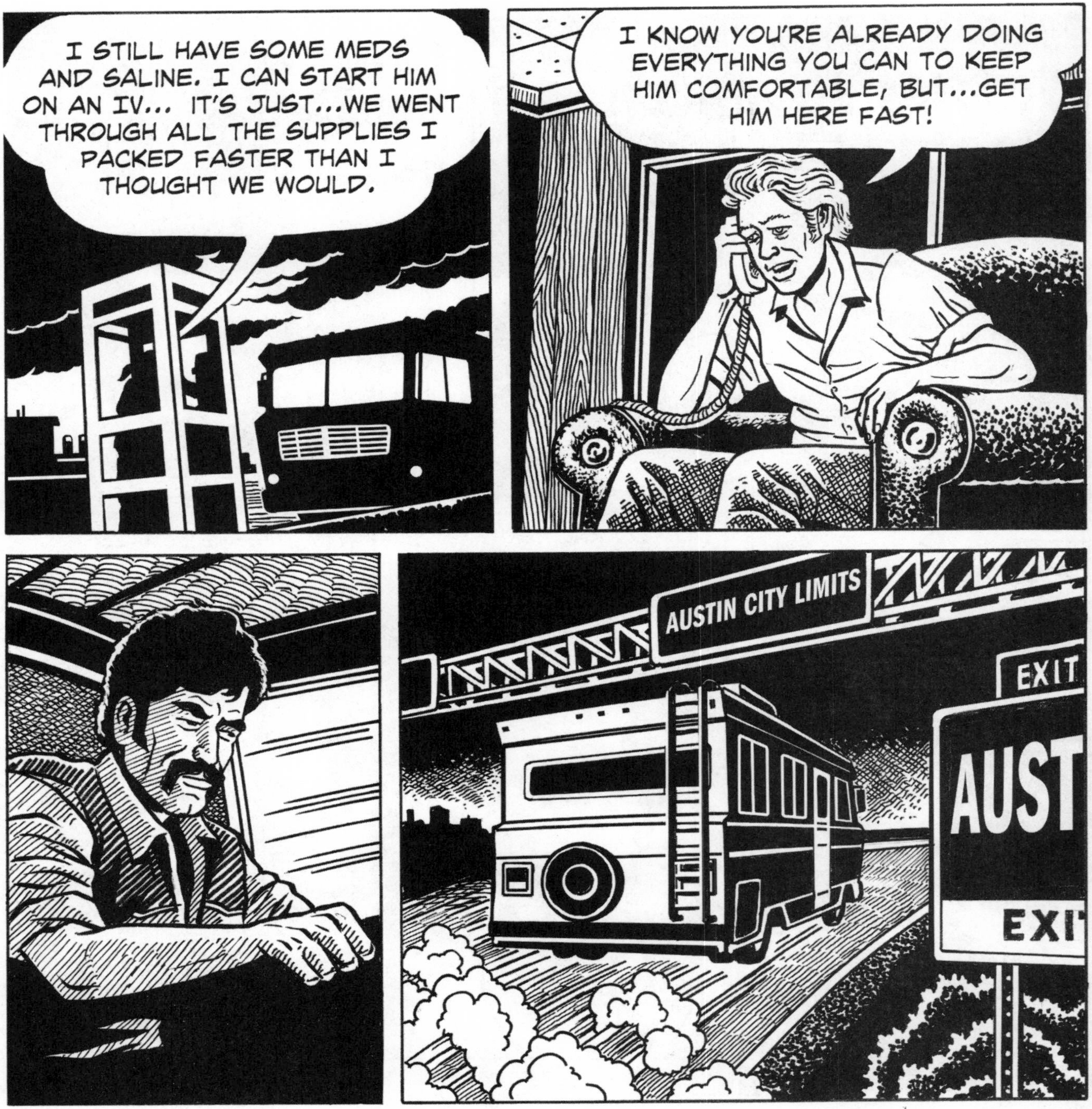
I STILL HAVE SOME MEDS AND SALINE. I CAN START HIM ON AN IV... IT'S JUST...WE WENT THROUGH ALL THE SUPPLIES I PACKED FASTER THAN I THOUGHT WE WOULD.
I KNOW YOU'RE ALREADY DOING EVERYTHING YOU CAN TO KEEP HIM COMFORTABLE, BUT...GET HIM HERE FAST!
AUSTIN CITY LIMITS
EXIT
AUST
EXIT

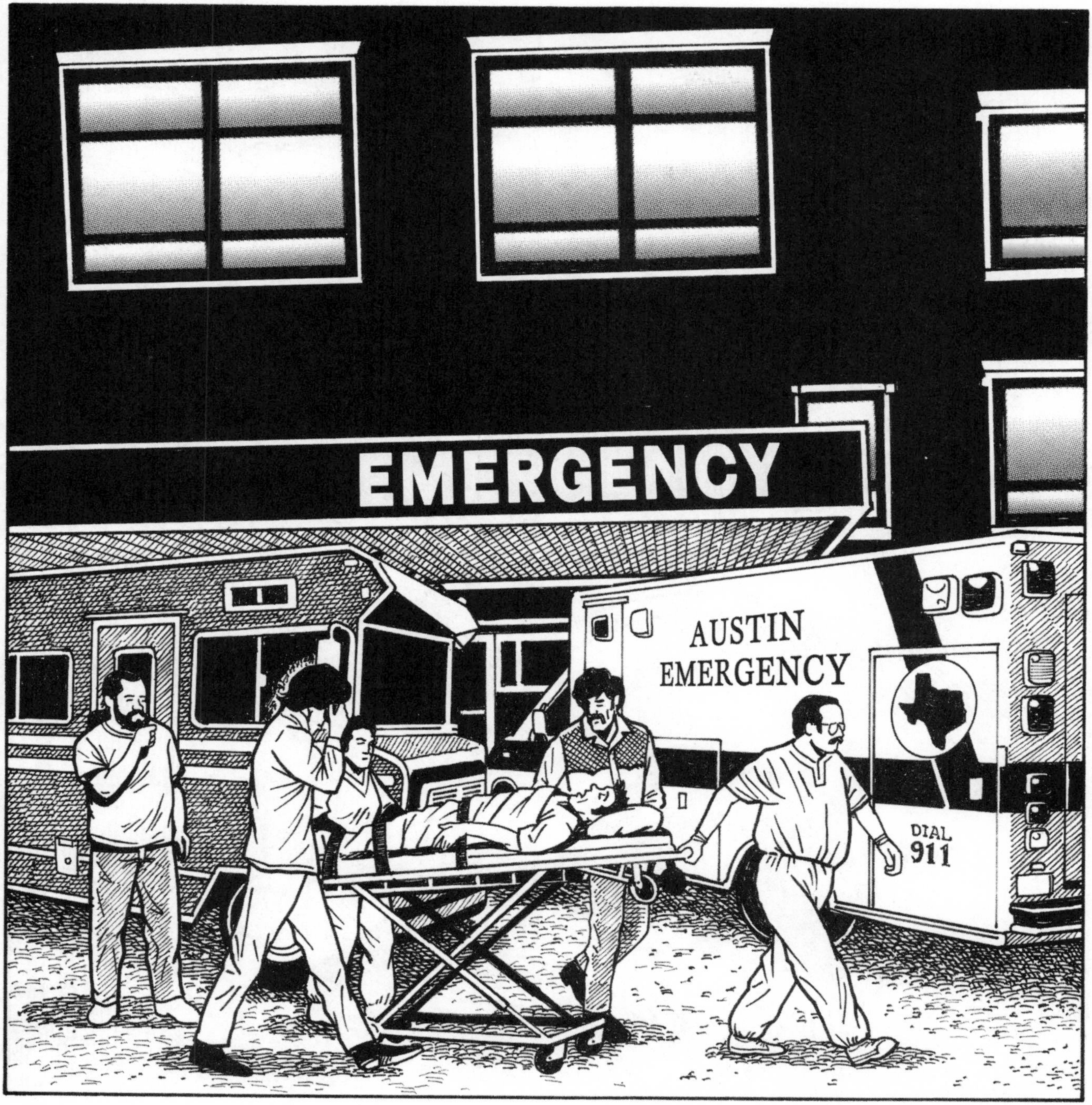
EMERGENCY
AUSTIN
EMERGENCY
DIAL
911

MRI

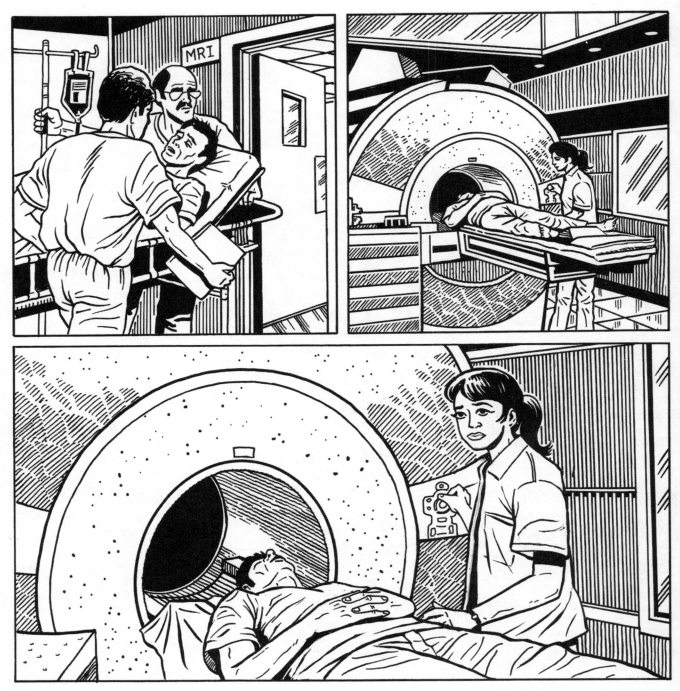

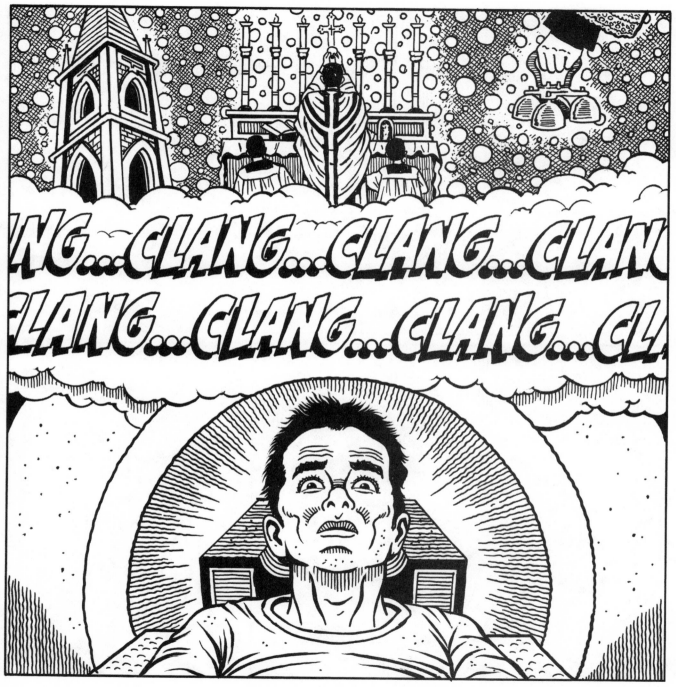

CLANG...CLANG...CLANG...CLAN
CLANG...CLANG...CLANG...CL

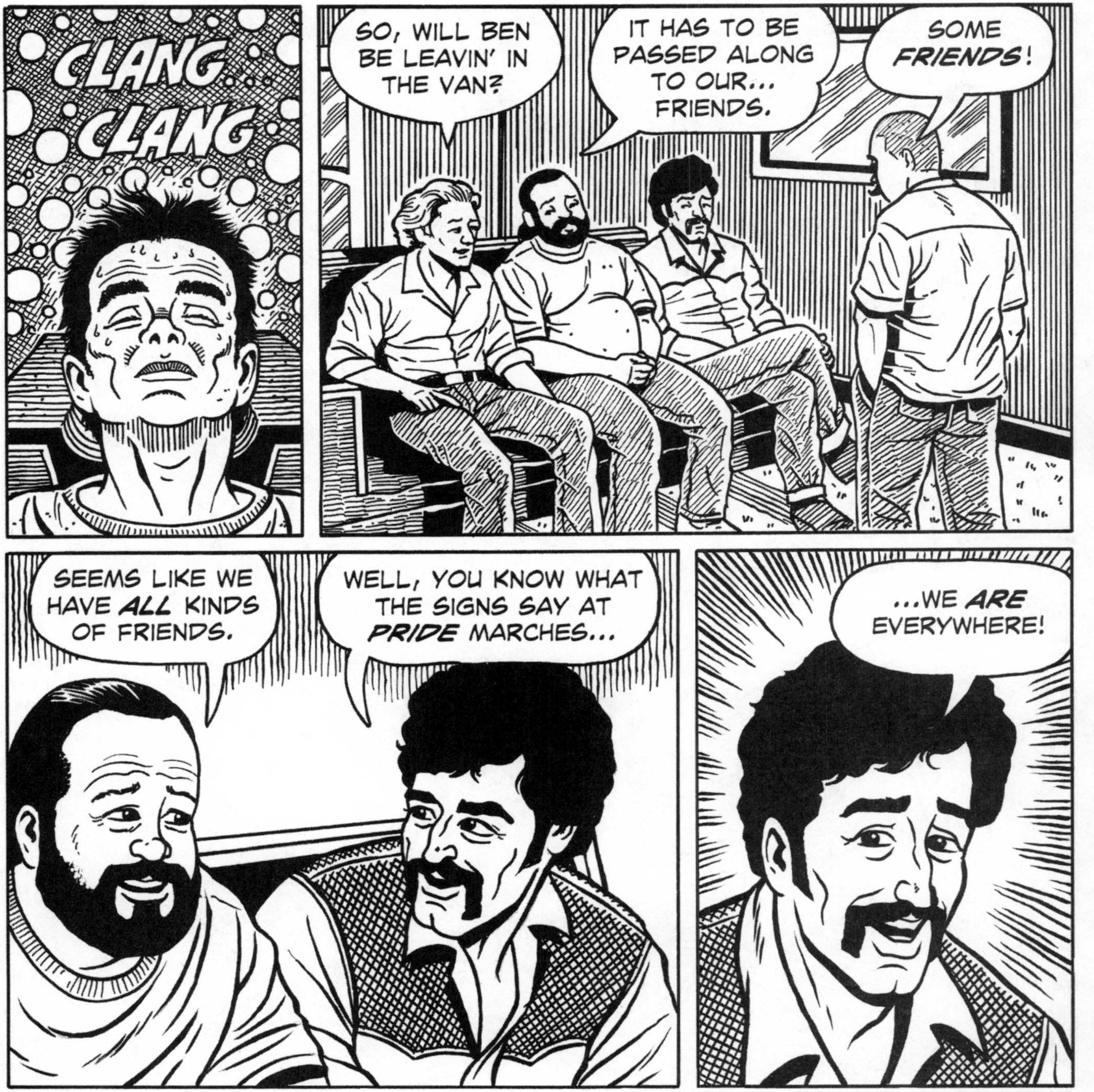
CLANG... CLANG
SO, WILL BEN BE LEAVIN' IN THE VAN?
IT HAS TO BE PASSED ALONG TO OUR... FRIENDS.
SOME FRIENDS!
SEEMS LIKE WE HAVE ALL KINDS OF FRIENDS.
WELL, YOU KNOW WHAT THE SIGNS SAY AT PRIDE MARCHES...
...WE ARE EVERYWHERE!

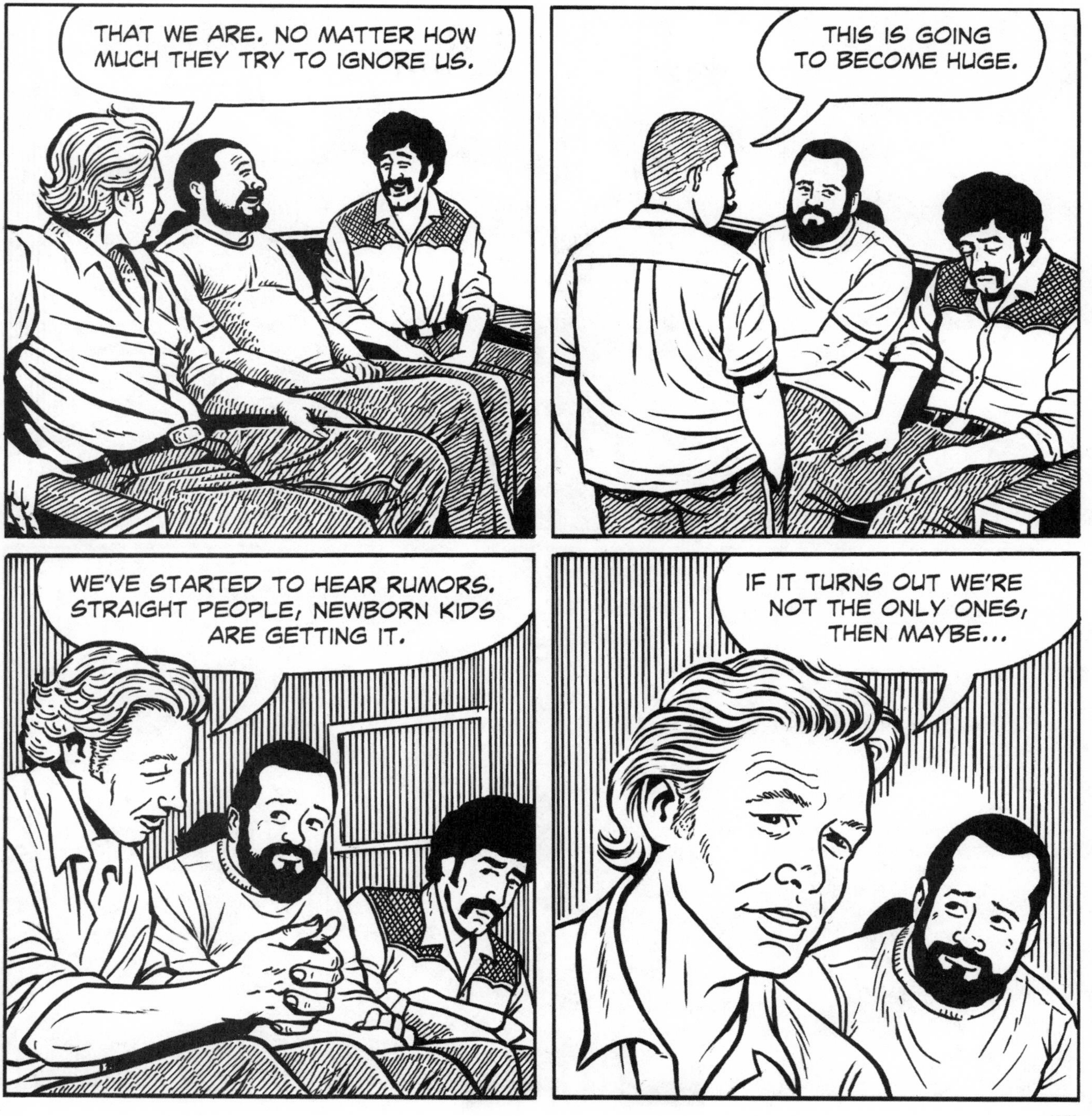
THAT WE ARE. NO MATTER HOW MUCH THEY TRY TO IGNORE US.
THIS IS GOING TO BECOME HUGE.
WE'VE STARTED TO HEAR RUMORS. STRAIGHT PEOPLE, NEWBORN KIDS ARE GETTING IT.
IF IT TURNS OUT WE'RE NOT THE ONLY ONES, THEN MAYBE...

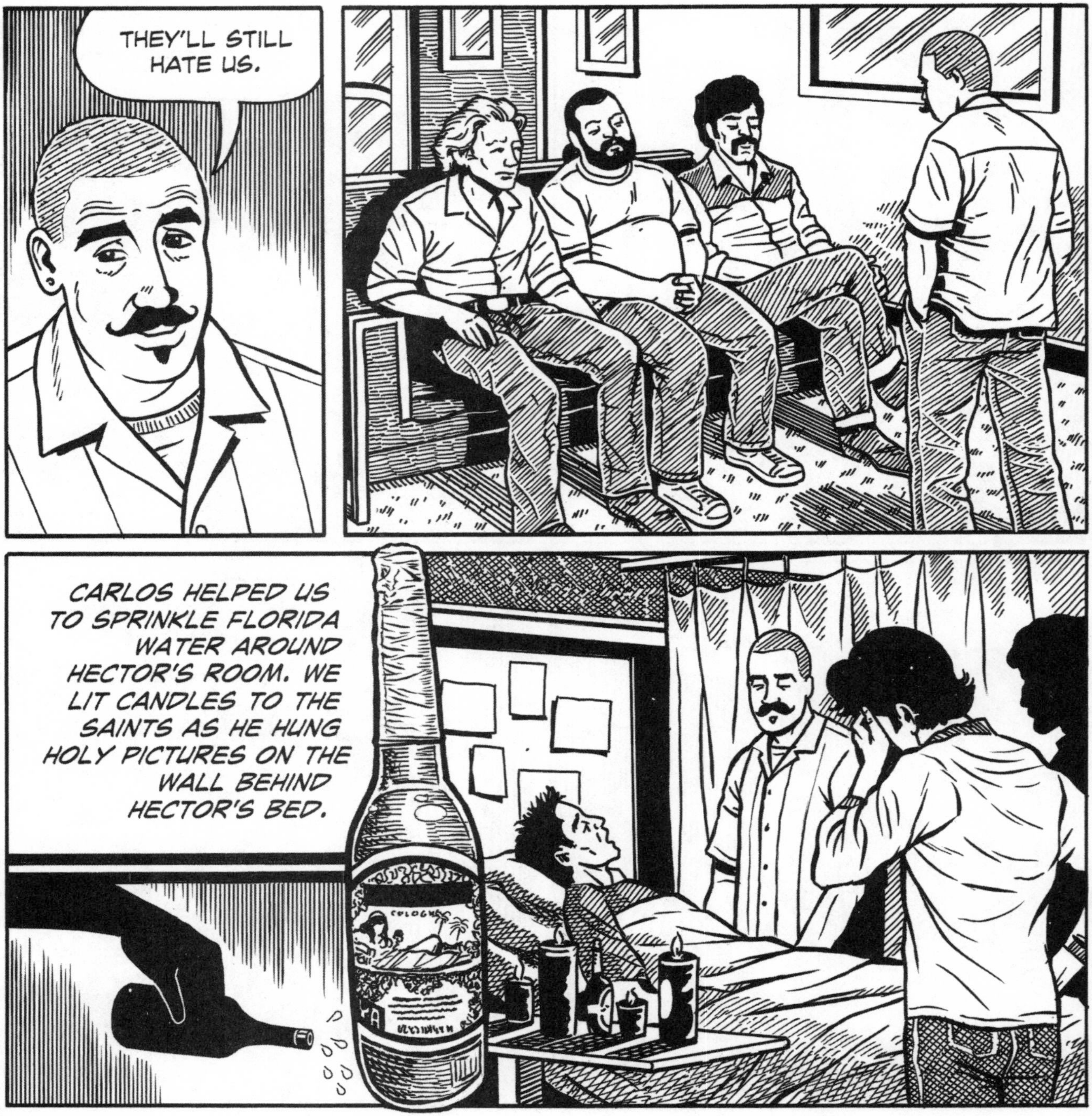
THEY'LL STILL HATE US.
CARLOS HELPED US TO SPRINKLE FLORIDA WATER AROUND HECTOR'S ROOM. WE LIT CANDLES TO THE SAINTS AS HE HUNG HOLY PICTURES ON THE WALL BEHIND HECTOR'S BED.

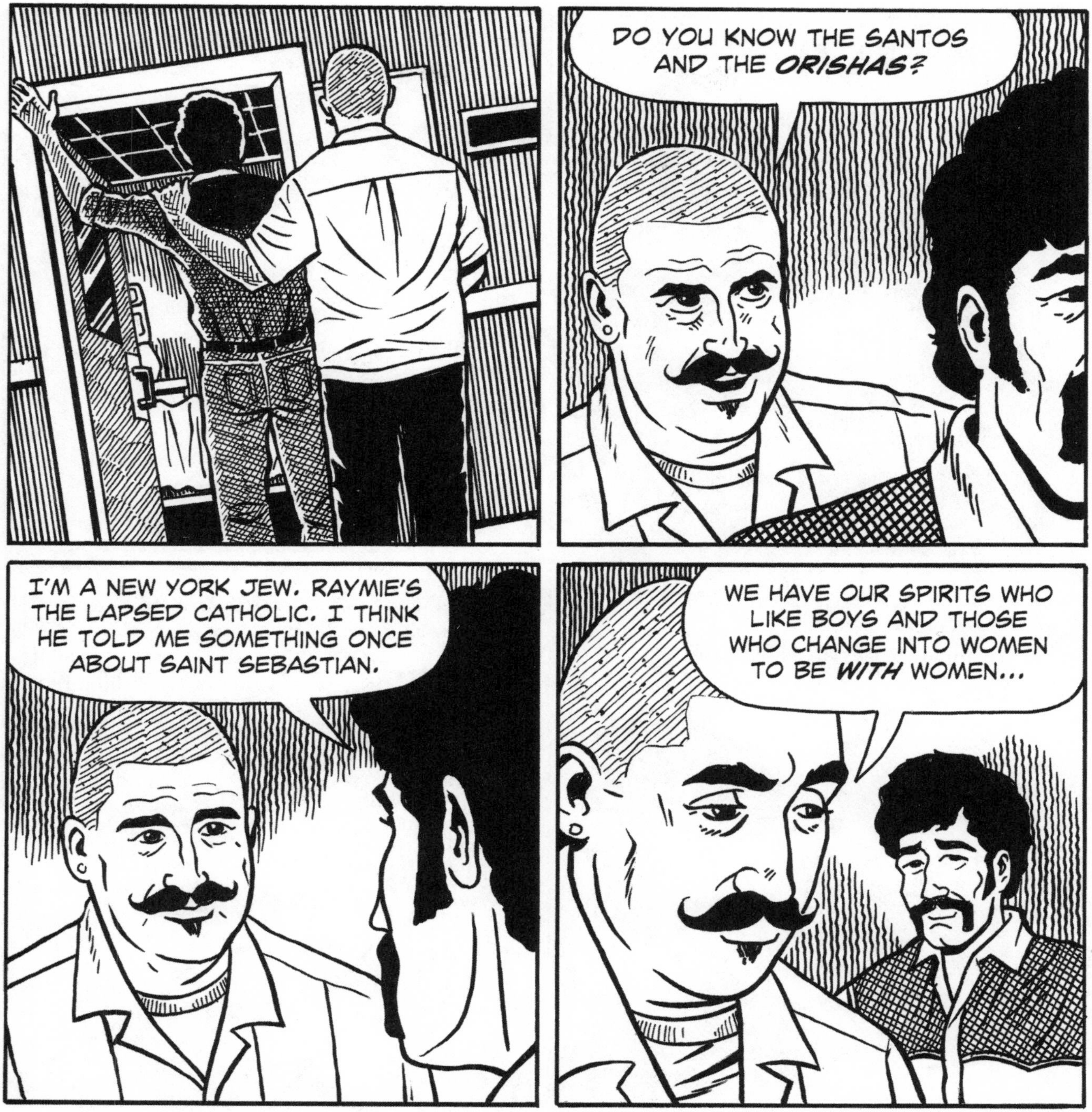
DO YOU KNOW THE SANTOS AND THE *ORISHAS*?
I'M A NEW YORK JEW. RAYMIE'S THE LAPSED CATHOLIC. I THINK HE TOLD ME SOMETHING ONCE ABOUT SAINT SEBASTIAN.
WE HAVE OUR SPIRITS WHO LIKE BOYS AND THOSE WHO CHANGE INTO WOMEN TO BE *WITH* WOMEN...

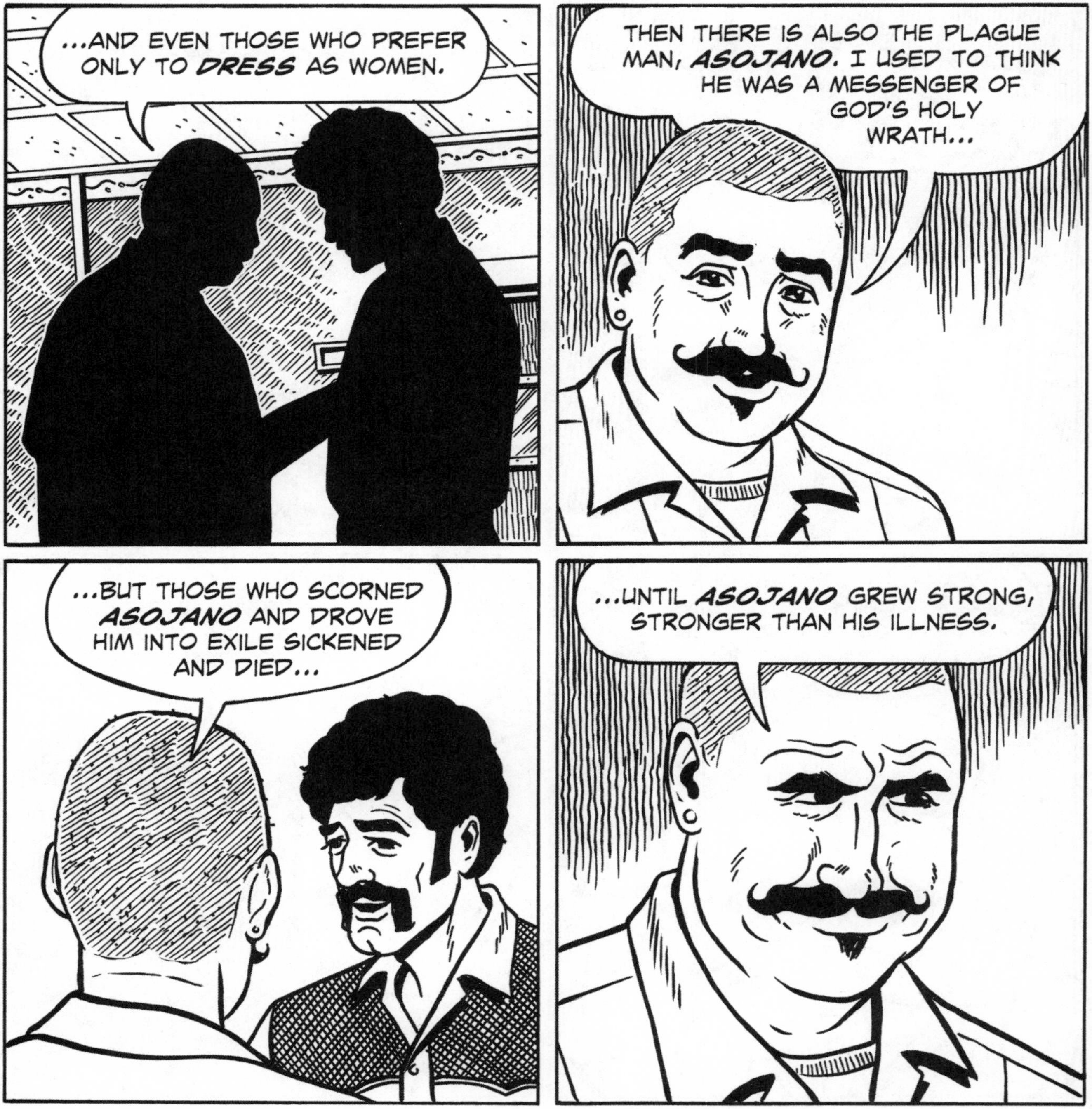
...AND EVEN THOSE WHO PREFER ONLY TO DRESS AS WOMEN.
THEN THERE IS ALSO THE PLAGUE MAN, ASOJANO. I USED TO THINK HE WAS A MESSENGER OF GOD'S HOLY WRATH...
...BUT THOSE WHO SCORNED ASOJANO AND DROVE HIM INTO EXILE SICKENED AND DIED...
...UNTIL ASOJANO GREW STRONG, STRONGER THAN HIS ILLNESS.

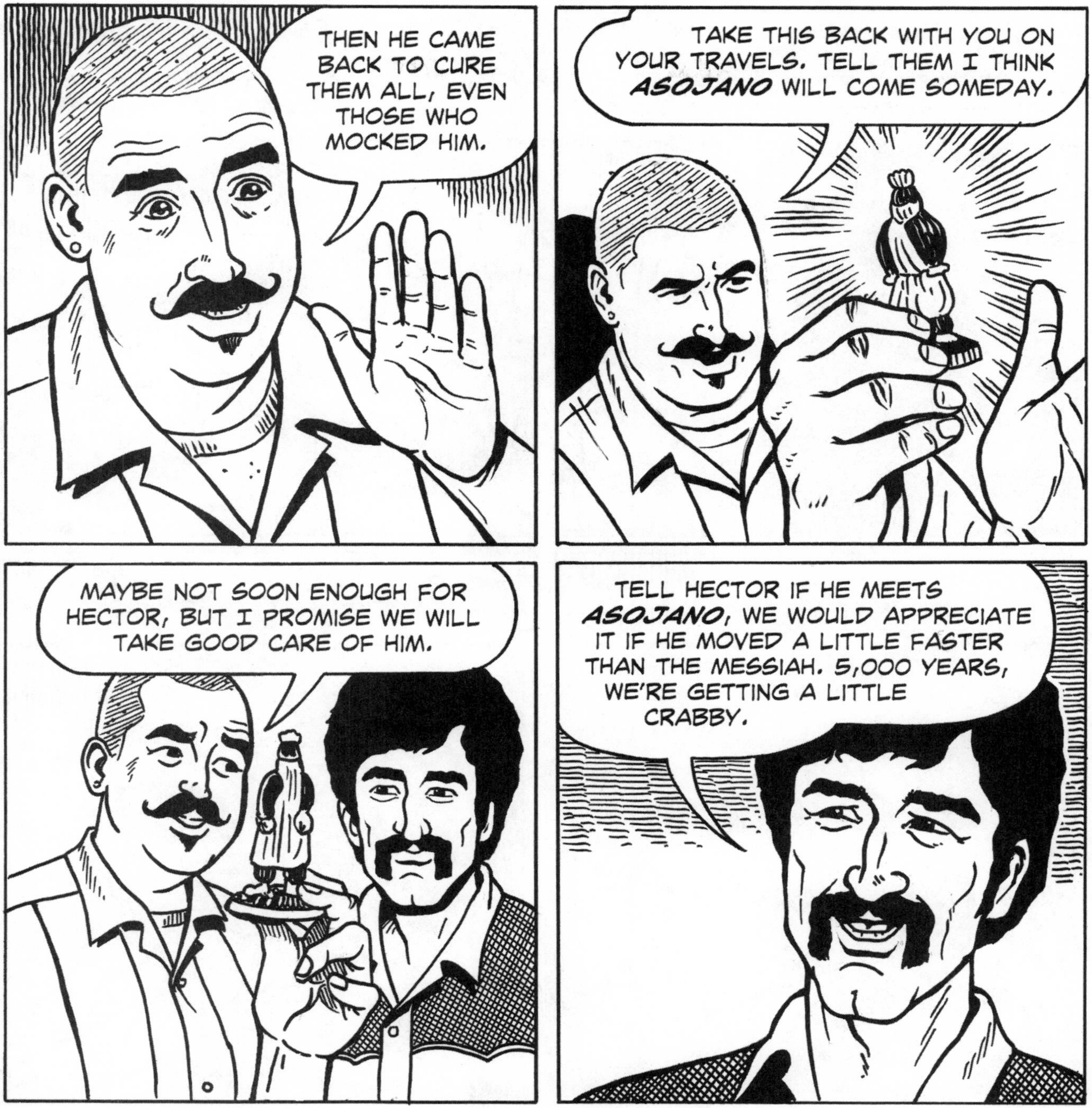
THEN HE CAME BACK TO CURE THEM ALL, EVEN THOSE WHO MOCKED HIM.
TAKE THIS BACK WITH YOU ON YOUR TRAVELS. TELL THEM I THINK *ASOJANO* WILL COME SOMEDAY.
MAYBE NOT SOON ENOUGH FOR HECTOR, BUT I PROMISE WE WILL TAKE GOOD CARE OF HIM.
TELL HECTOR IF HE MEETS *ASOJANO*, WE WOULD APPRECIATE IT IF HE MOVED A LITTLE FASTER THAN THE MESSIAH. 5,000 YEARS, WE'RE GETTING A LITTLE CRABBY.

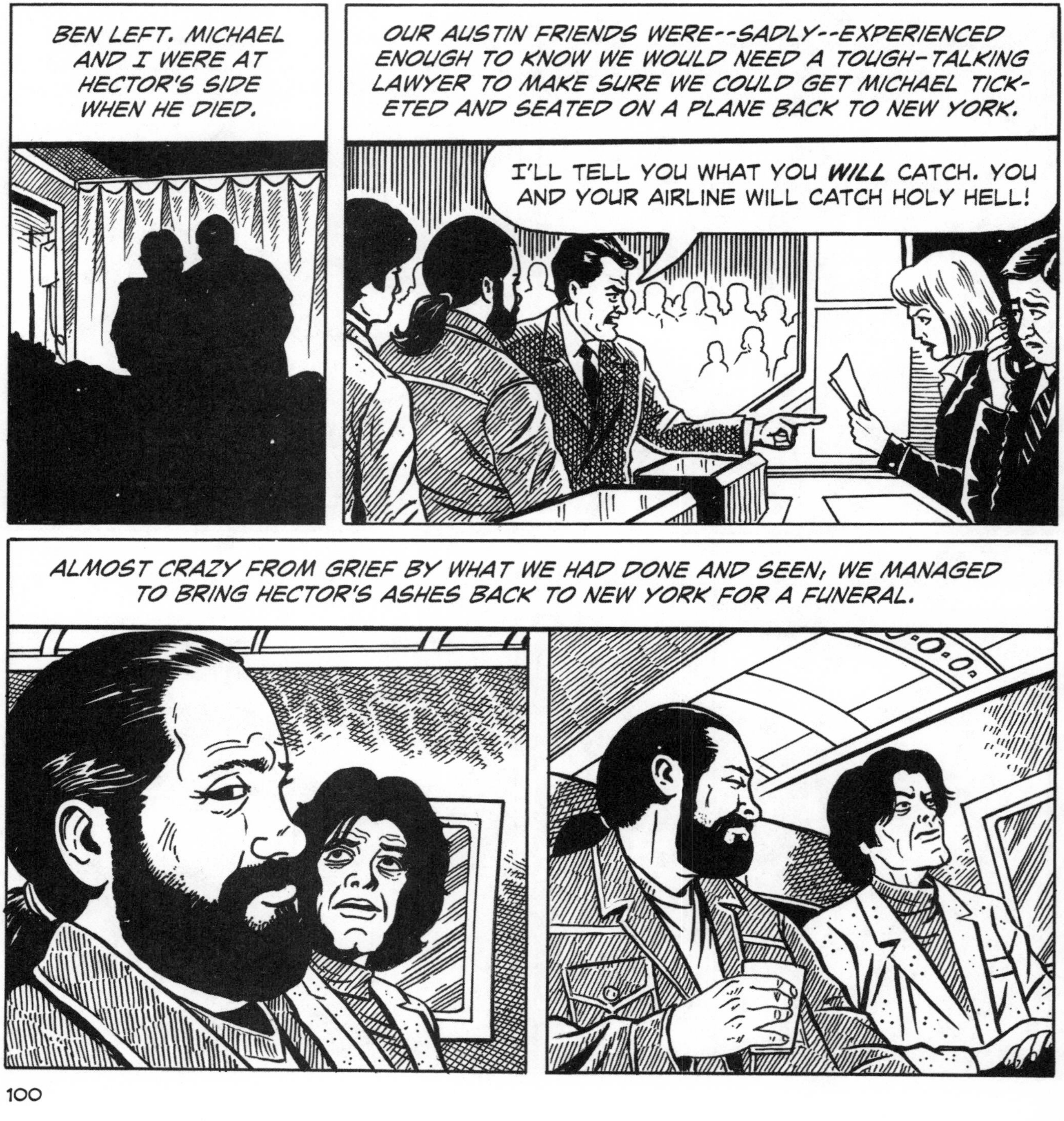
BEN LEFT. MICHAEL AND I WERE AT HECTOR'S SIDE WHEN HE DIED.
OUR AUSTIN FRIENDS WERE--SADLY--EXPERIENCED ENOUGH TO KNOW WE WOULD NEED A TOUGH-TALKING LAWYER TO MAKE SURE WE COULD GET MICHAEL TICKETED AND SEATED ON A PLANE BACK TO NEW YORK.
I'LL TELL YOU WHAT YOU WILL CATCH. YOU AND YOUR AIRLINE WILL CATCH HOLY HELL!
ALMOST CRAZY FROM GRIEF BY WHAT WE HAD DONE AND SEEN, WE MANAGED TO BRING HECTOR'S ASHES BACK TO NEW YORK FOR A FUNERAL.

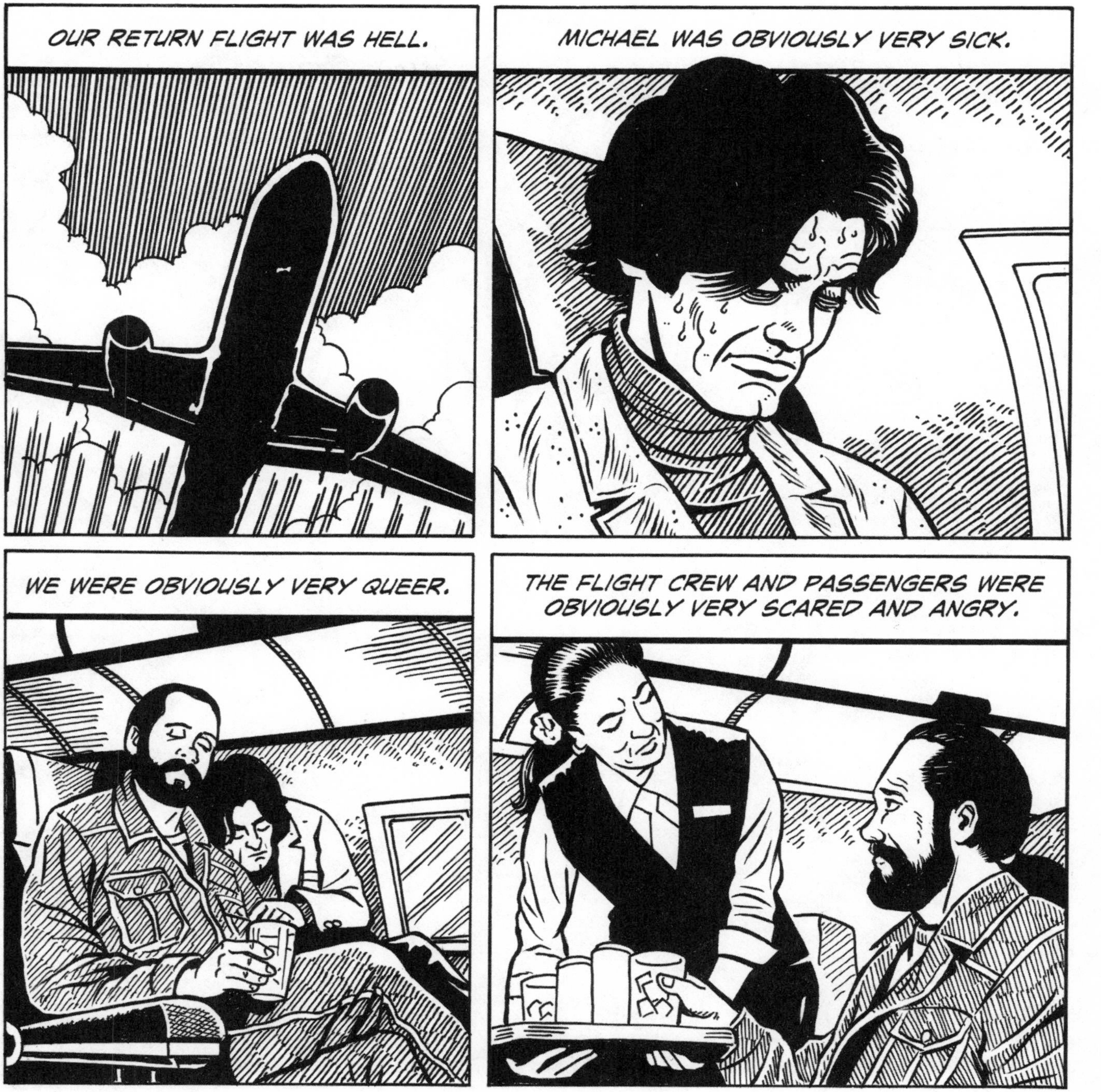
OUR RETURN FLIGHT WAS HELL.
MICHAEL WAS OBVIOUSLY VERY SICK.
WE WERE OBVIOUSLY VERY QUEER.
THE FLIGHT CREW AND PASSENGERS WERE OBVIOUSLY VERY SCARED AND ANGRY.

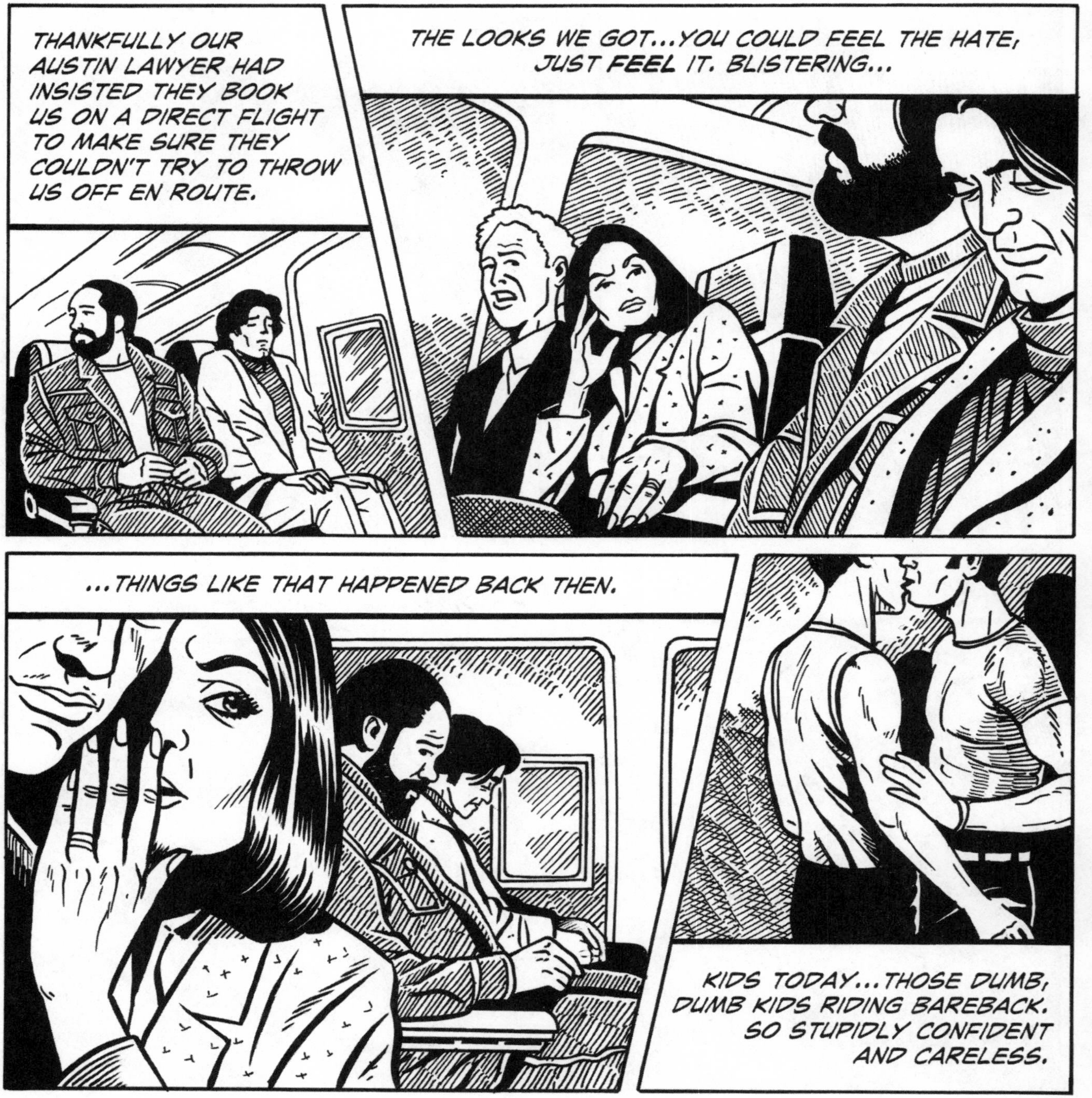
THANKFULLY OUR AUSTIN LAWYER HAD INSISTED THEY BOOK US ON A DIRECT FLIGHT TO MAKE SURE THEY COULDN'T TRY TO THROW US OFF EN ROUTE.
THE LOOKS WE GOT...YOU COULD FEEL THE HATE, JUST FEEL IT. BLISTERING...
...THINGS LIKE THAT HAPPENED BACK THEN.
KIDS TODAY...THOSE DUMB, DUMB KIDS RIDING BAREBACK. SO STUPIDLY CONFIDENT AND CARELESS.

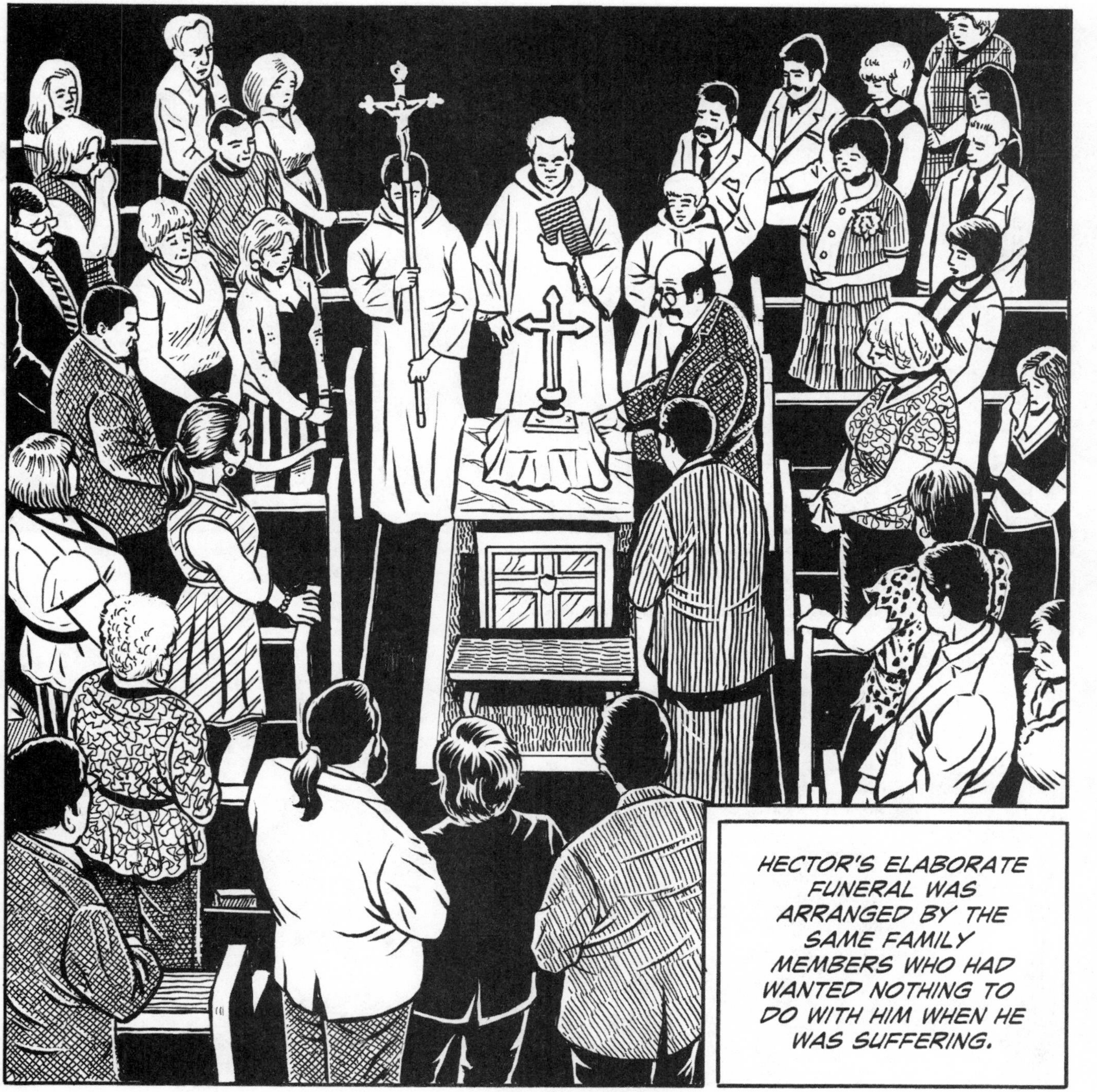
HECTOR'S ELABORATE FUNERAL WAS ARRANGED BY THE SAME FAMILY MEMBERS WHO HAD WANTED NOTHING TO DO WITH HIM WHEN HE WAS SUFFERING.

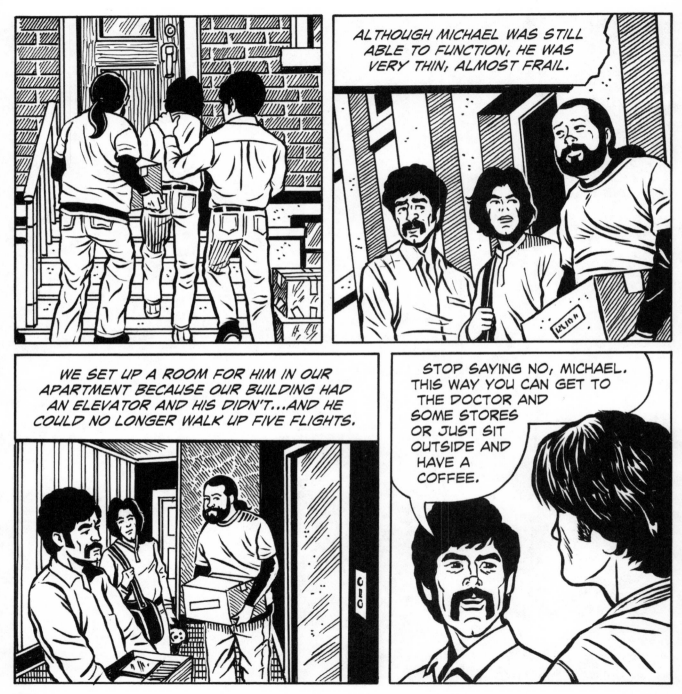

ALTHOUGH MICHAEL WAS STILL ABLE TO FUNCTION, HE WAS VERY THIN, ALMOST FRAIL.

WE SET UP A ROOM FOR HIM IN OUR APARTMENT BECAUSE OUR BUILDING HAD AN ELEVATOR AND HIS DIDN'T...AND HE COULD NO LONGER WALK UP FIVE FLIGHTS.

STOP SAYING NO, MICHAEL. THIS WAY YOU CAN GET TO THE DOCTOR AND SOME STORES OR JUST SIT OUTSIDE AND HAVE A COFFEE.

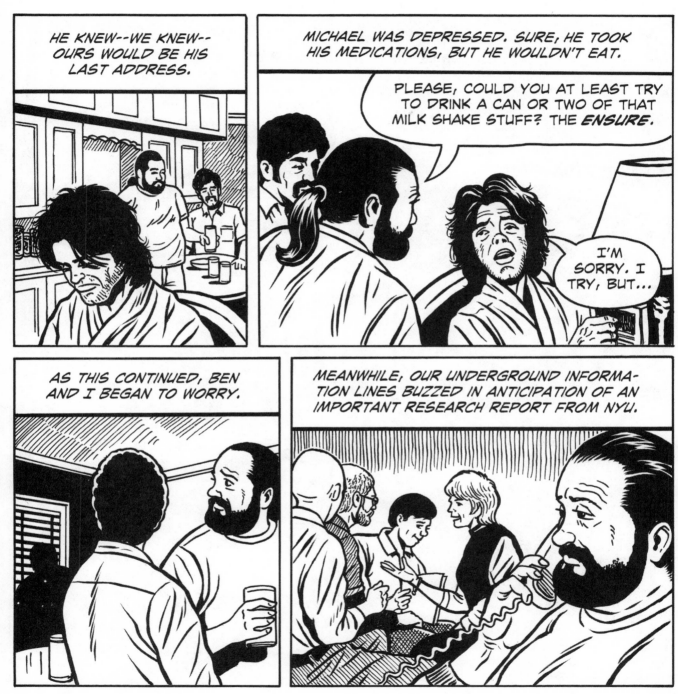

HE KNEW--WE KNEW--OURS WOULD BE HIS LAST ADDRESS.

MICHAEL WAS DEPRESSED. SURE, HE TOOK HIS MEDICATIONS, BUT HE WOULDN'T EAT.

PLEASE, COULD YOU AT LEAST TRY TO DRINK A CAN OR TWO OF THAT MILK SHAKE STUFF? THE *ENSURE*.

I'M SORRY. I TRY, BUT...

AS THIS CONTINUED, BEN AND I BEGAN TO WORRY.

MEANWHILE, OUR UNDERGROUND INFORMATION LINES BUZZED IN ANTICIPATION OF AN IMPORTANT RESEARCH REPORT FROM NYU.

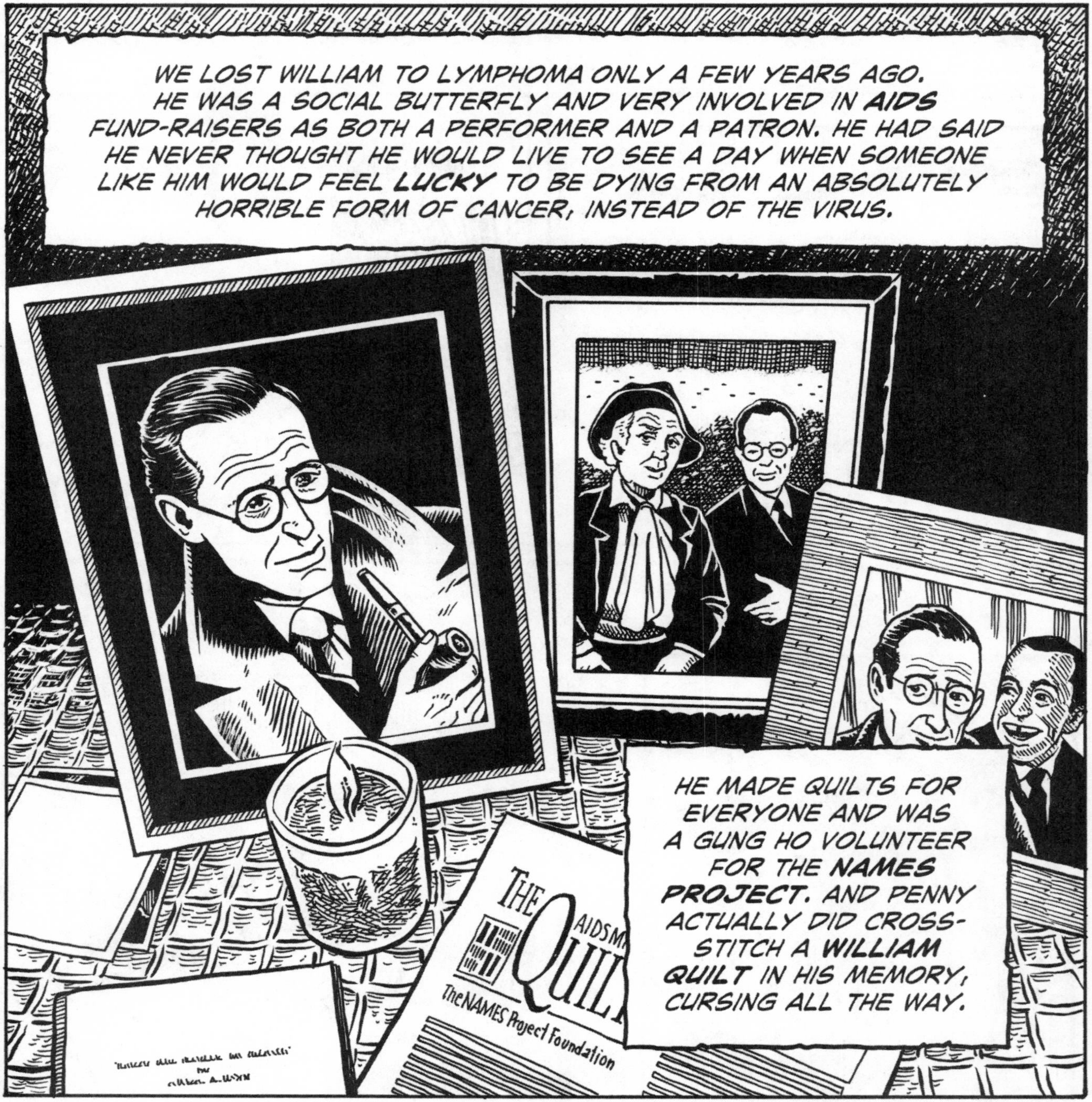
WE LOST WILLIAM TO LYMPHOMA ONLY A FEW YEARS AGO. HE WAS A SOCIAL BUTTERFLY AND VERY INVOLVED IN **AIDS** FUND-RAISERS AS BOTH A PERFORMER AND A PATRON. HE HAD SAID HE NEVER THOUGHT HE WOULD LIVE TO SEE A DAY WHEN SOMEONE LIKE HIM WOULD FEEL **LUCKY** TO BE DYING FROM AN ABSOLUTELY HORRIBLE FORM OF CANCER, INSTEAD OF THE VIRUS.
THE AIDS M QUILT
The NAMES Project Foundation
HE MADE QUILTS FOR EVERYONE AND WAS A GUNG HO VOLUNTEER FOR THE **NAMES PROJECT**. AND PENNY ACTUALLY DID CROSS-STITCH A **WILLIAM QUILT** IN HIS MEMORY, CURSING ALL THE WAY.

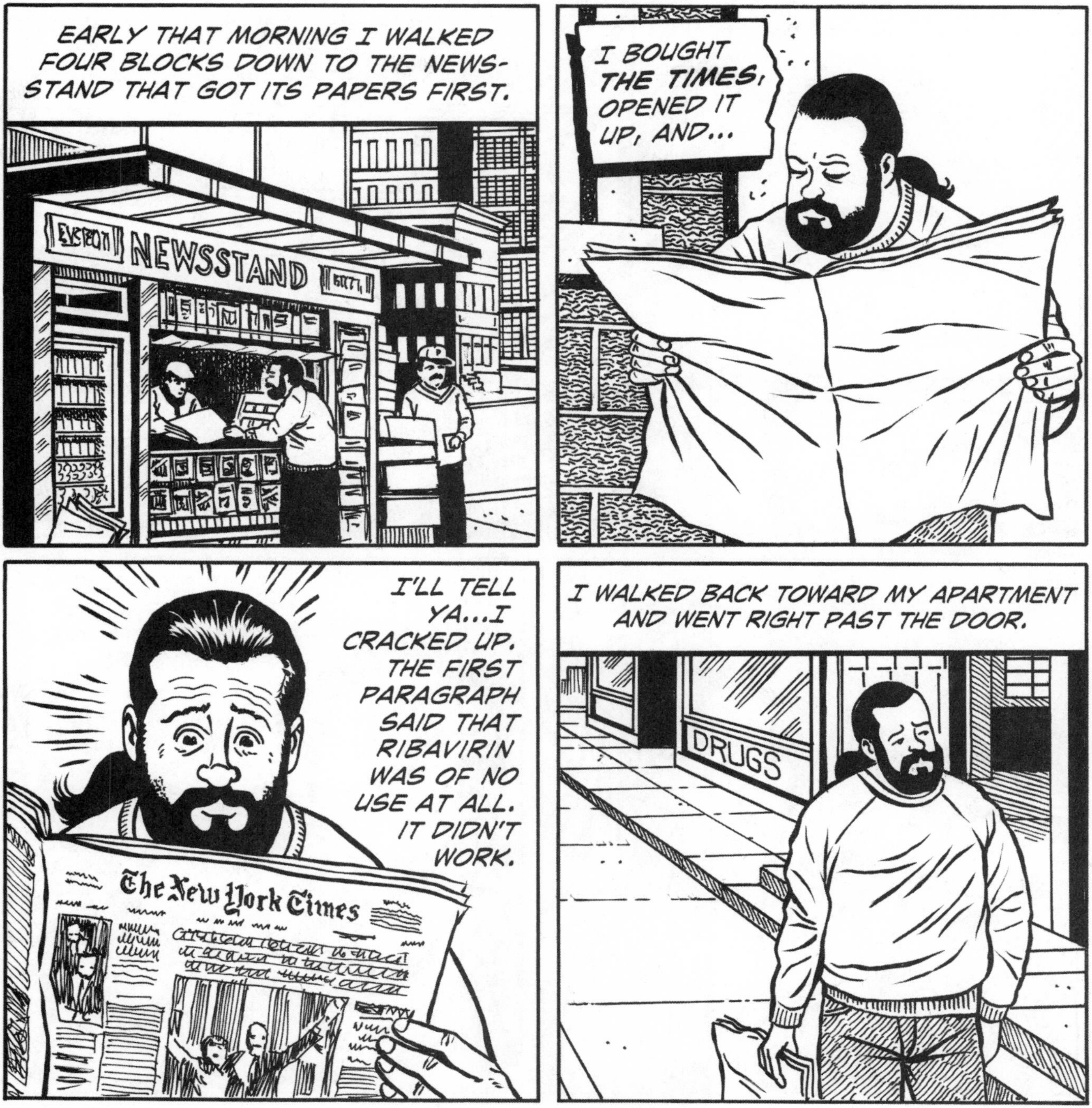
EARLY THAT MORNING I WALKED FOUR BLOCKS DOWN TO THE NEWS-STAND THAT GOT ITS PAPERS FIRST.
NEWSSTAND
I BOUGHT **THE TIMES**, OPENED IT UP, AND...
I'LL TELL YA...I CRACKED UP. THE FIRST PARAGRAPH SAID THAT RIBAVIRIN WAS OF NO USE AT ALL. IT DIDN'T WORK.
The New York Times
I WALKED BACK TOWARD MY APARTMENT AND WENT RIGHT PAST THE DOOR.
DRUGS

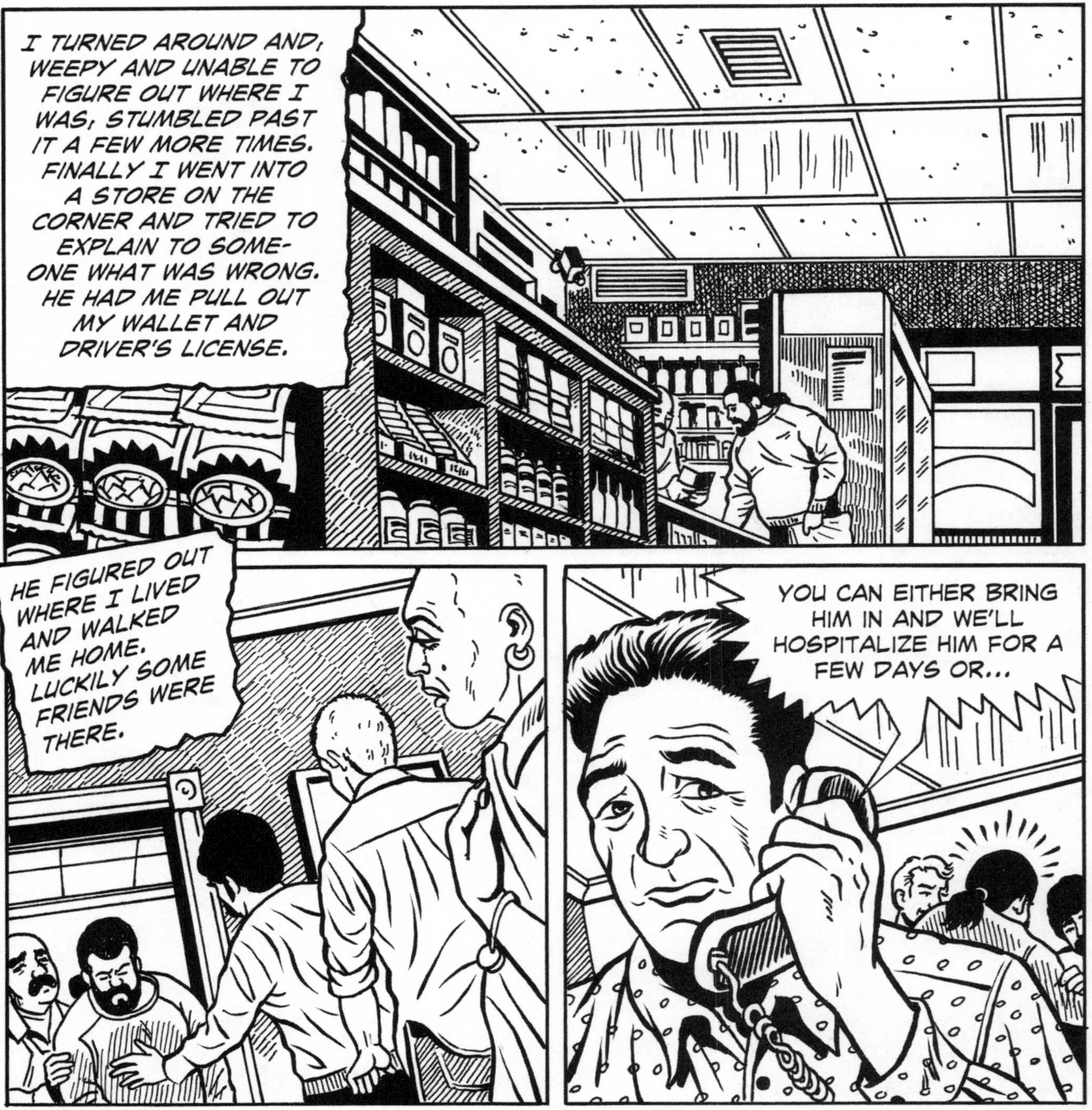
I TURNED AROUND AND, WEEPY AND UNABLE TO FIGURE OUT WHERE I WAS, STUMBLED PAST IT A FEW MORE TIMES. FINALLY I WENT INTO A STORE ON THE CORNER AND TRIED TO EXPLAIN TO SOME-ONE WHAT WAS WRONG. HE HAD ME PULL OUT MY WALLET AND DRIVER'S LICENSE.
HE FIGURED OUT WHERE I LIVED AND WALKED ME HOME. LUCKILY SOME FRIENDS WERE THERE.
YOU CAN EITHER BRING HIM IN AND WE'LL HOSPITALIZE HIM FOR A FEW DAYS OR...

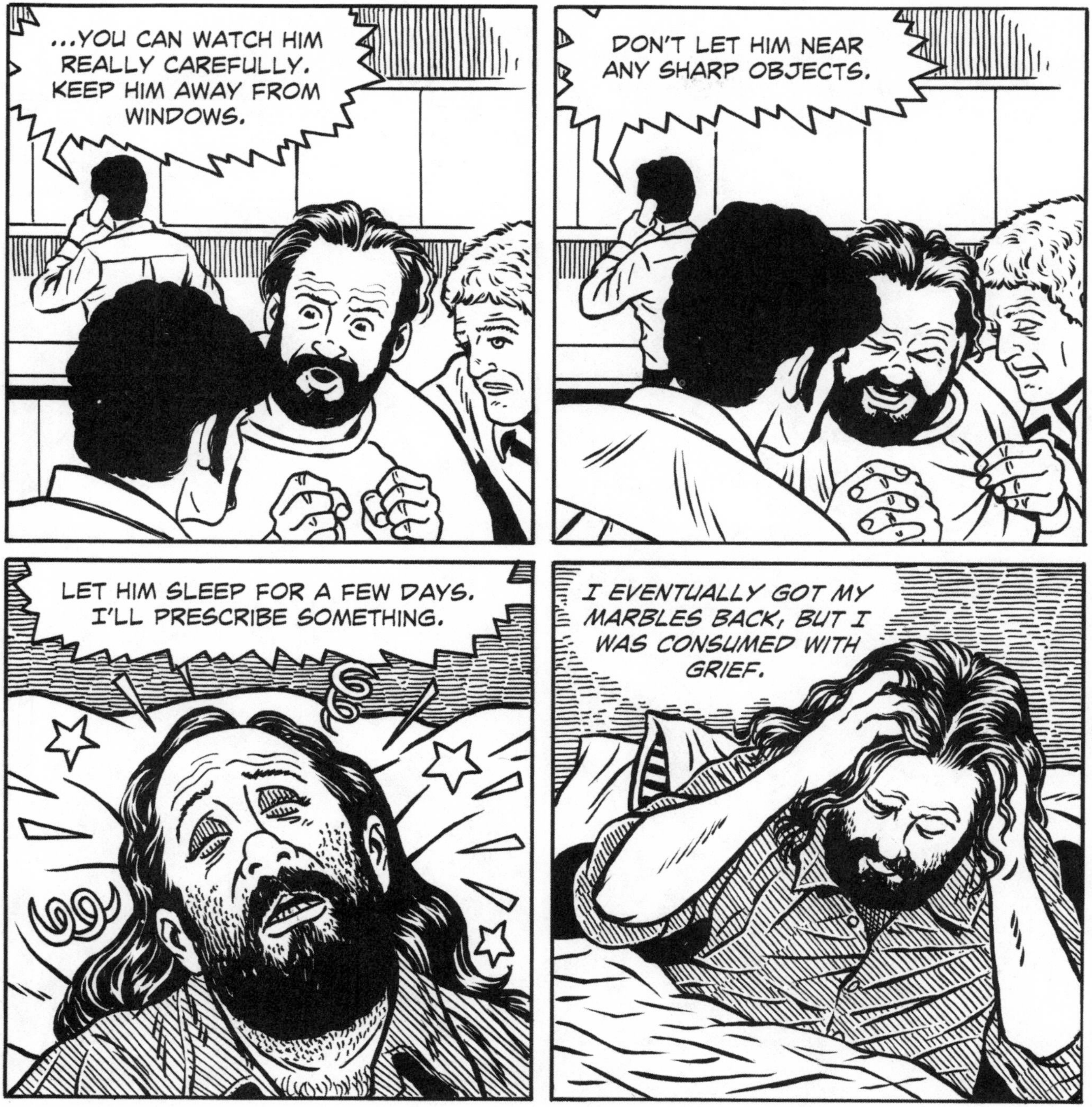
...YOU CAN WATCH HIM REALLY CAREFULLY. KEEP HIM AWAY FROM WINDOWS.
DON'T LET HIM NEAR ANY SHARP OBJECTS.
LET HIM SLEEP FOR A FEW DAYS. I'LL PRESCRIBE SOMETHING.
I EVENTUALLY GOT MY MARBLES BACK, BUT I WAS CONSUMED WITH GRIEF.

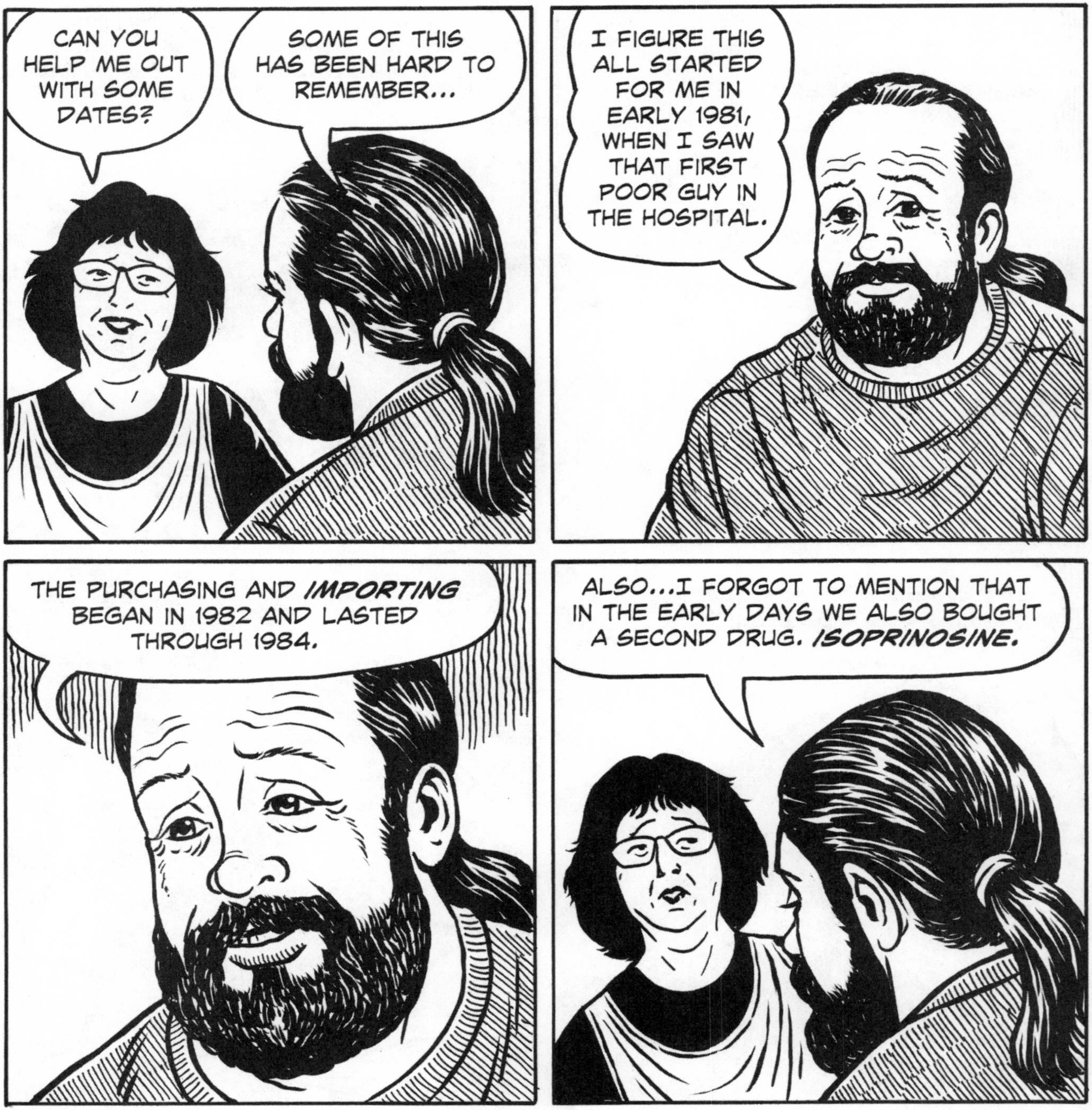
CAN YOU HELP ME OUT WITH SOME DATES?
SOME OF THIS HAS BEEN HARD TO REMEMBER...
I FIGURE THIS ALL STARTED FOR ME IN EARLY 1981, WHEN I SAW THAT FIRST POOR GUY IN THE HOSPITAL.
THE PURCHASING AND *IMPORTING* BEGAN IN 1982 AND LASTED THROUGH 1984.
ALSO...I FORGOT TO MENTION THAT IN THE EARLY DAYS WE ALSO BOUGHT A SECOND DRUG. *ISOPRINOSINE.*

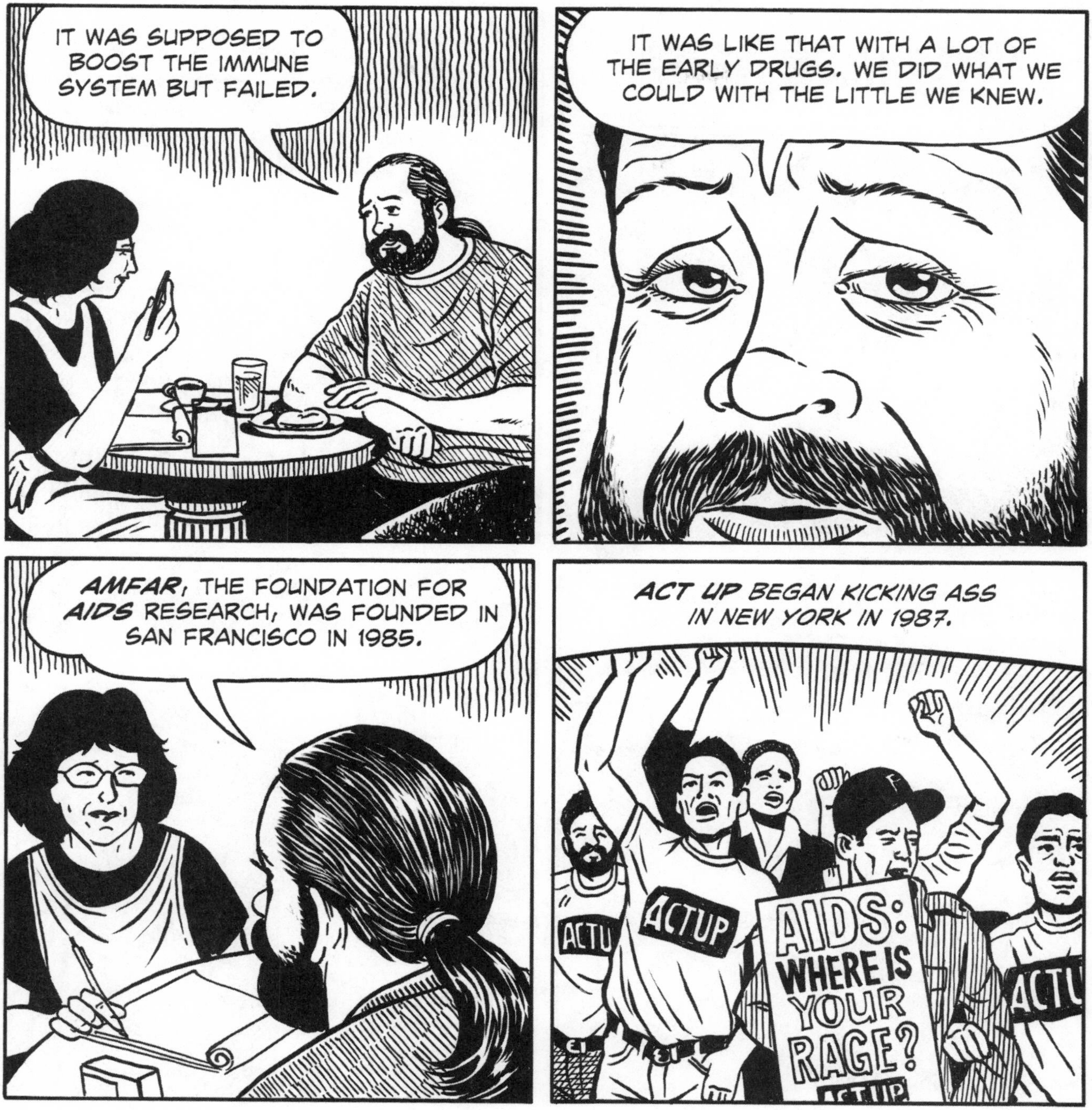
IT WAS SUPPOSED TO BOOST THE IMMUNE SYSTEM BUT FAILED.
IT WAS LIKE THAT WITH A LOT OF THE EARLY DRUGS. WE DID WHAT WE COULD WITH THE LITTLE WE KNEW.
AMFAR, THE FOUNDATION FOR AIDS RESEARCH, WAS FOUNDED IN SAN FRANCISCO IN 1985.
ACT UP BEGAN KICKING ASS IN NEW YORK IN 1987.
ACTUP
AIDS: WHERE IS YOUR RAGE?

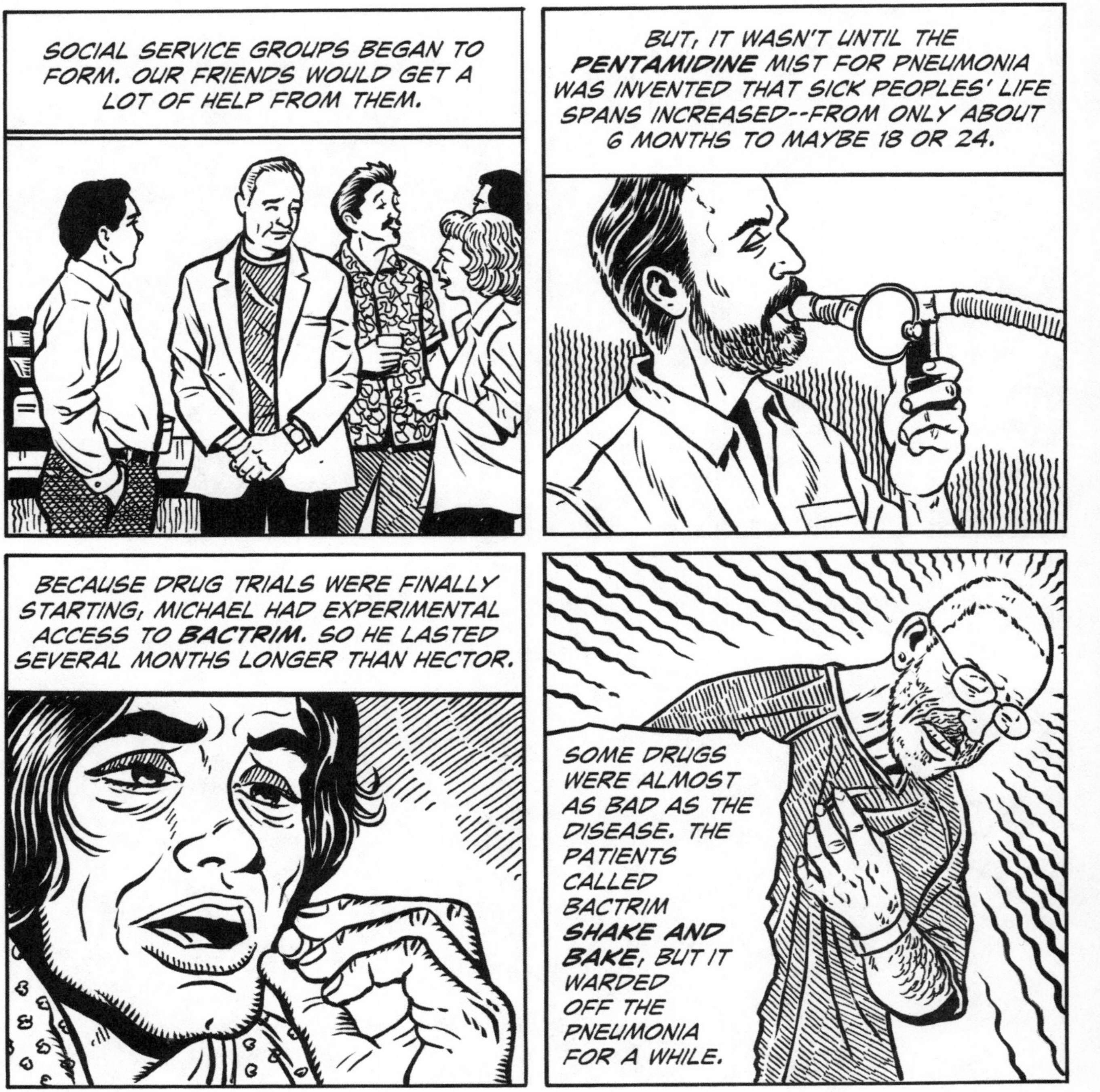
SOCIAL SERVICE GROUPS BEGAN TO FORM. OUR FRIENDS WOULD GET A LOT OF HELP FROM THEM.
BUT, IT WASN'T UNTIL THE **PENTAMIDINE** MIST FOR PNEUMONIA WAS INVENTED THAT SICK PEOPLES' LIFE SPANS INCREASED--FROM ONLY ABOUT 6 MONTHS TO MAYBE 18 OR 24.
BECAUSE DRUG TRIALS WERE FINALLY STARTING, MICHAEL HAD EXPERIMENTAL ACCESS TO **BACTRIM**. SO HE LASTED SEVERAL MONTHS LONGER THAN HECTOR.
SOME DRUGS WERE ALMOST AS BAD AS THE DISEASE. THE PATIENTS CALLED BACTRIM **SHAKE AND BAKE**, BUT IT WARDED OFF THE PNEUMONIA FOR A WHILE.

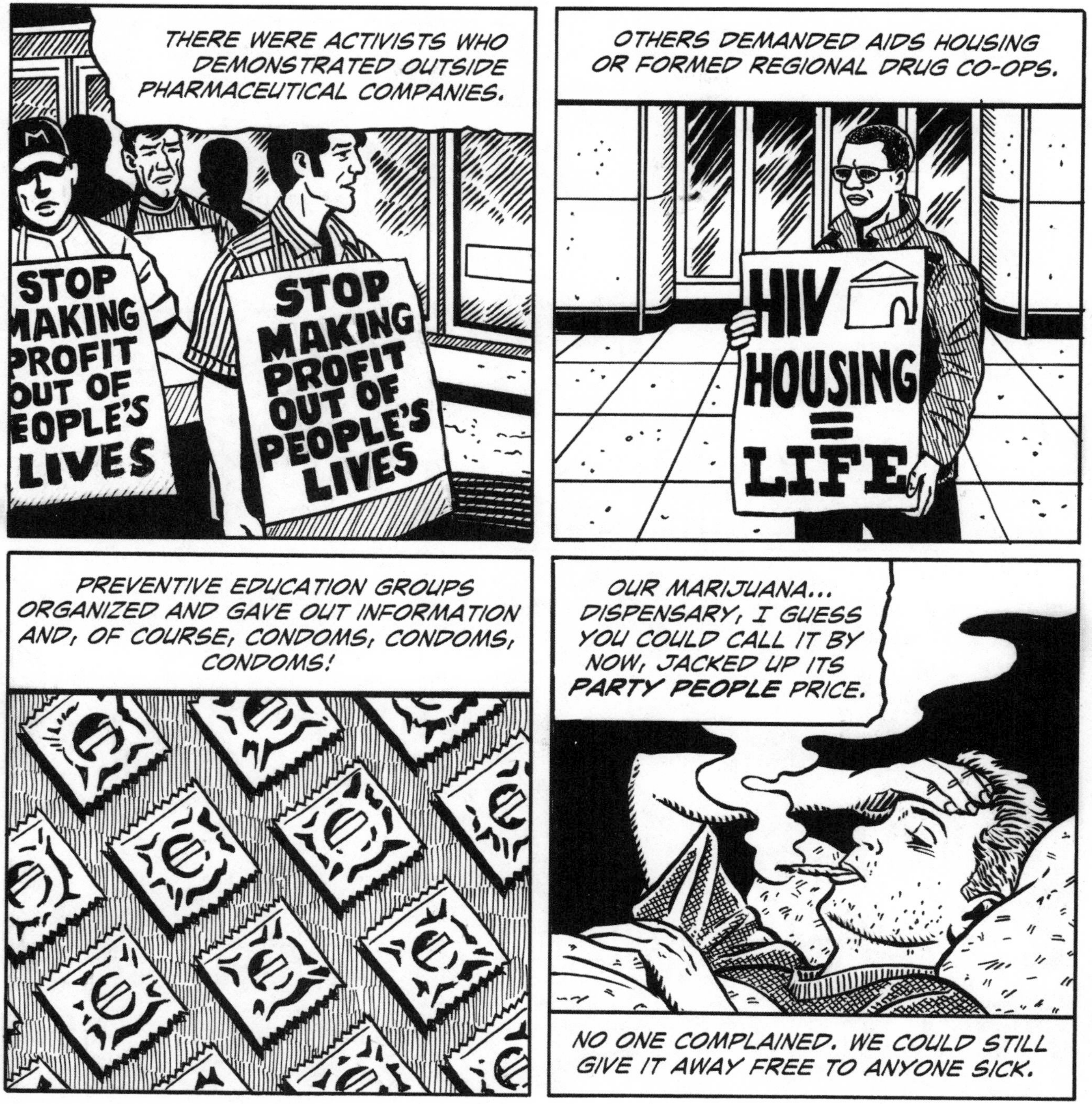
THERE WERE ACTIVISTS WHO DEMONSTRATED OUTSIDE PHARMACEUTICAL COMPANIES.
STOP MAKING PROFIT OUT OF PEOPLE'S LIVES
STOP MAKING PROFIT OUT OF PEOPLE'S LIVES
OTHERS DEMANDED AIDS HOUSING OR FORMED REGIONAL DRUG CO-OPS.
HIV HOUSING = LIFE
PREVENTIVE EDUCATION GROUPS ORGANIZED AND GAVE OUT INFORMATION AND, OF COURSE, CONDOMS, CONDOMS, CONDOMS!
OUR MARIJUANA... DISPENSARY, I GUESS YOU COULD CALL IT BY NOW, JACKED UP ITS PARTY PEOPLE PRICE.
NO ONE COMPLAINED. WE COULD STILL GIVE IT AWAY FREE TO ANYONE SICK.

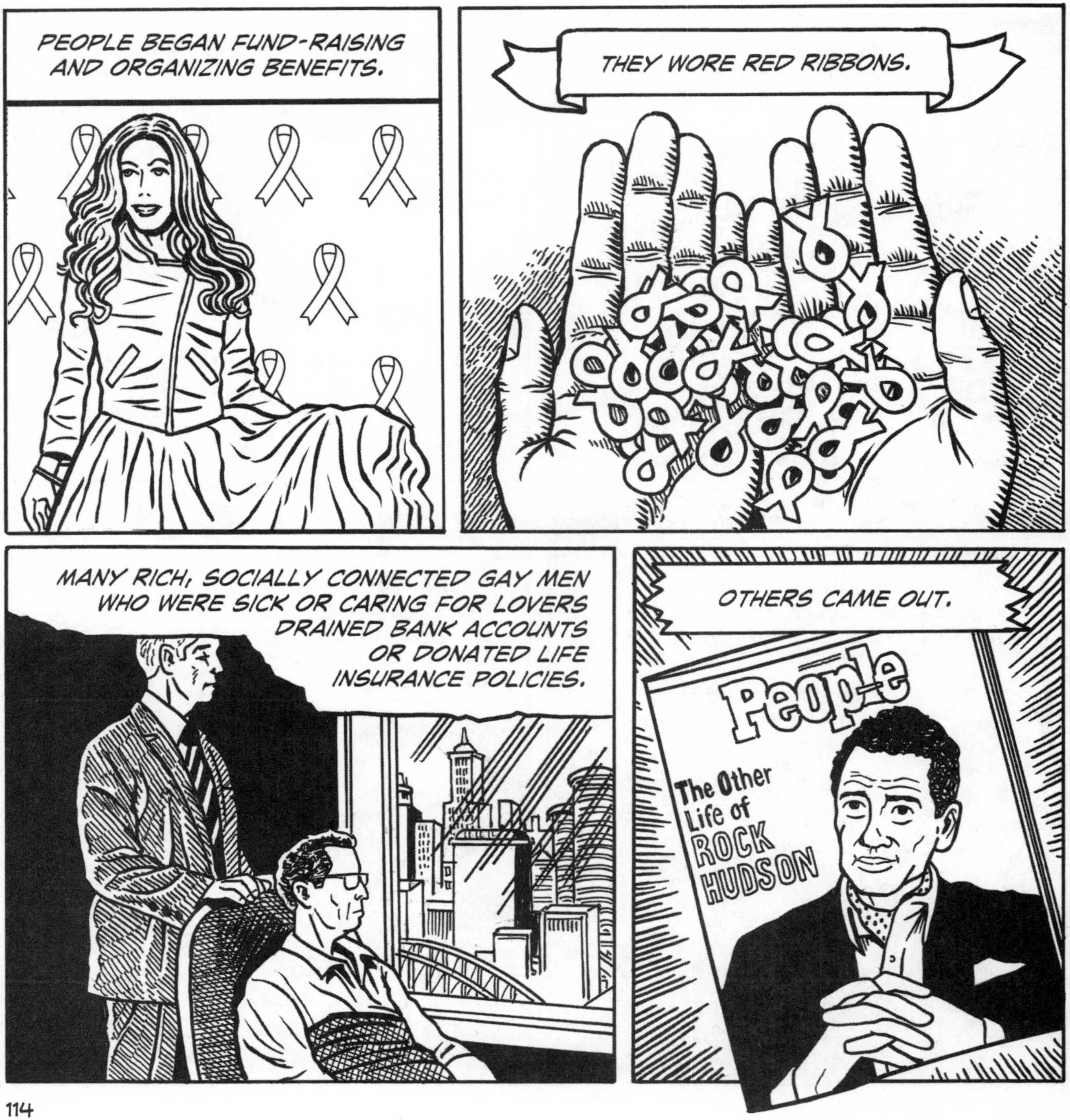
PEOPLE BEGAN FUND-RAISING AND ORGANIZING BENEFITS.
THEY WORE RED RIBBONS.
MANY RICH, SOCIALLY CONNECTED GAY MEN WHO WERE SICK OR CARING FOR LOVERS DRAINED BANK ACCOUNTS OR DONATED LIFE INSURANCE POLICIES.
OTHERS CAME OUT.
People
The Other Life of ROCK HUDSON

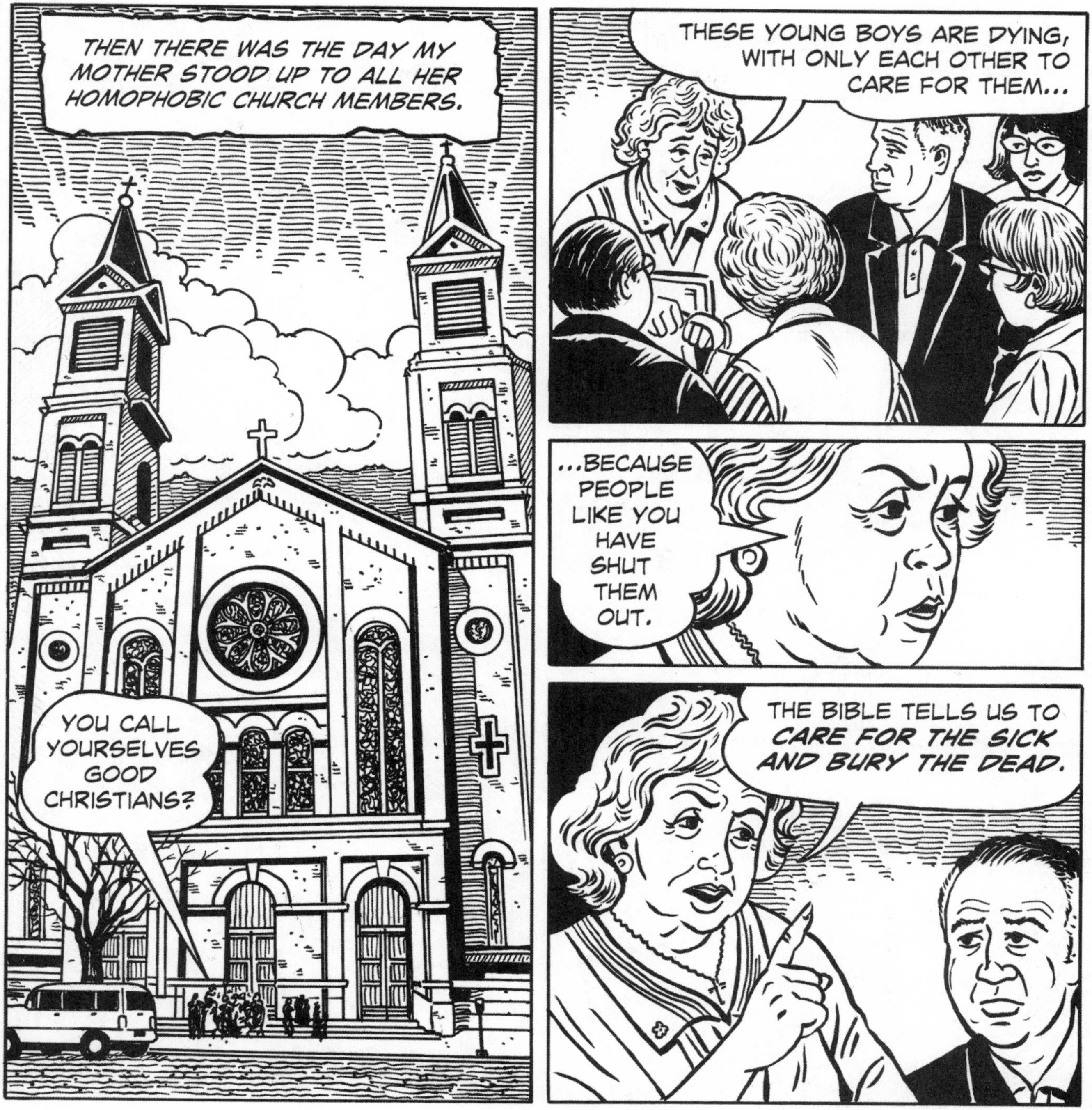
THEN THERE WAS THE DAY MY MOTHER STOOD UP TO ALL HER HOMOPHOBIC CHURCH MEMBERS.
YOU CALL YOURSELVES GOOD CHRISTIANS?
THESE YOUNG BOYS ARE DYING, WITH ONLY EACH OTHER TO CARE FOR THEM...
...BECAUSE PEOPLE LIKE YOU HAVE SHUT THEM OUT.
THE BIBLE TELLS US TO *CARE FOR THE SICK AND BURY THE DEAD.*

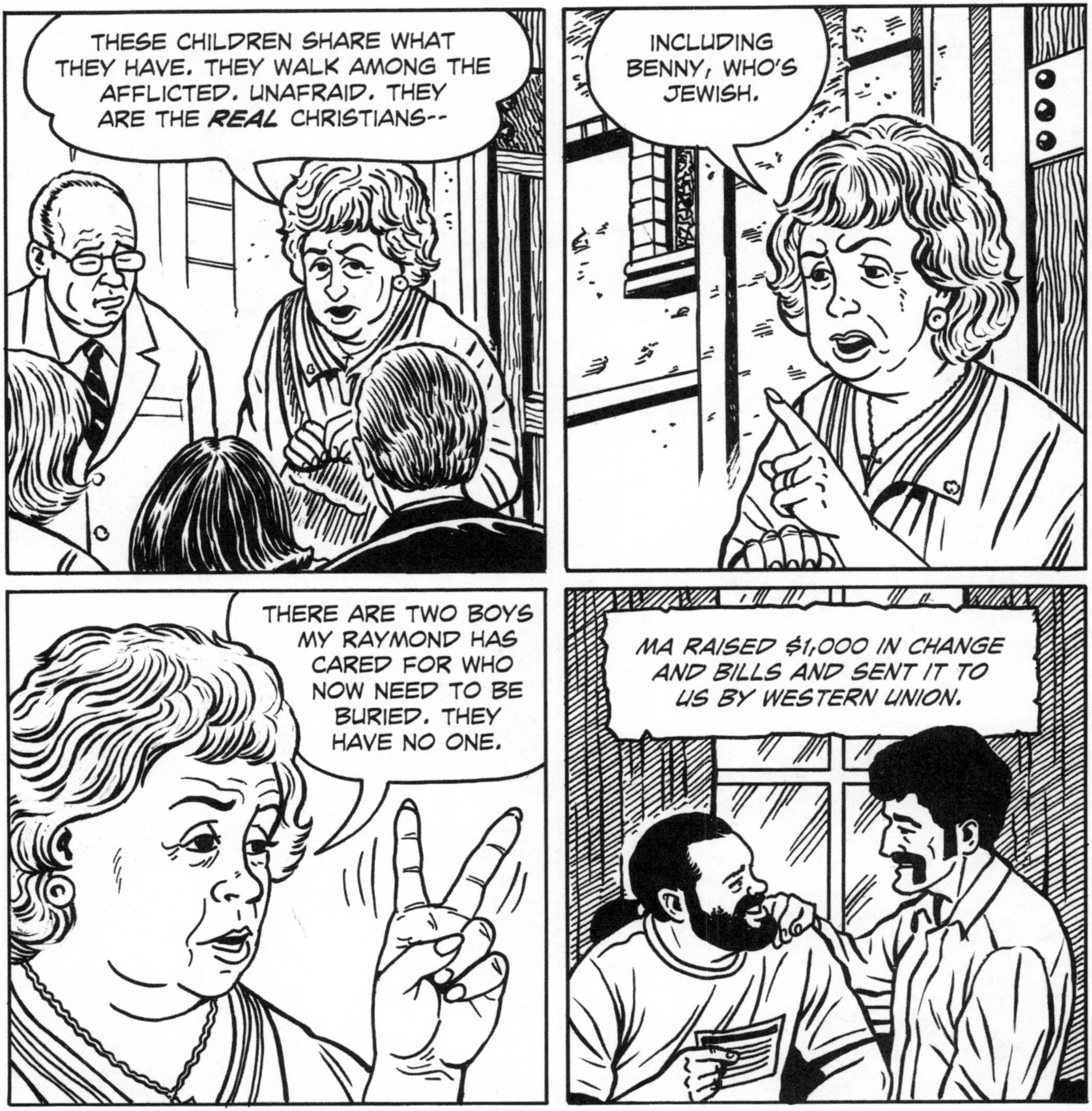
THESE CHILDREN SHARE WHAT THEY HAVE. THEY WALK AMONG THE AFFLICTED. UNAFRAID. THEY ARE THE *REAL* CHRISTIANS--
INCLUDING BENNY, WHO'S JEWISH.
THERE ARE TWO BOYS MY RAYMOND HAS CARED FOR WHO NOW NEED TO BE BURIED. THEY HAVE NO ONE.
MA RAISED $1,000 IN CHANGE AND BILLS AND SENT IT TO US BY WESTERN UNION.

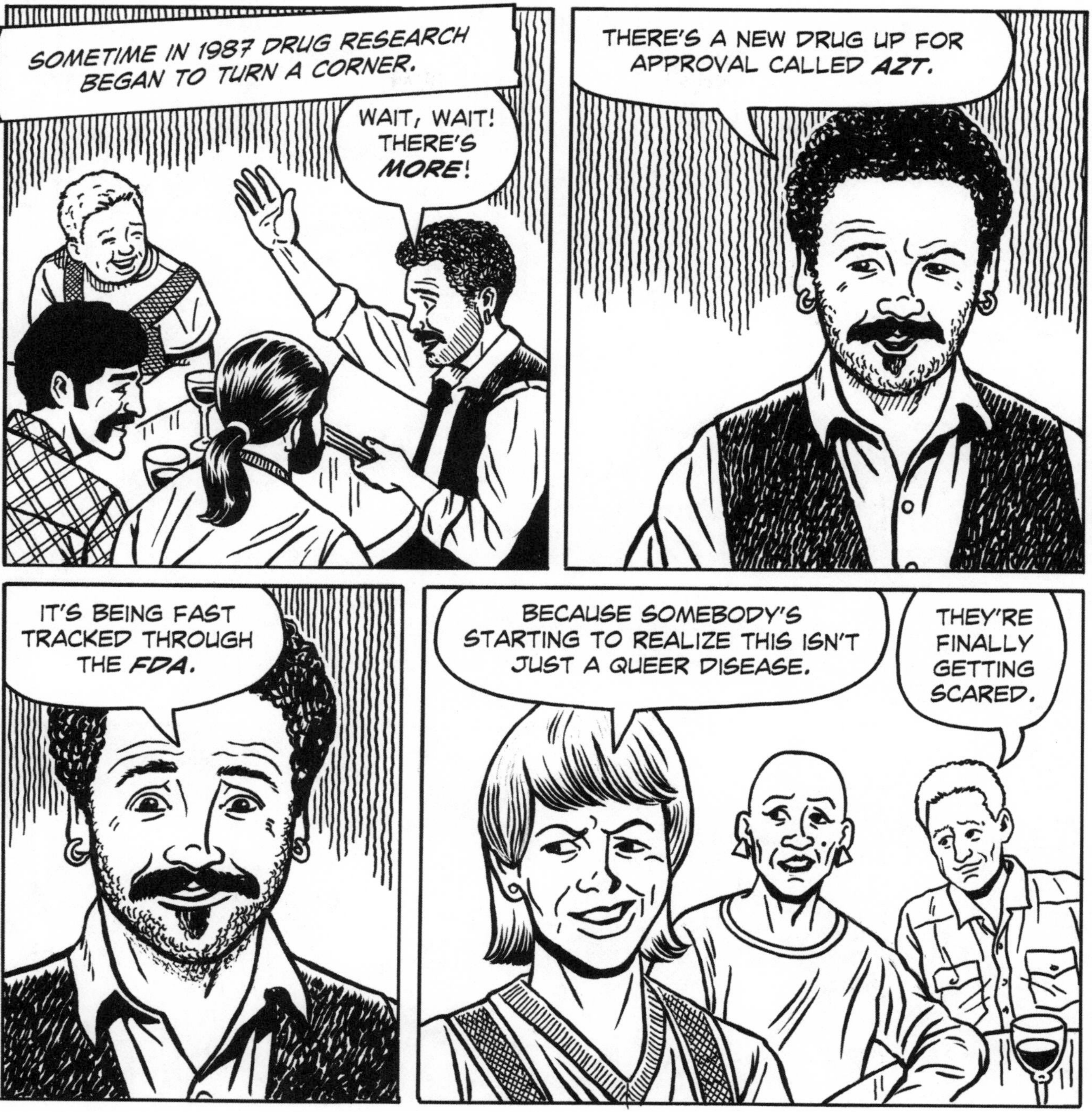
SOMETIME IN 1987 DRUG RESEARCH BEGAN TO TURN A CORNER.
WAIT, WAIT! THERE'S *MORE*!
THERE'S A NEW DRUG UP FOR APPROVAL CALLED *AZT*.
IT'S BEING FAST TRACKED THROUGH THE *FDA*.
BECAUSE SOMEBODY'S STARTING TO REALIZE THIS ISN'T JUST A QUEER DISEASE.
THEY'RE FINALLY GETTING SCARED.

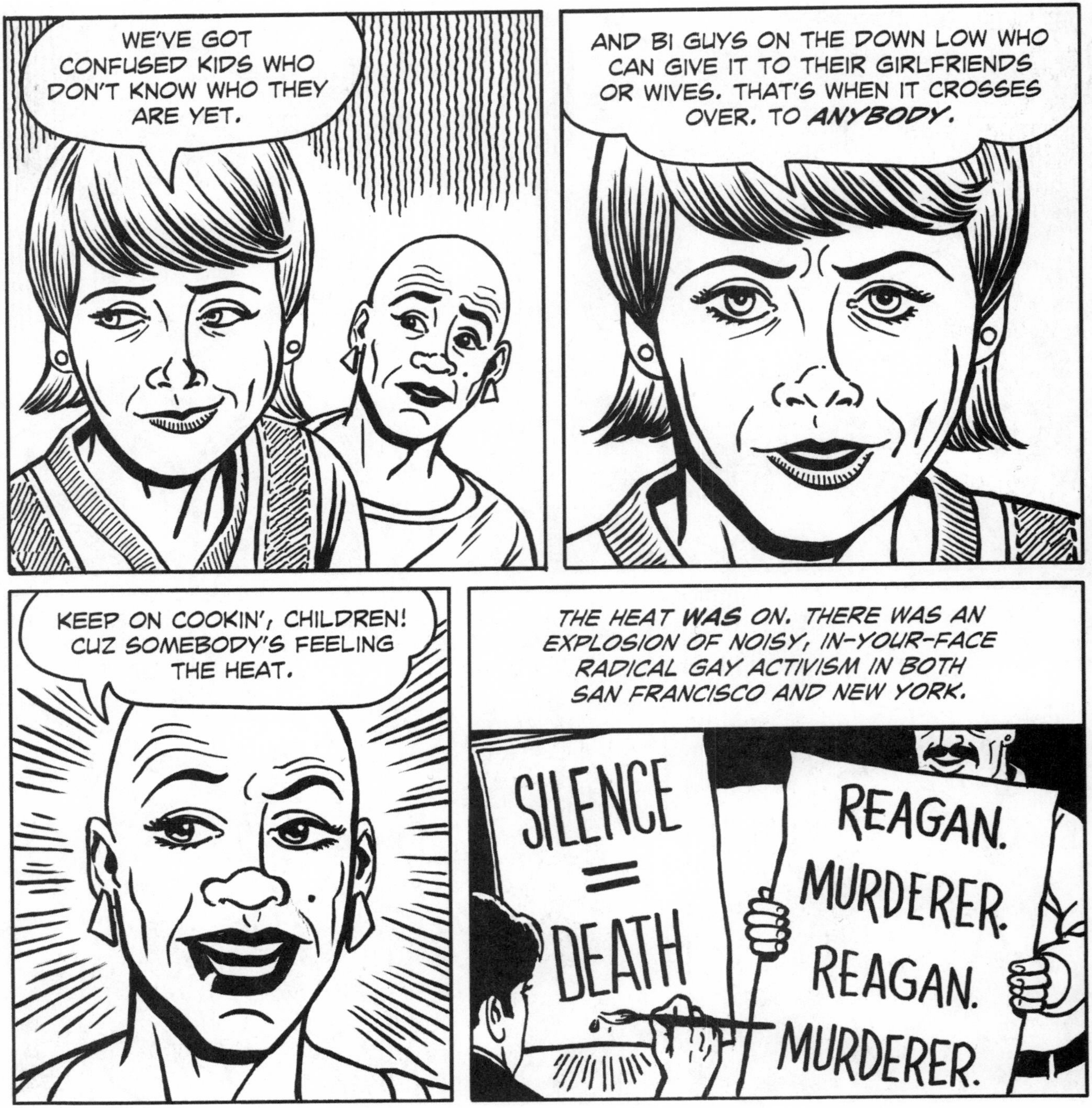
WE'VE GOT CONFUSED KIDS WHO DON'T KNOW WHO THEY ARE YET.
AND BI GUYS ON THE DOWN LOW WHO CAN GIVE IT TO THEIR GIRLFRIENDS OR WIVES. THAT'S WHEN IT CROSSES OVER. TO *ANYBODY*.
KEEP ON COOKIN', CHILDREN! CUZ SOMEBODY'S FEELING THE HEAT.
*THE HEAT **WAS** ON. THERE WAS AN EXPLOSION OF NOISY, IN-YOUR-FACE RADICAL GAY ACTIVISM IN BOTH SAN FRANCISCO AND NEW YORK.*
SILENCE = DEATH
REAGAN. MURDERER. REAGAN. MURDERER.

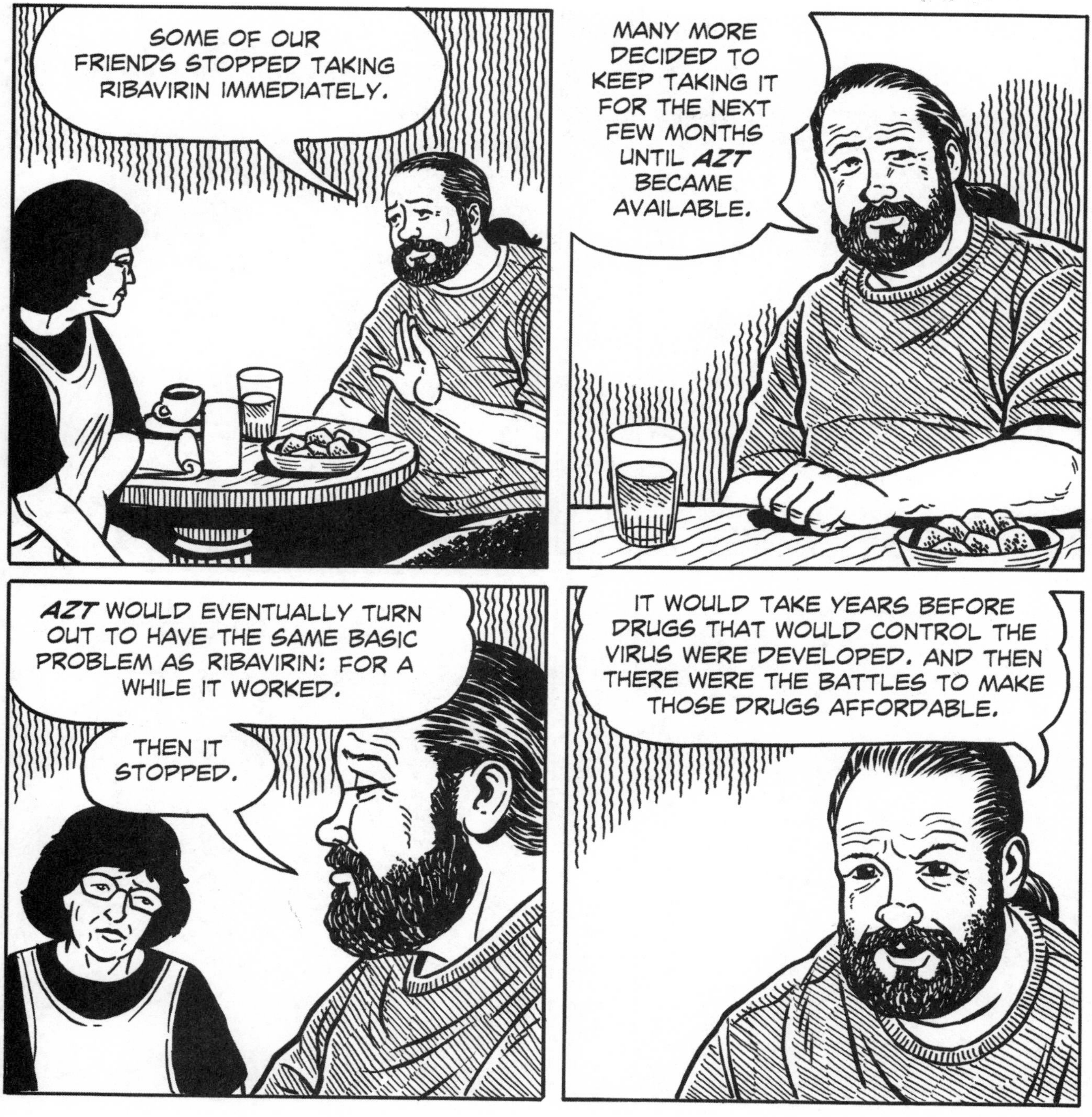
SOME OF OUR FRIENDS STOPPED TAKING RIBAVIRIN IMMEDIATELY.
MANY MORE DECIDED TO KEEP TAKING IT FOR THE NEXT FEW MONTHS UNTIL AZT BECAME AVAILABLE.
AZT WOULD EVENTUALLY TURN OUT TO HAVE THE SAME BASIC PROBLEM AS RIBAVIRIN: FOR A WHILE IT WORKED.
THEN IT STOPPED.
IT WOULD TAKE YEARS BEFORE DRUGS THAT WOULD CONTROL THE VIRUS WERE DEVELOPED. AND THEN THERE WERE THE BATTLES TO MAKE THOSE DRUGS AFFORDABLE.

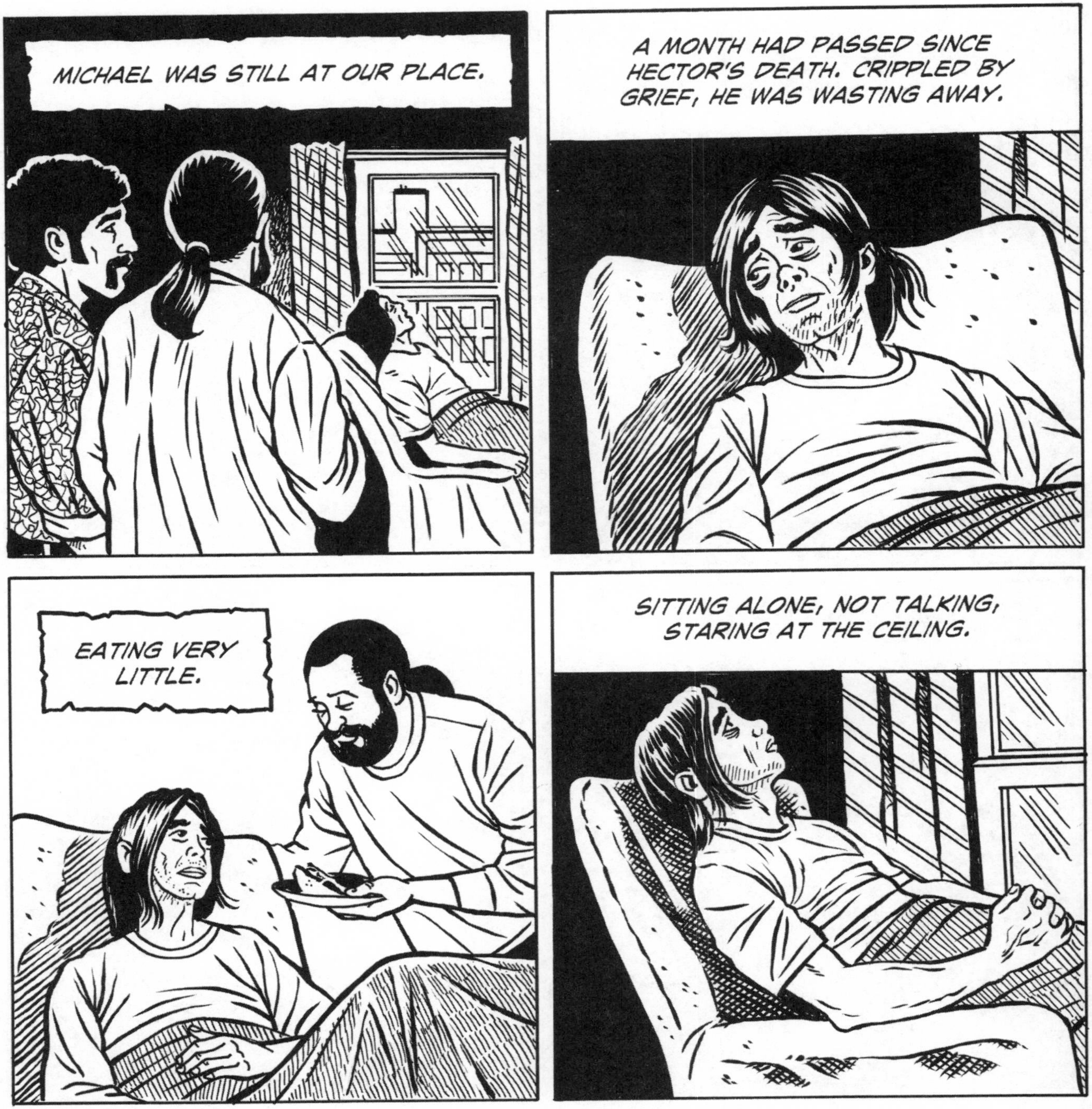
MICHAEL WAS STILL AT OUR PLACE.
A MONTH HAD PASSED SINCE HECTOR'S DEATH. CRIPPLED BY GRIEF, HE WAS WASTING AWAY.
EATING VERY LITTLE.
SITTING ALONE, NOT TALKING, STARING AT THE CEILING.

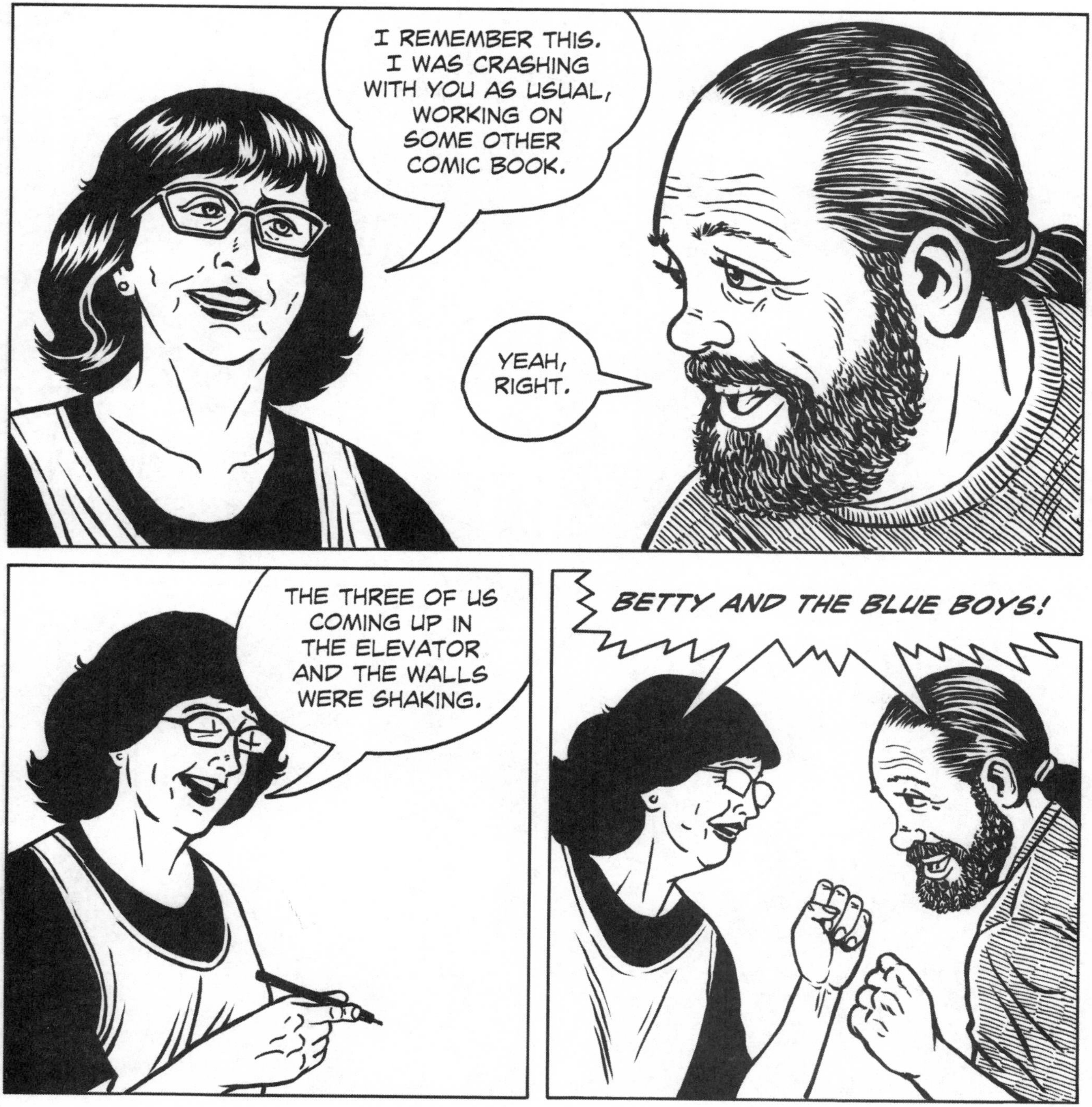
I REMEMBER THIS. I WAS CRASHING WITH YOU AS USUAL, WORKING ON SOME OTHER COMIC BOOK.
YEAH, RIGHT.
THE THREE OF US COMING UP IN THE ELEVATOR AND THE WALLS WERE SHAKING.
BETTY AND THE BLUE BOYS!

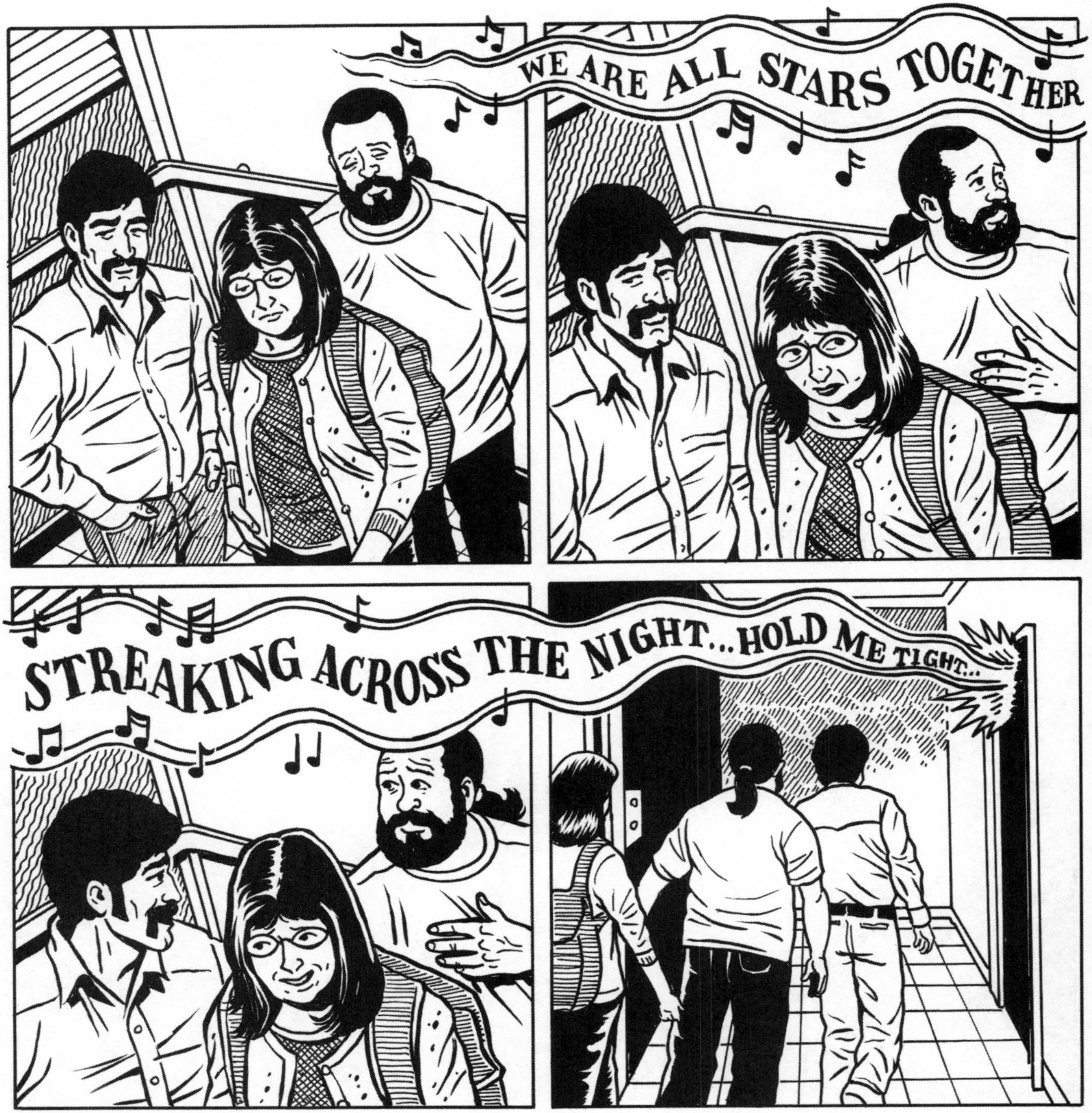
WE ARE ALL STARS TOGETHER
STREAKING ACROSS THE NIGHT... HOLD ME TIGHT...

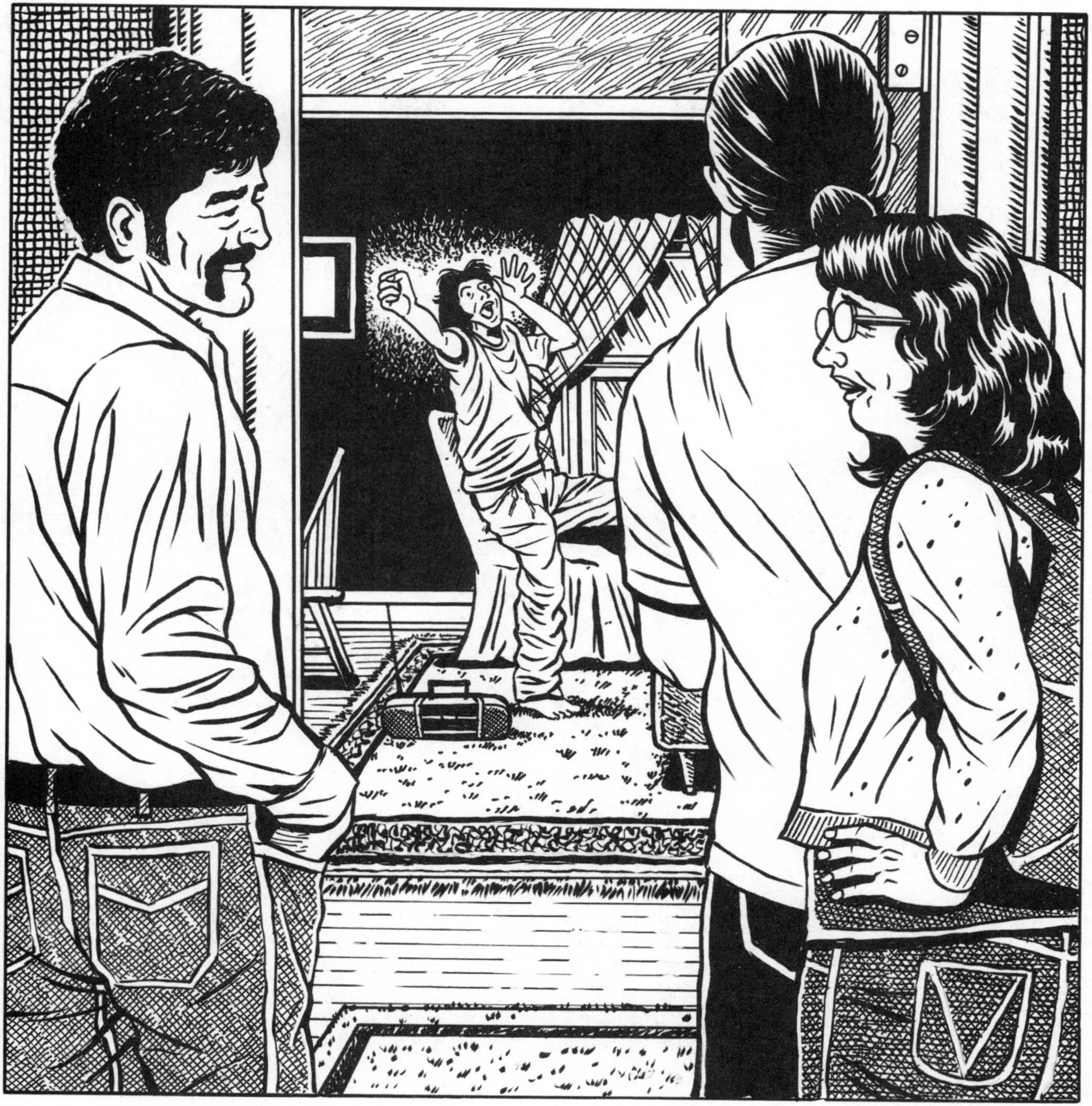

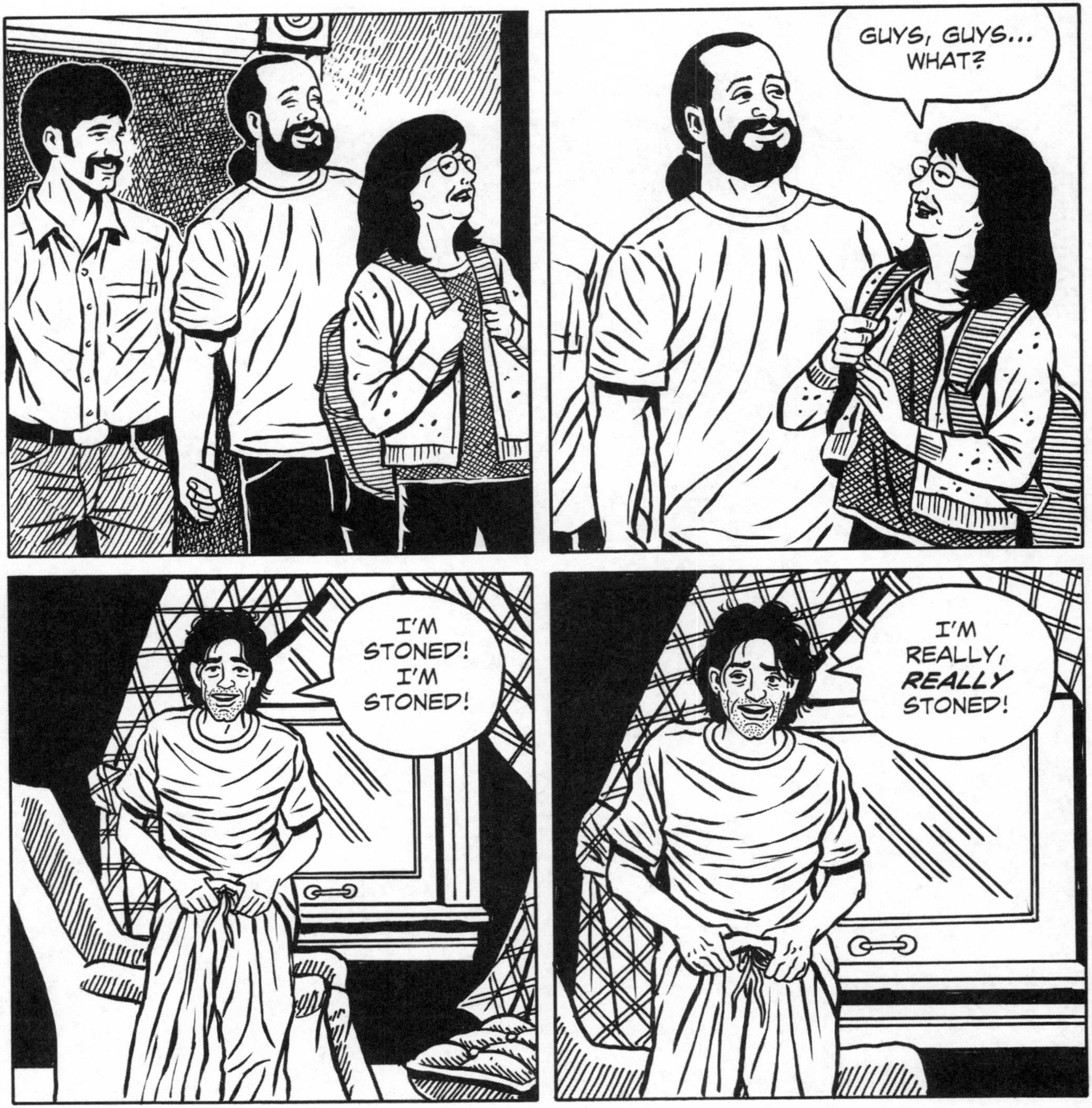
GUYS, GUYS... WHAT?
I'M STONED! I'M STONED!
I'M REALLY, *REALLY* STONED!

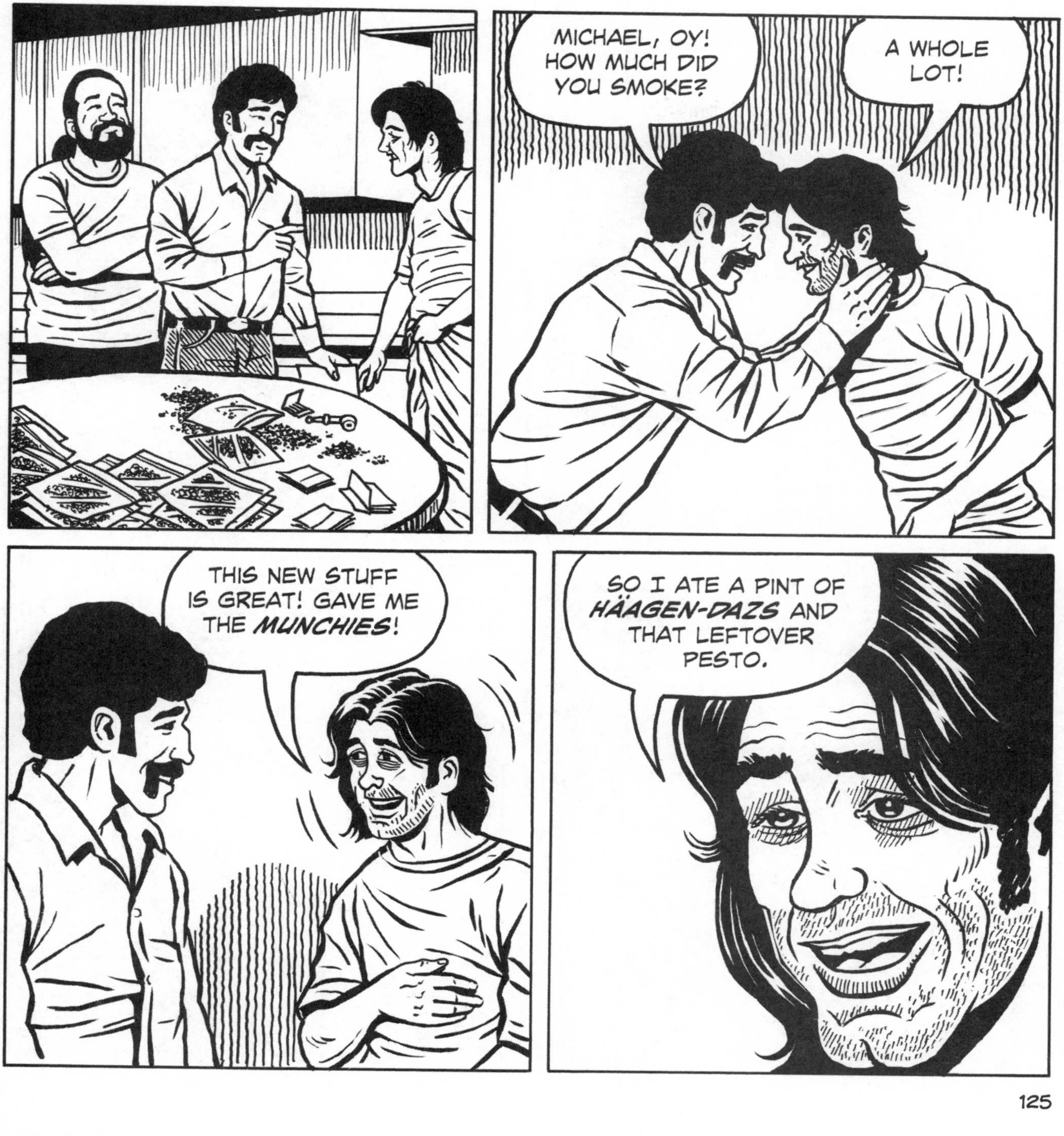
MICHAEL, OY! HOW MUCH DID YOU SMOKE?
A WHOLE LOT!
THIS NEW STUFF IS GREAT! GAVE ME THE *MUNCHIES*!
SO I ATE A PINT OF *HÄAGEN-DAZS* AND THAT LEFTOVER PESTO.

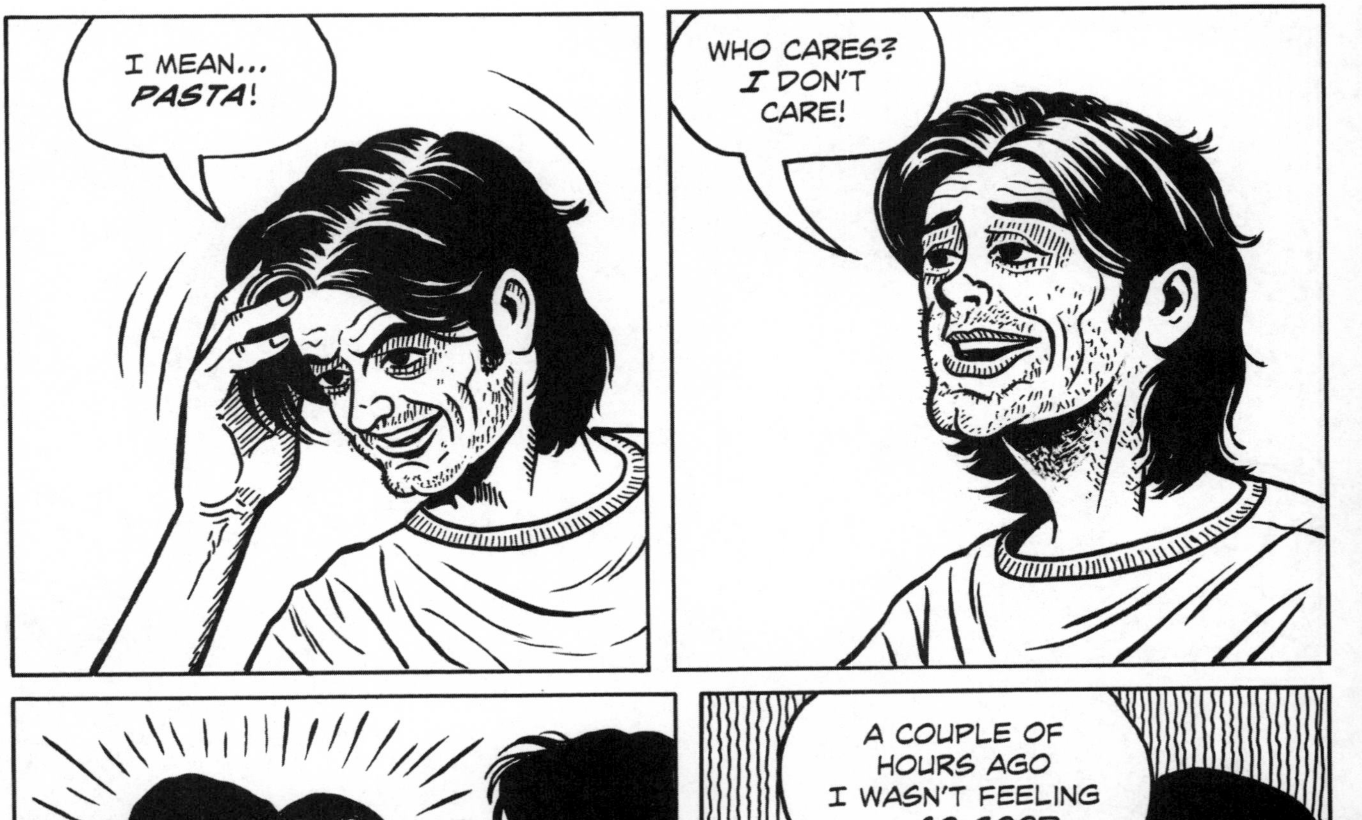
I MEAN... PASTA!
WHO CARES? I DON'T CARE!
A COUPLE OF HOURS AGO I WASN'T FEELING SO GOOD.

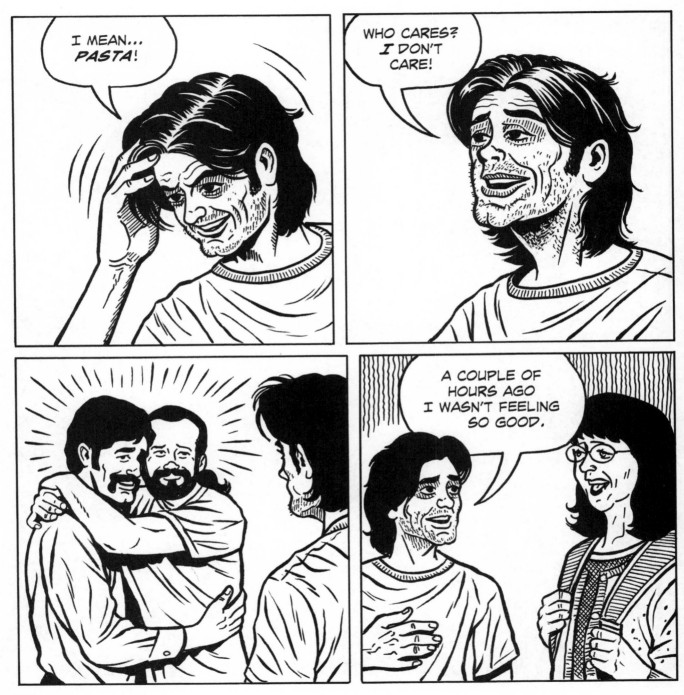

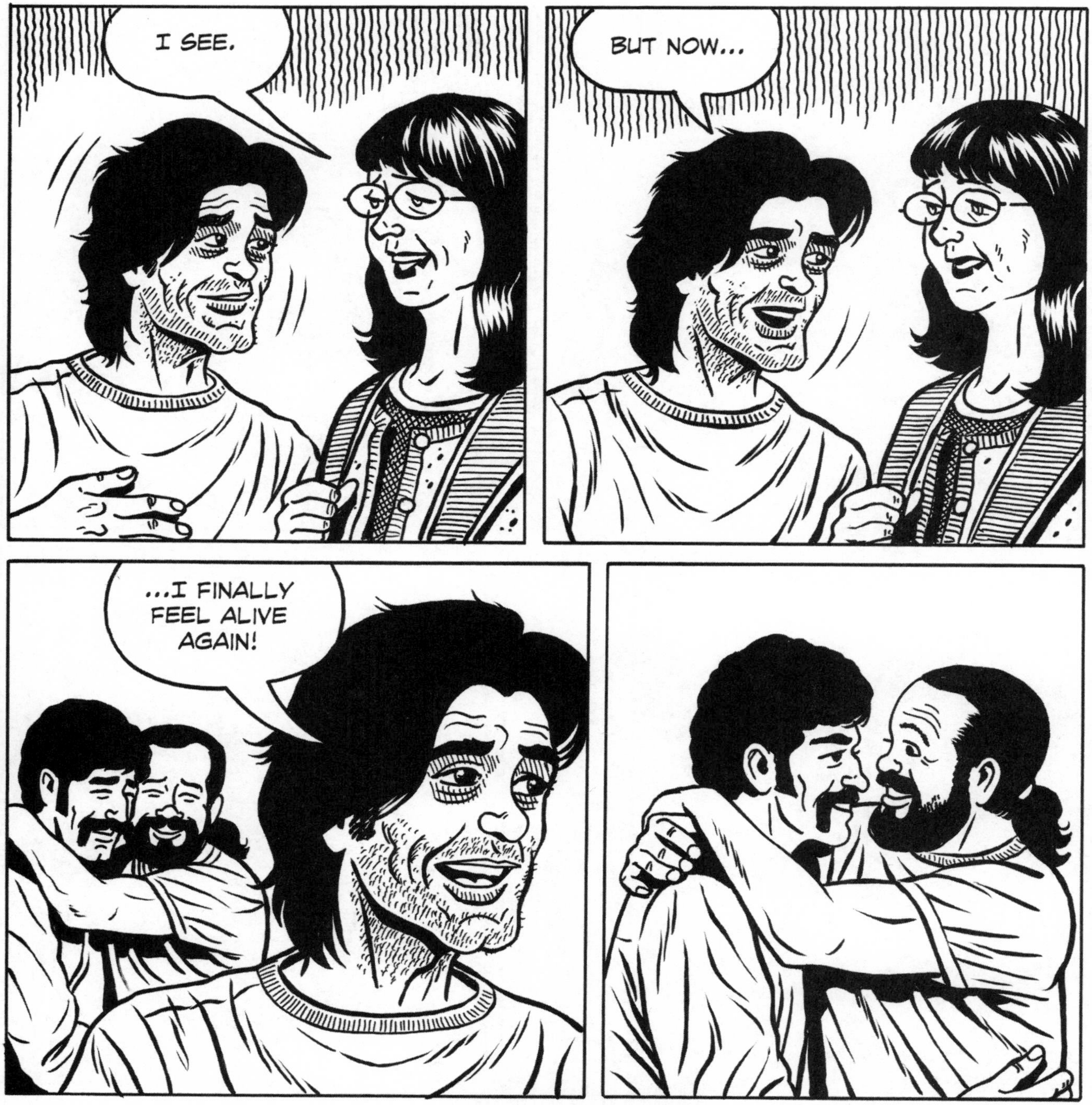
I SEE.
BUT NOW...
...I FINALLY FEEL ALIVE AGAIN!

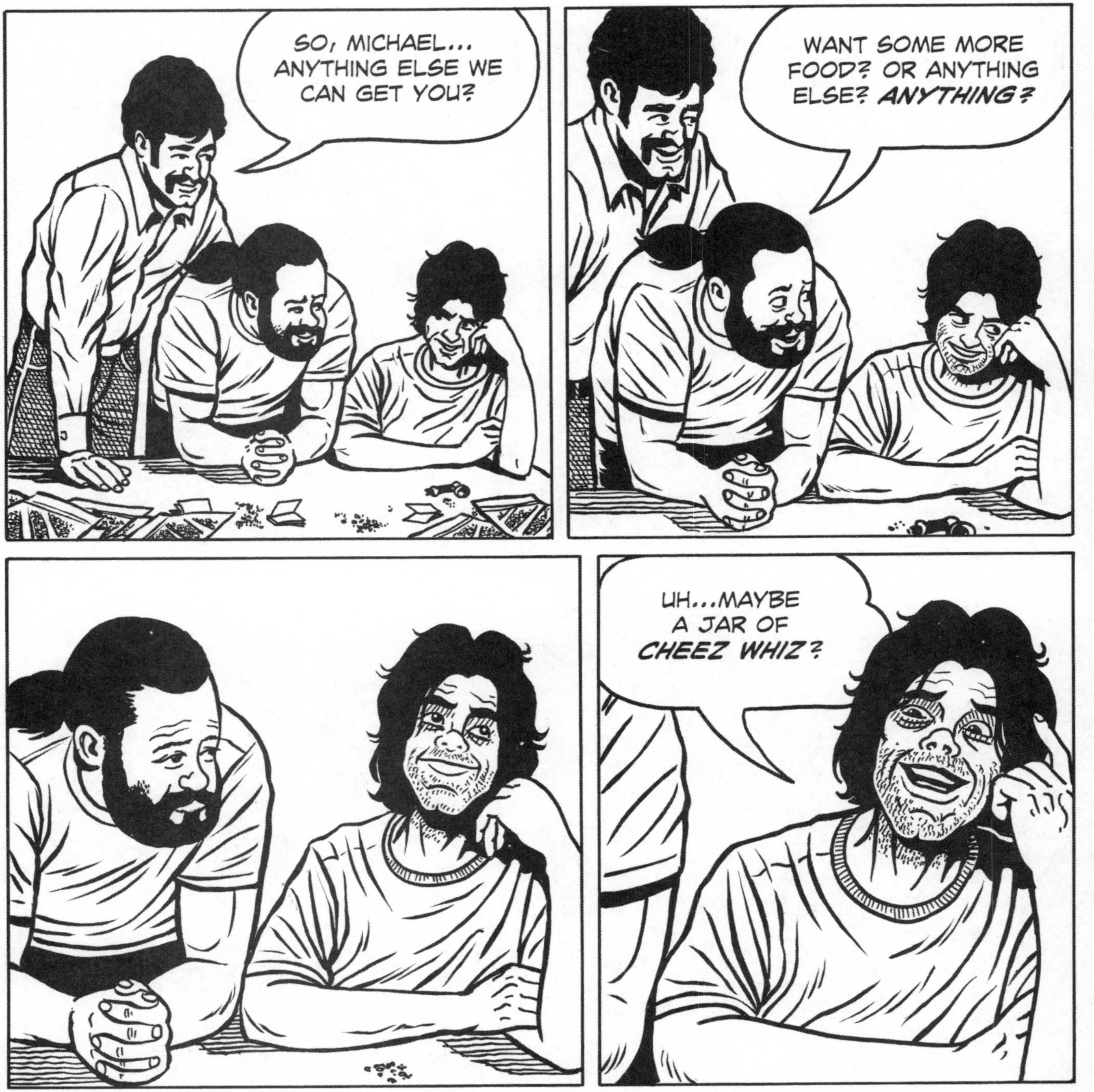
SO, MICHAEL... ANYTHING ELSE WE CAN GET YOU?
WANT SOME MORE FOOD? OR ANYTHING ELSE? *ANYTHING?*
UH...MAYBE A JAR OF *CHEEZ WHIZ?*

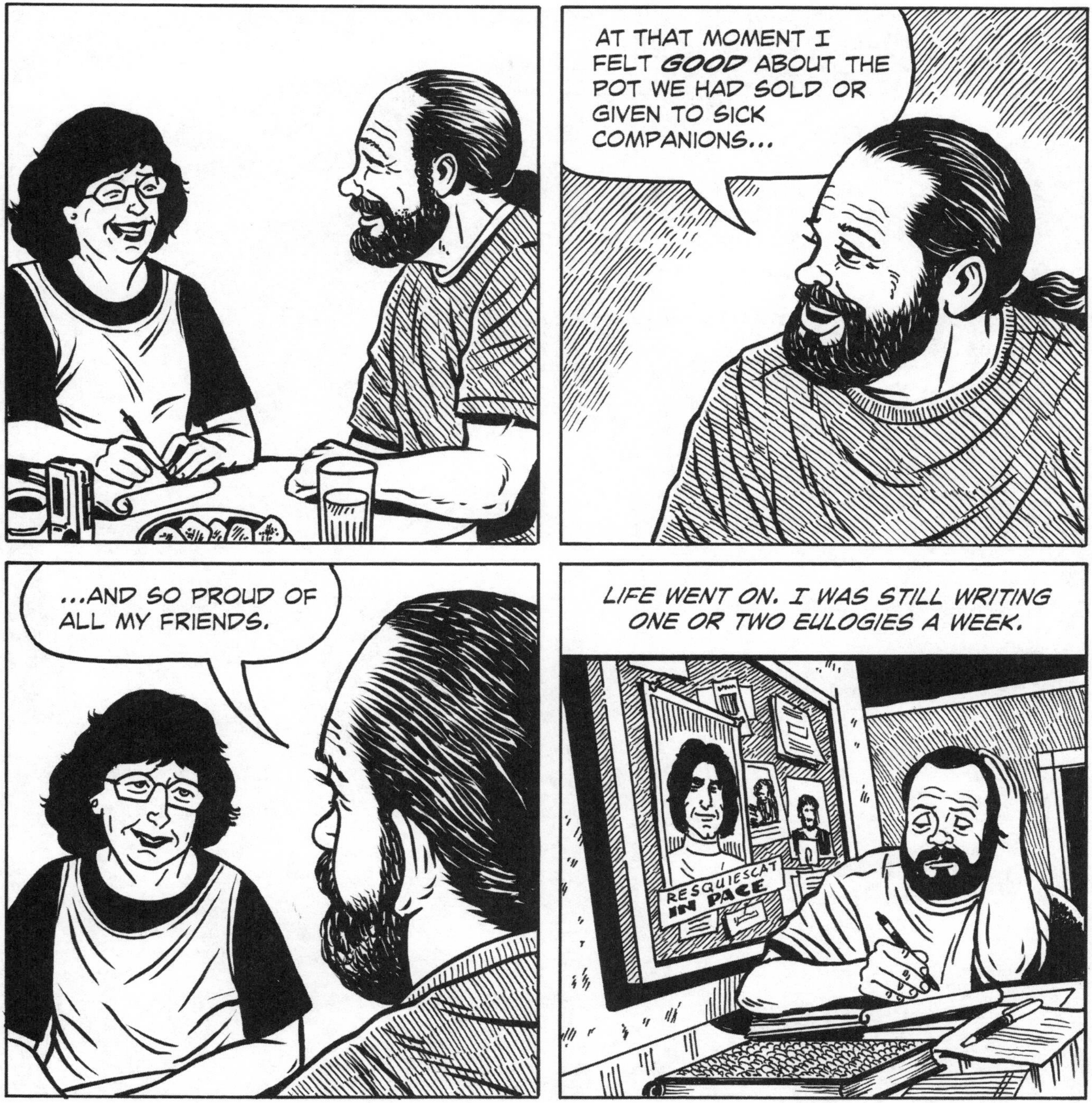
AT THAT MOMENT I FELT GOOD ABOUT THE POT WE HAD SOLD OR GIVEN TO SICK COMPANIONS...
...AND SO PROUD OF ALL MY FRIENDS.
LIFE WENT ON. I WAS STILL WRITING ONE OR TWO EULOGIES A WEEK.
RESQUIESCAT IN PACE

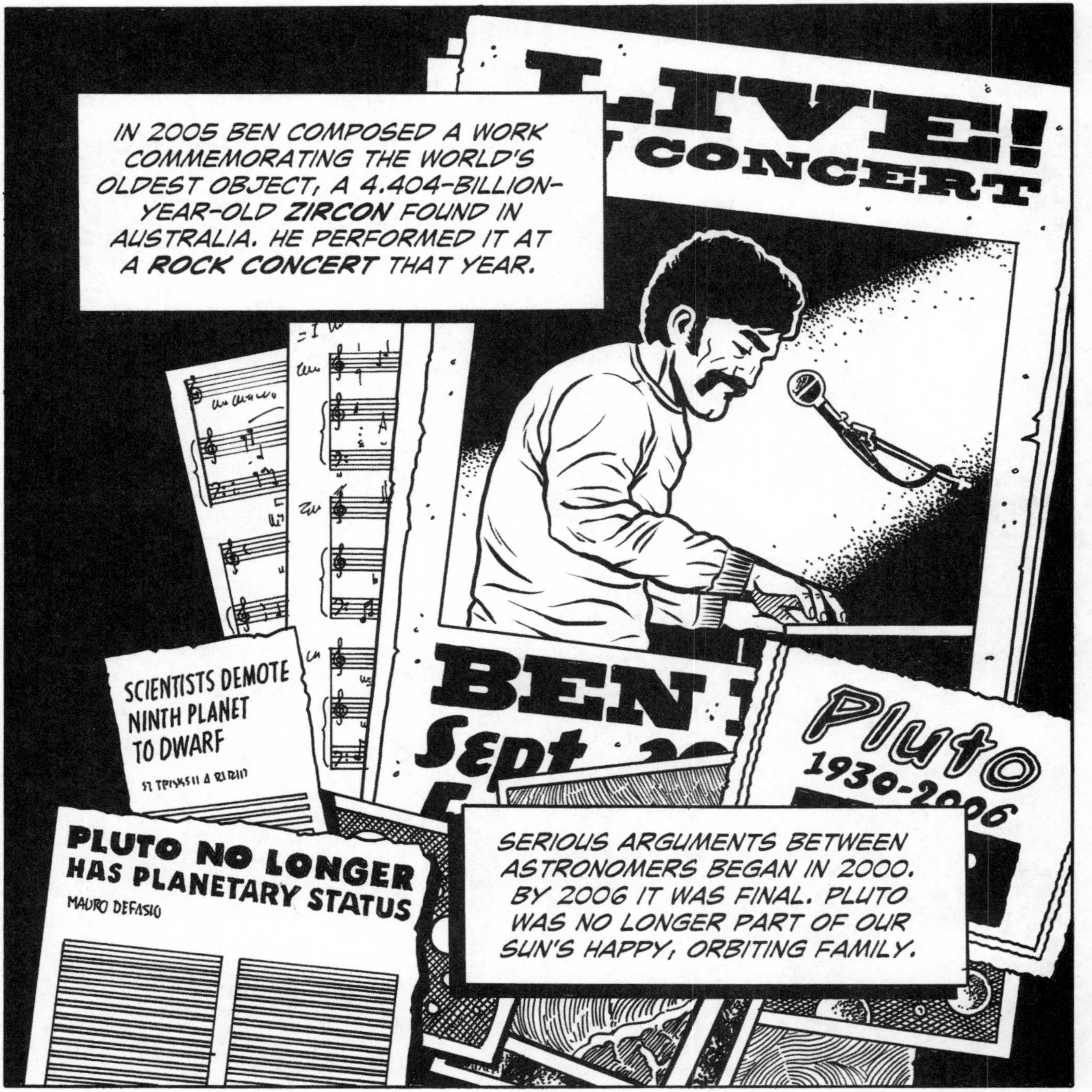
IN 2005 BEN COMPOSED A WORK COMMEMORATING THE WORLD'S OLDEST OBJECT, A 4.404-BILLION-YEAR-OLD ZIRCON FOUND IN AUSTRALIA. HE PERFORMED IT AT A ROCK CONCERT THAT YEAR.
LIVE!
CONCERT
BEN
Sept
SCIENTISTS DEMOTE NINTH PLANET TO DWARF
Pluto
1930-2006
PLUTO NO LONGER HAS PLANETARY STATUS
MAURO DEFASIO
SERIOUS ARGUMENTS BETWEEN ASTRONOMERS BEGAN IN 2000. BY 2006 IT WAS FINAL. PLUTO WAS NO LONGER PART OF OUR SUN'S HAPPY, ORBITING FAMILY.

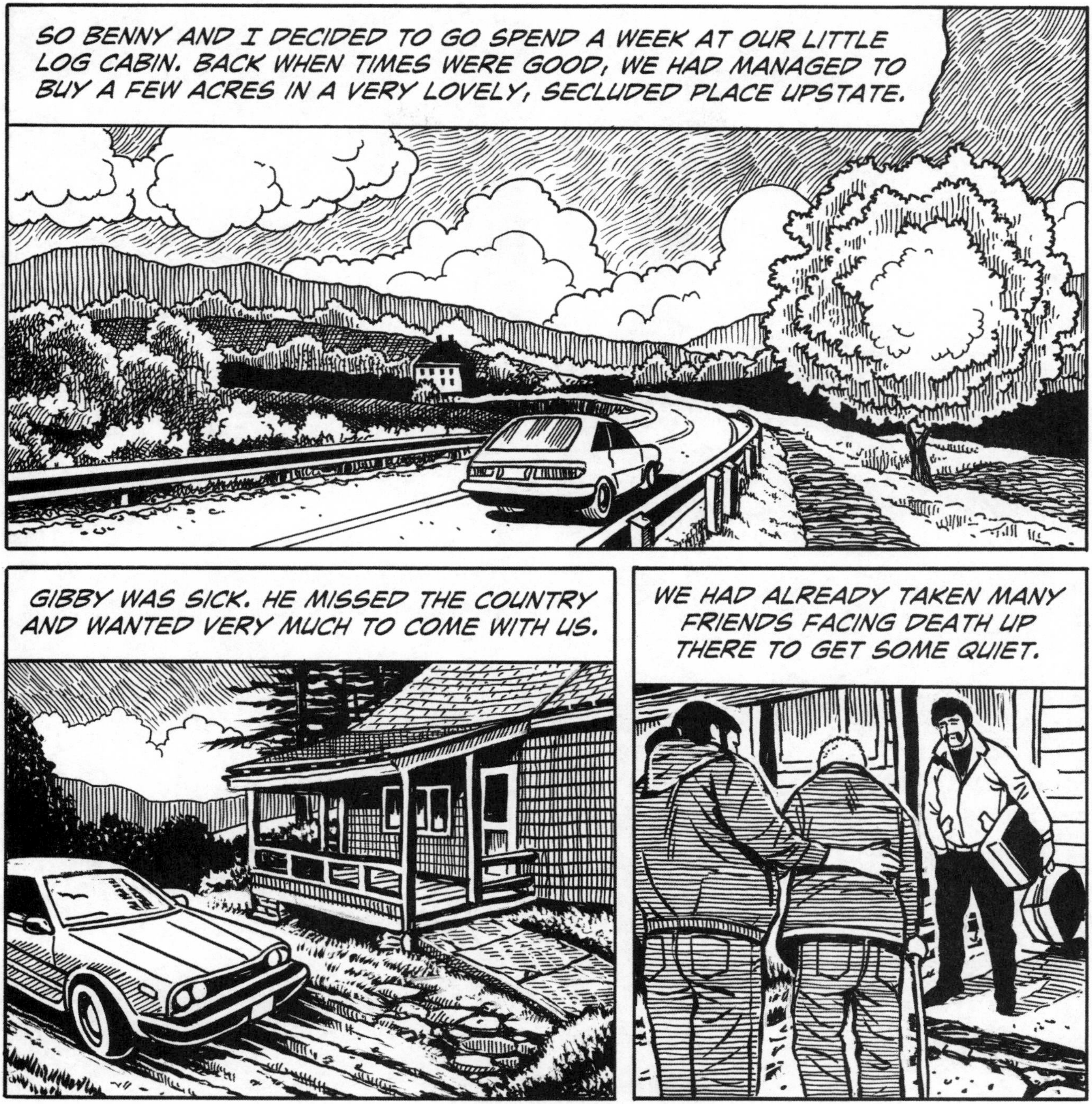
SO BENNY AND I DECIDED TO GO SPEND A WEEK AT OUR LITTLE LOG CABIN. BACK WHEN TIMES WERE GOOD, WE HAD MANAGED TO BUY A FEW ACRES IN A VERY LOVELY, SECLUDED PLACE UPSTATE.
GIBBY WAS SICK. HE MISSED THE COUNTRY AND WANTED VERY MUCH TO COME WITH US.
WE HAD ALREADY TAKEN MANY FRIENDS FACING DEATH UP THERE TO GET SOME QUIET.

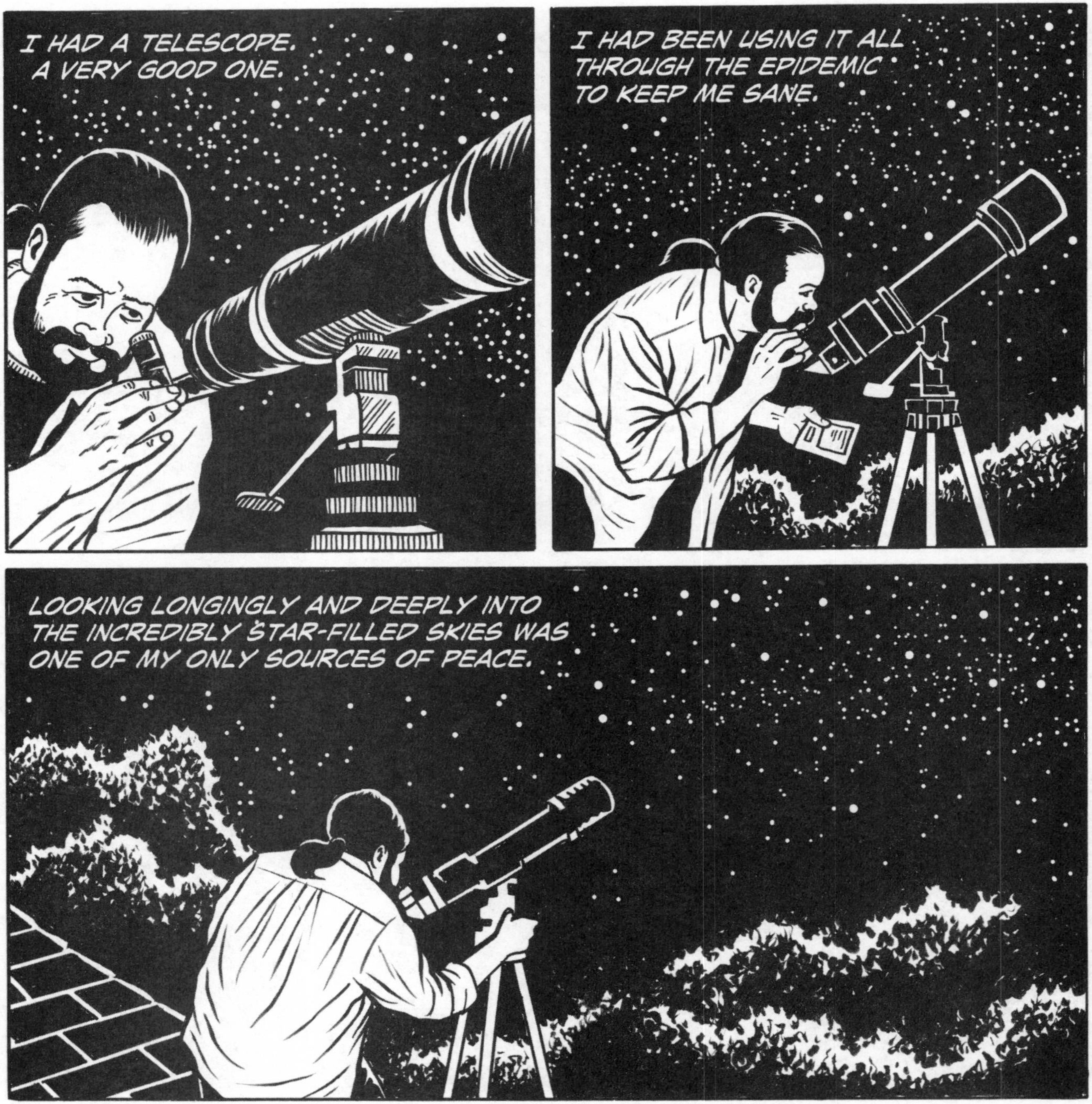
I HAD A TELESCOPE. A VERY GOOD ONE.
I HAD BEEN USING IT ALL THROUGH THE EPIDEMIC TO KEEP ME SANE.
LOOKING LONGINGLY AND DEEPLY INTO THE INCREDIBLY STAR-FILLED SKIES WAS ONE OF MY ONLY SOURCES OF PEACE.

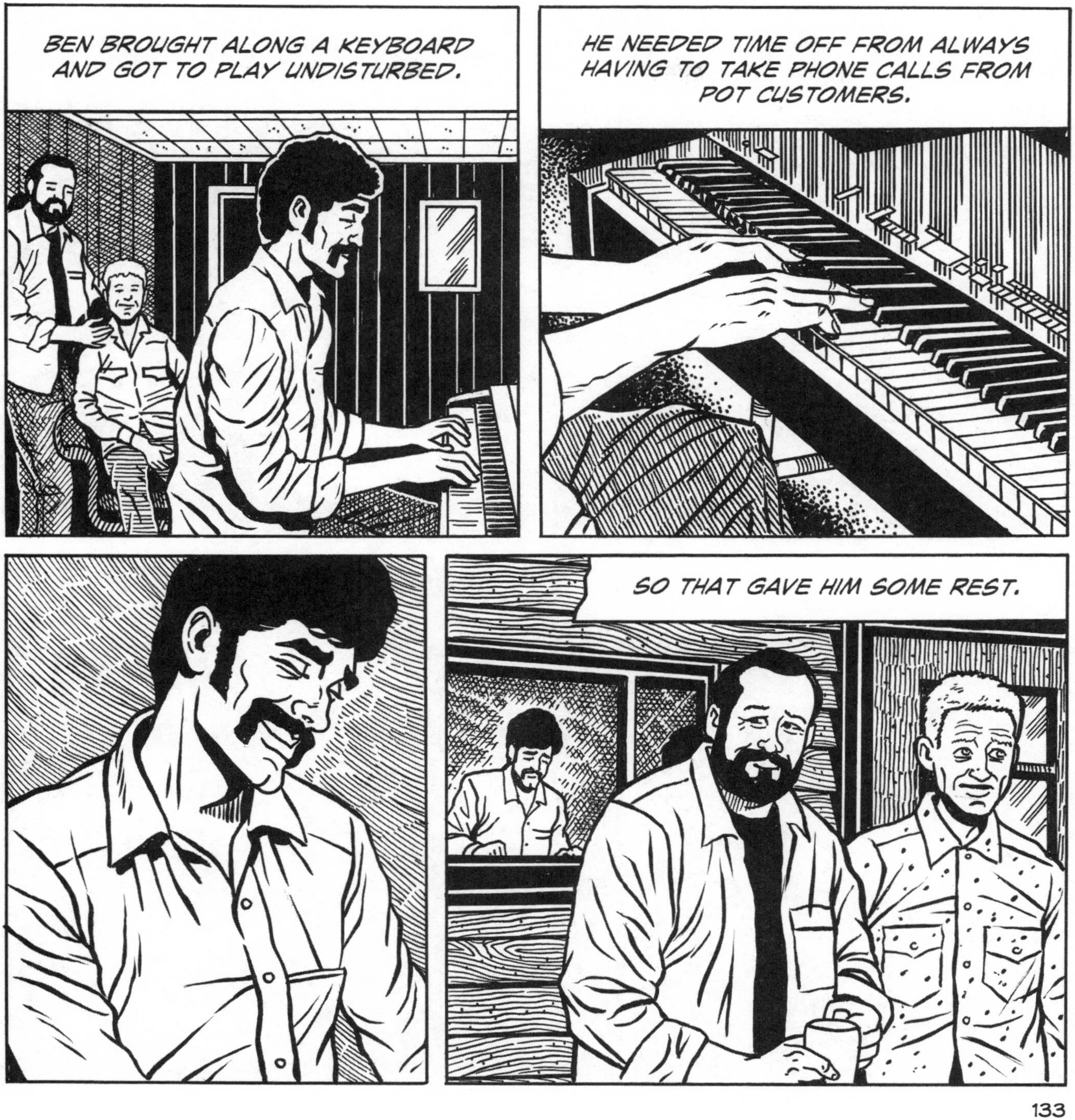
BEN BROUGHT ALONG A KEYBOARD AND GOT TO PLAY UNDISTURBED.
HE NEEDED TIME OFF FROM ALWAYS HAVING TO TAKE PHONE CALLS FROM POT CUSTOMERS.
SO THAT GAVE HIM SOME REST.

ONE OF THOSE NIGHTS I SHOWED GIBBY AROUND THE SKY.
BEN WAS PLAYING A MIX OF SCALES AND SONGS SOFTLY ON THE PIANO.
SO THAT'S THE MOON...IT'S SO BIG!
THERE ARE JUPITER'S MOONS... AND SATURN'S RINGS.

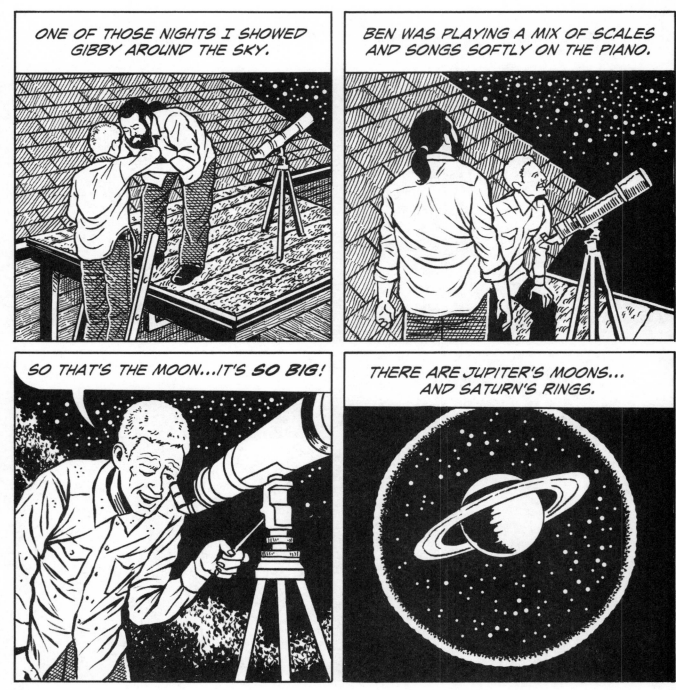

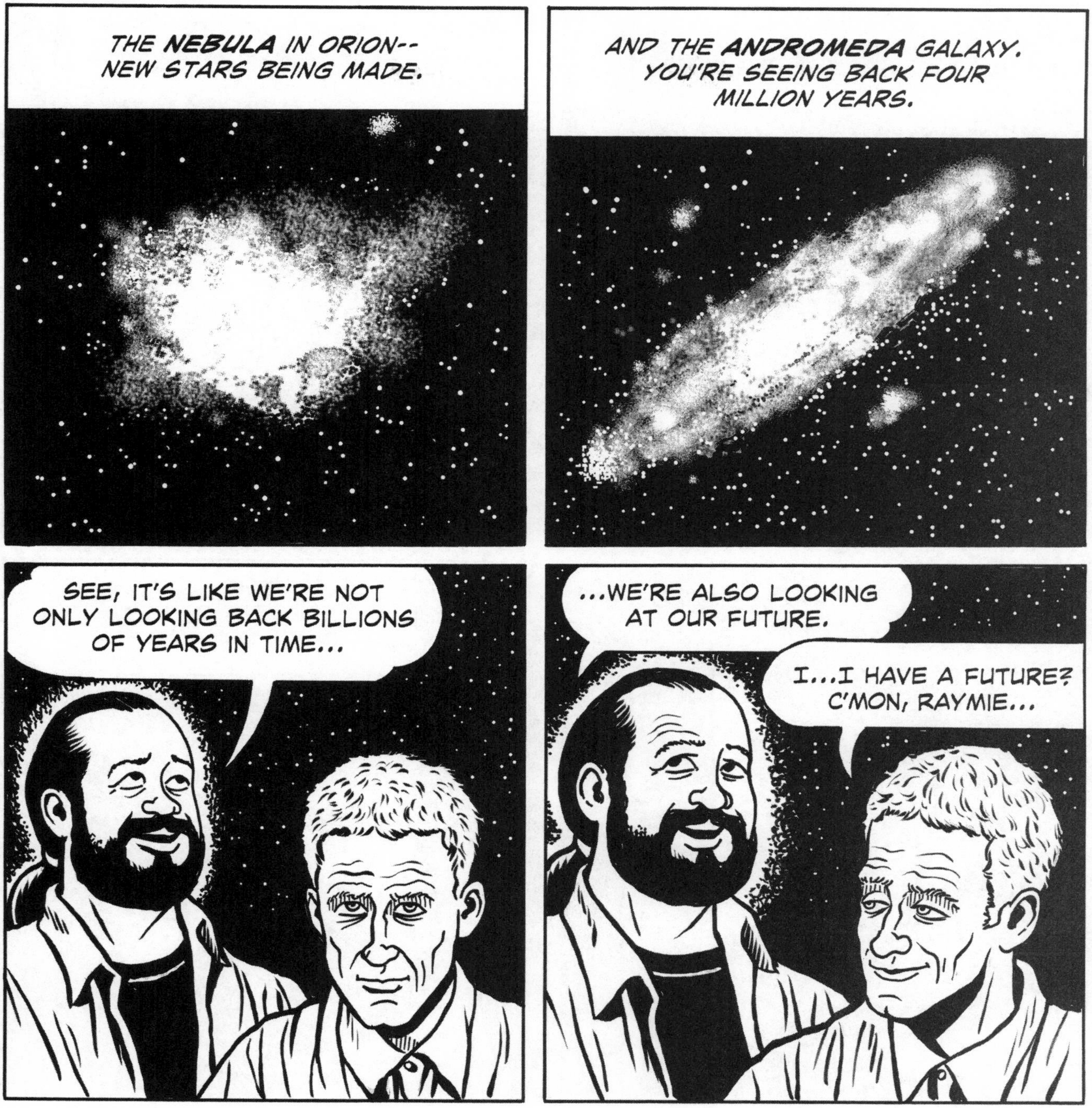
THE NEBULA IN ORION--
NEW STARS BEING MADE.
AND THE ANDROMEDA GALAXY.
YOU'RE SEEING BACK FOUR
MILLION YEARS.
SEE, IT'S LIKE WE'RE NOT ONLY LOOKING BACK BILLIONS OF YEARS IN TIME...
...WE'RE ALSO LOOKING AT OUR FUTURE.
I...I HAVE A FUTURE? C'MON, RAYMIE...

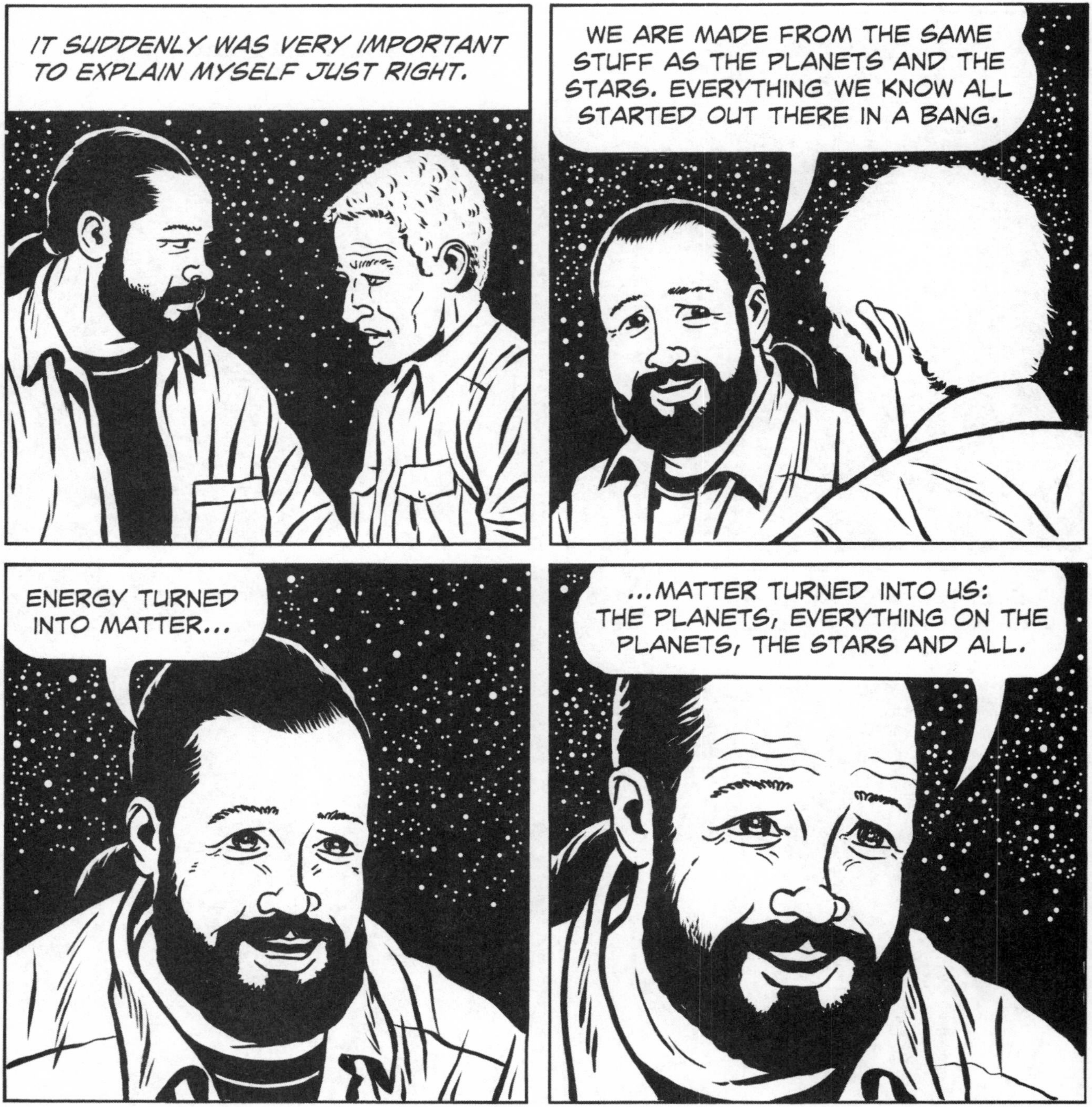
IT SUDDENLY WAS VERY IMPORTANT TO EXPLAIN MYSELF JUST RIGHT.
WE ARE MADE FROM THE SAME STUFF AS THE PLANETS AND THE STARS. EVERYTHING WE KNOW ALL STARTED OUT THERE IN A BANG.
ENERGY TURNED INTO MATTER...
...MATTER TURNED INTO US: THE PLANETS, EVERYTHING ON THE PLANETS, THE STARS AND ALL.

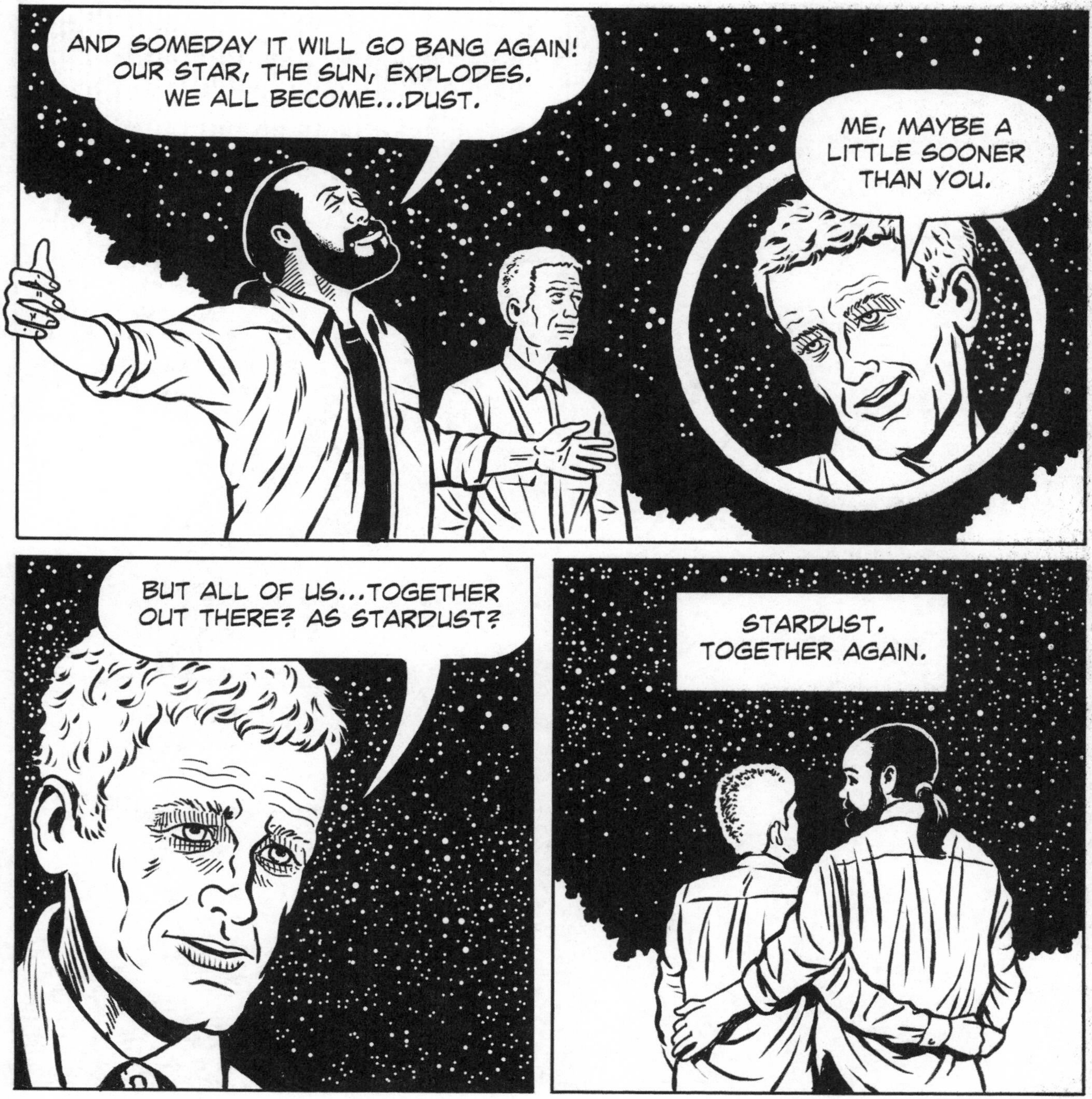
AND SOMEDAY IT WILL GO BANG AGAIN! OUR STAR, THE SUN, EXPLODES. WE ALL BECOME...DUST.
ME, MAYBE A LITTLE SOONER THAN YOU.
BUT ALL OF US...TOGETHER OUT THERE? AS STARDUST?
STARDUST. TOGETHER AGAIN.

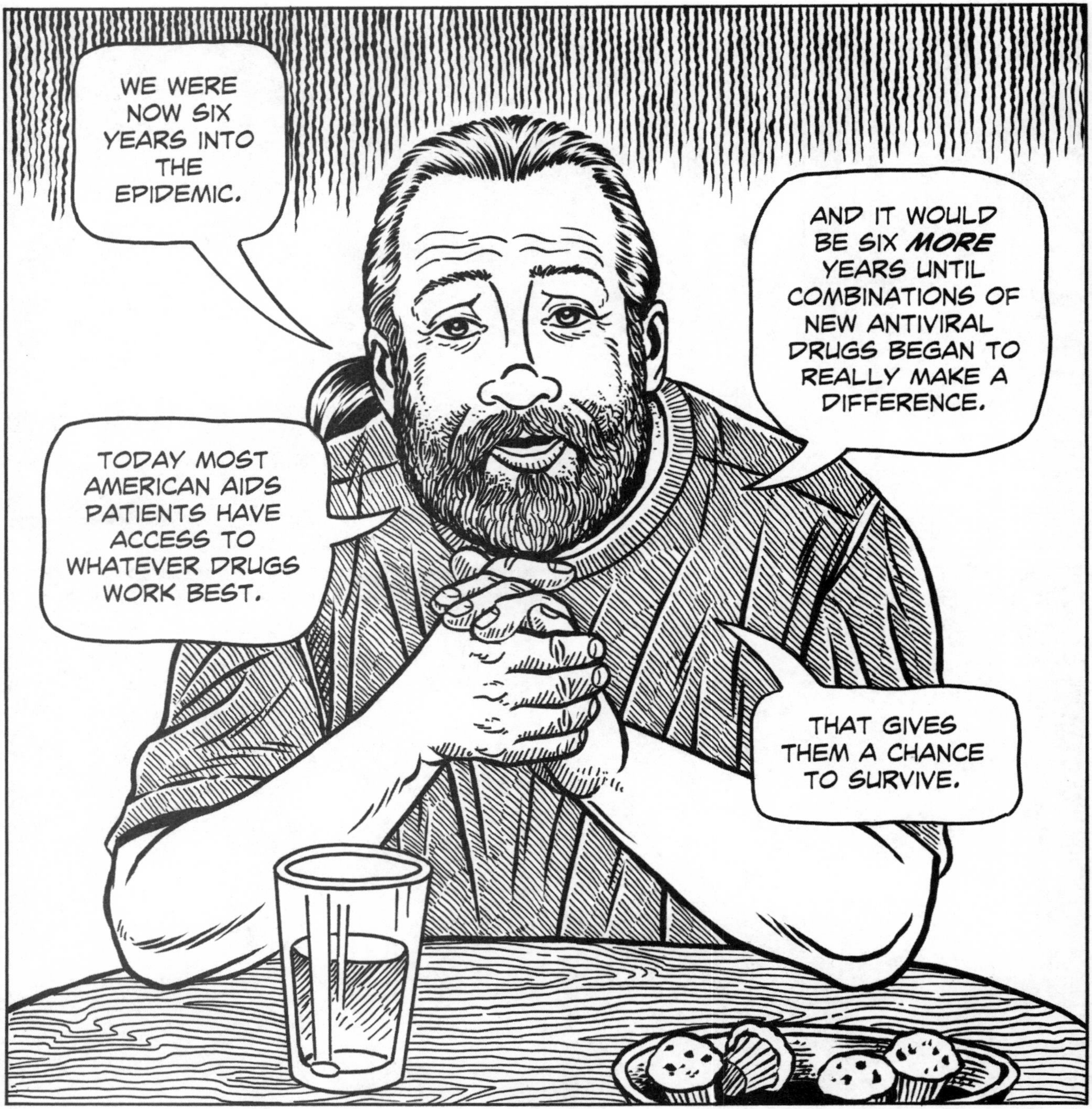
WE WERE NOW SIX YEARS INTO THE EPIDEMIC.
AND IT WOULD BE SIX *MORE* YEARS UNTIL COMBINATIONS OF NEW ANTIVIRAL DRUGS BEGAN TO REALLY MAKE A DIFFERENCE.
TODAY MOST AMERICAN AIDS PATIENTS HAVE ACCESS TO WHATEVER DRUGS WORK BEST.
THAT GIVES THEM A CHANCE TO SURVIVE.

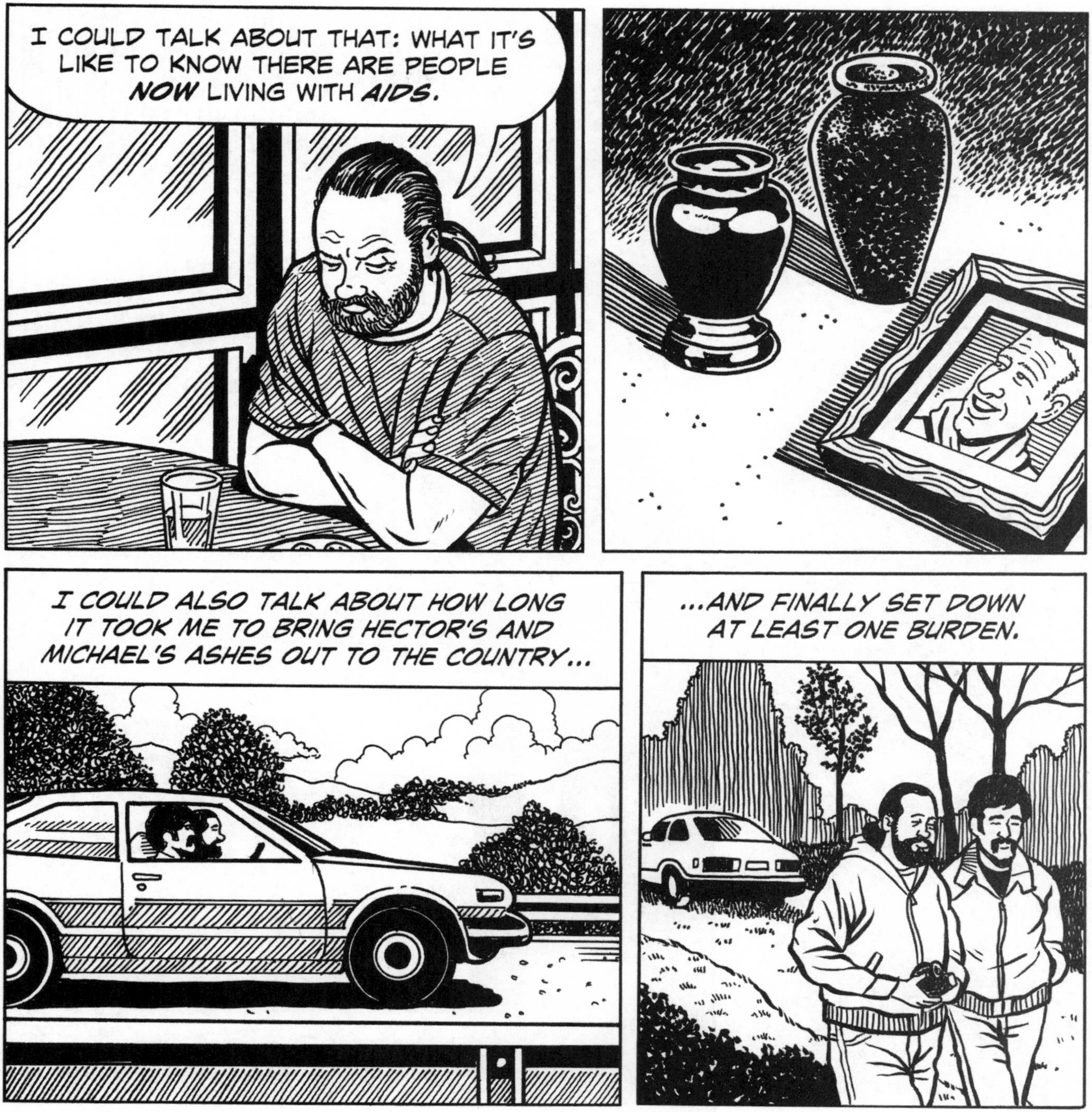
I COULD TALK ABOUT THAT: WHAT IT'S LIKE TO KNOW THERE ARE PEOPLE *NOW* LIVING WITH *AIDS*.
I COULD ALSO TALK ABOUT HOW LONG IT TOOK ME TO BRING HECTOR'S AND MICHAEL'S ASHES OUT TO THE COUNTRY...
...AND FINALLY SET DOWN AT LEAST ONE BURDEN.

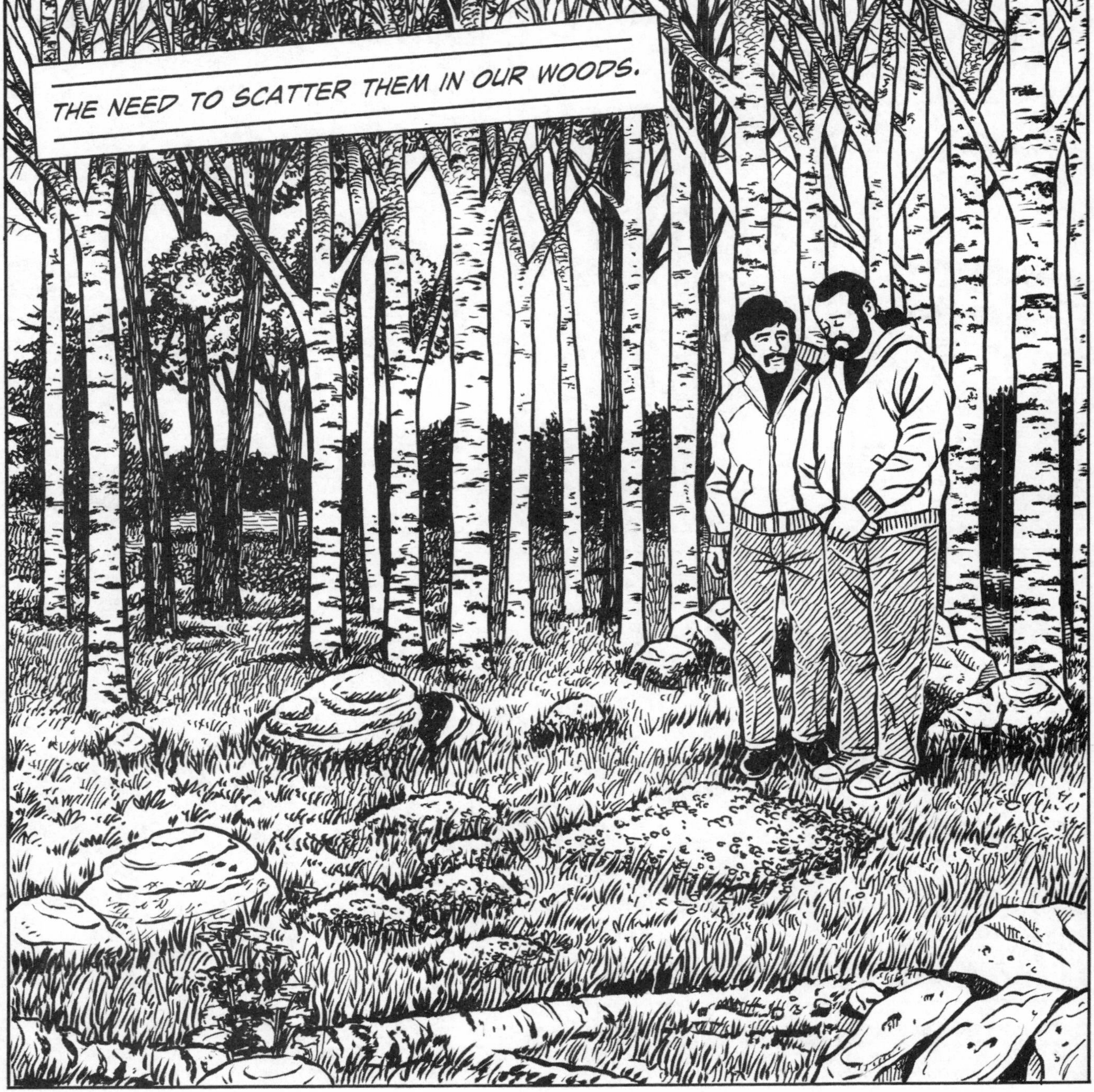
THE NEED TO SCATTER THEM IN OUR WOODS.

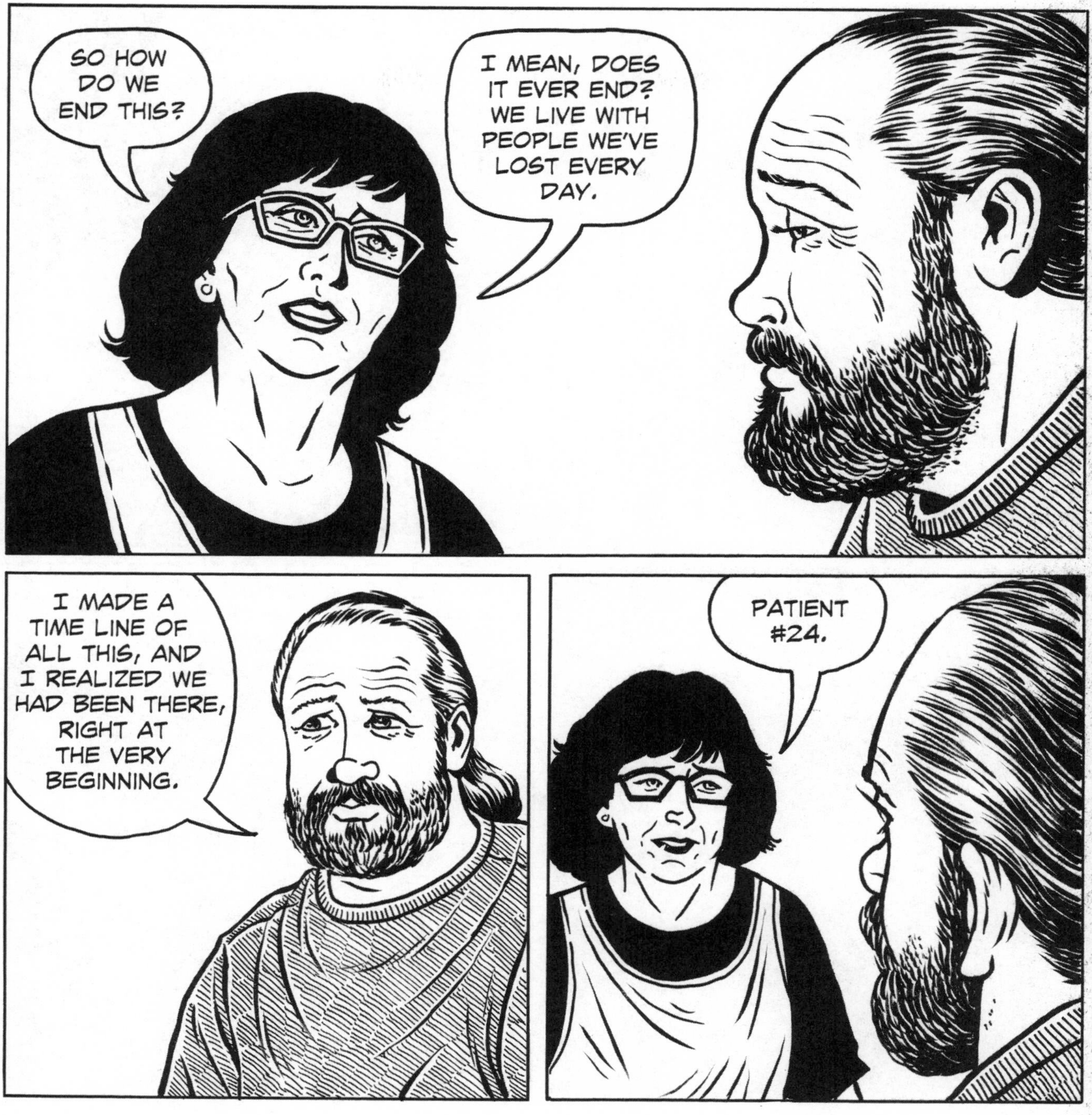
SO HOW DO WE END THIS?
I MEAN, DOES IT EVER END? WE LIVE WITH PEOPLE WE'VE LOST EVERY DAY.
I MADE A TIME LINE OF ALL THIS, AND I REALIZED WE HAD BEEN THERE, RIGHT AT THE VERY BEGINNING.
PATIENT #24.

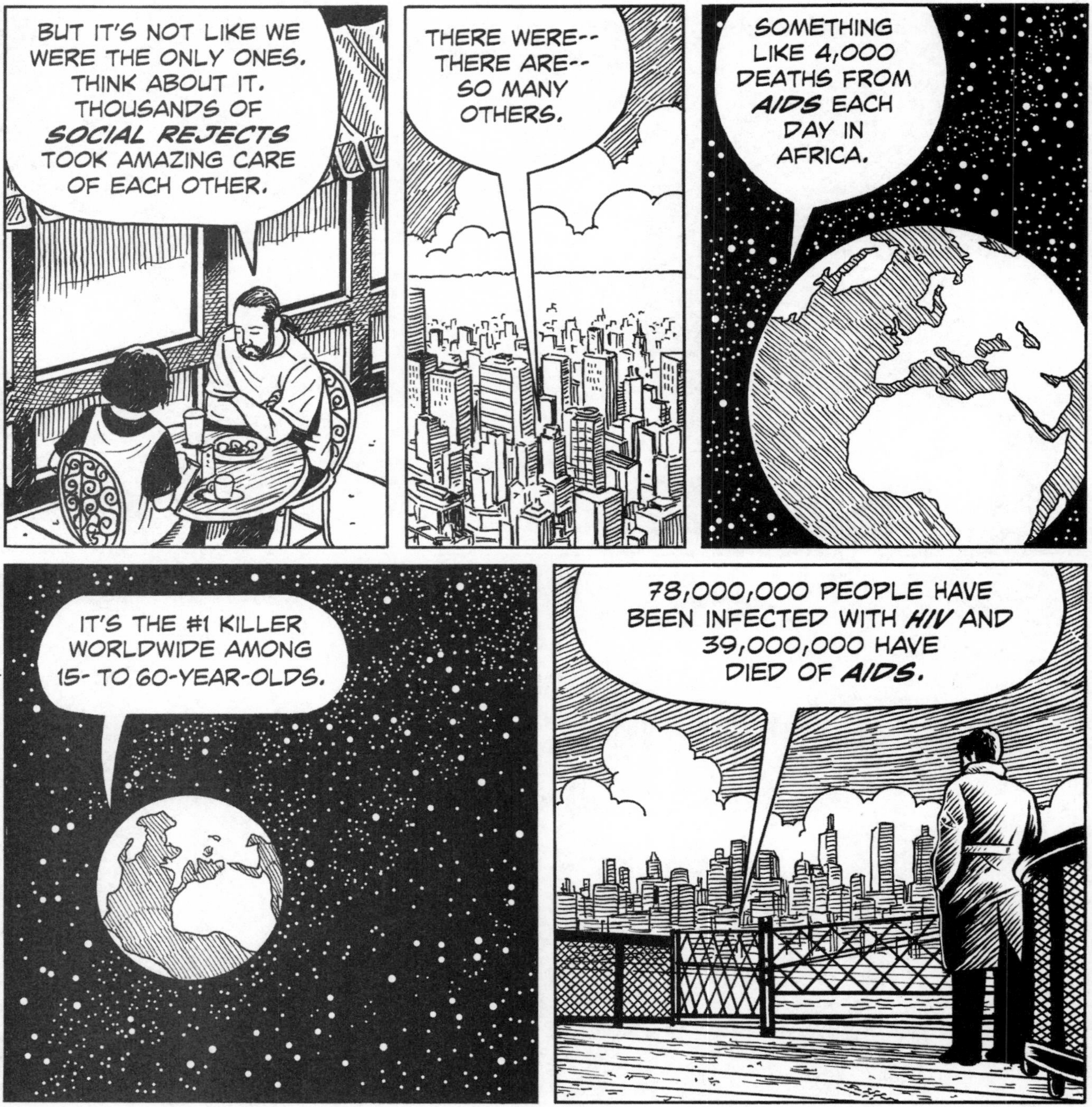
BUT IT'S NOT LIKE WE WERE THE ONLY ONES. THINK ABOUT IT. THOUSANDS OF SOCIAL REJECTS TOOK AMAZING CARE OF EACH OTHER.
THERE WERE-- THERE ARE-- SO MANY OTHERS.
SOMETHING LIKE 4,000 DEATHS FROM AIDS EACH DAY IN AFRICA.
IT'S THE #1 KILLER WORLDWIDE AMONG 15- TO 60-YEAR-OLDS.
78,000,000 PEOPLE HAVE BEEN INFECTED WITH HIV AND 39,000,000 HAVE DIED OF AIDS.

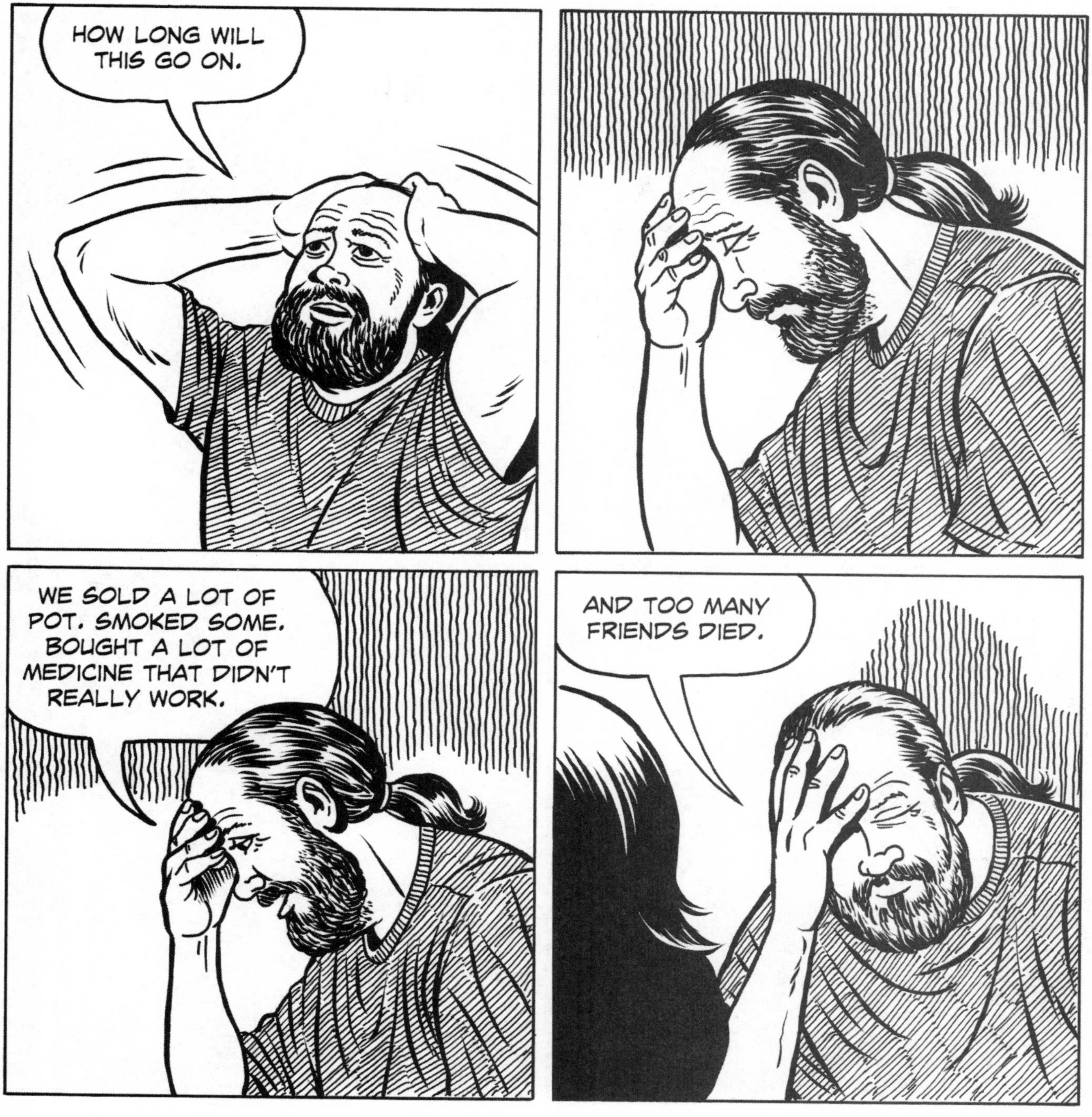
HOW LONG WILL THIS GO ON.
WE SOLD A LOT OF POT. SMOKED SOME. BOUGHT A LOT OF MEDICINE THAT DIDN'T REALLY WORK.
AND TOO MANY FRIENDS DIED.

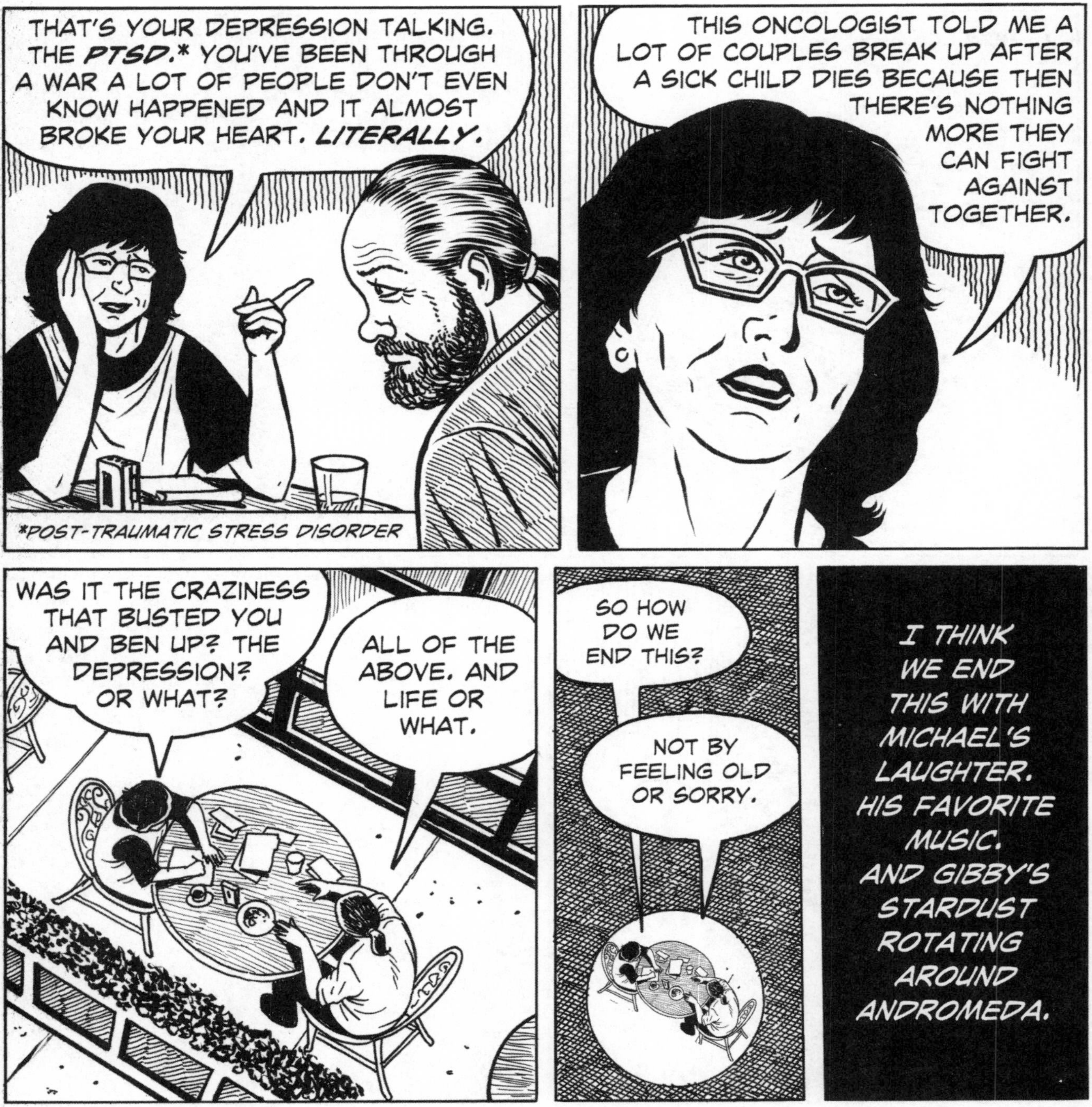

THAT'S YOUR DEPRESSION TALKING. THE PTSD.* YOU'VE BEEN THROUGH A WAR A LOT OF PEOPLE DON'T EVEN KNOW HAPPENED AND IT ALMOST BROKE YOUR HEART. LITERALLY.
*POST-TRAUMATIC STRESS DISORDER
THIS ONCOLOGIST TOLD ME A LOT OF COUPLES BREAK UP AFTER A SICK CHILD DIES BECAUSE THEN THERE'S NOTHING MORE THEY CAN FIGHT AGAINST TOGETHER.
WAS IT THE CRAZINESS THAT BUSTED YOU AND BEN UP? THE DEPRESSION? OR WHAT?
ALL OF THE ABOVE. AND LIFE OR WHAT.
SO HOW DO WE END THIS?
NOT BY FEELING OLD OR SORRY.
I THINK WE END THIS WITH MICHAEL'S LAUGHTER. HIS FAVORITE MUSIC. AND GIBBY'S STARDUST ROTATING AROUND ANDROMEDA.

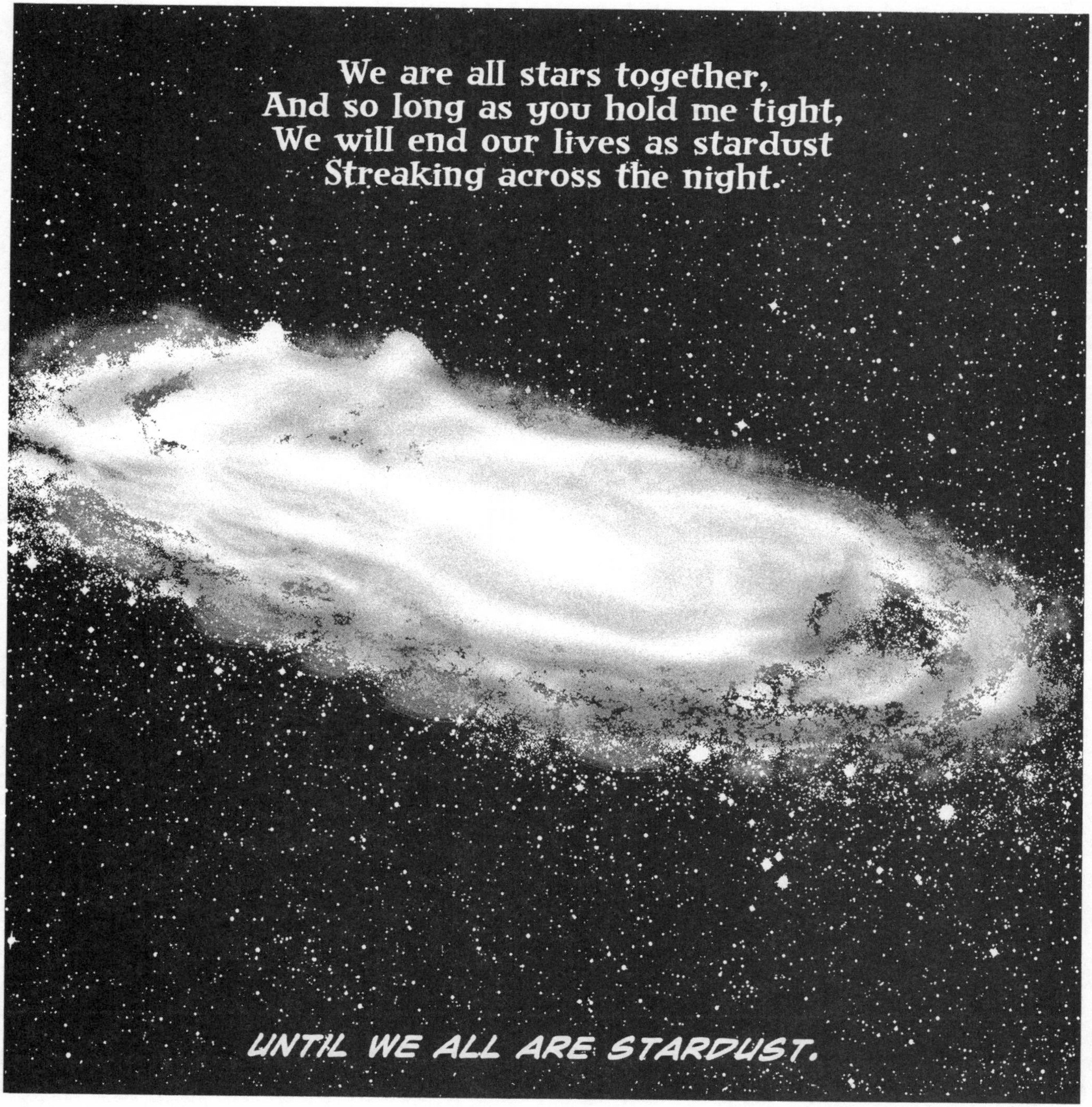
We are all stars together,
And so long as you hold me tight,
We will end our lives as stardust
Streaking across the night.
UNTIL WE ALL ARE STARDUST.

Acknowledgments

This is a true story, although we changed names, likenesses, certain locations, and a few other details to protect those still vulnerable.

Besides always wanting to write a "gang of misfits" caper, I really started this in 2006 because I saw another generation of outcast artists and young punks growing up without affordable health care and trying to take care of each other. Nothing brings that home to me more than the little pamphlets, comix, and self-published zines you will not have seen by such folk, many of which I found through Portland's Joe Biel at Microcosm Publishing. Find, read, and support.

Danielle and Lee, thanks for looking after me. And thank you Thomas LeBien (who said yes) and my late husband, Harvey Pekar, who said, "Of course!"

A Note About the Author and Illustrator

Joyce Brabner

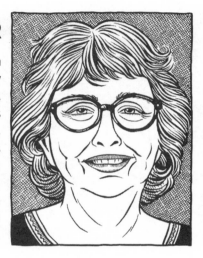

is an award-winning author of nonfiction comics about tough social issues. She frequently collaborated with her late husband, Harvey Pekar, on his *American Splendor* series. Her own titles include the *Real War Stories* series, *Activists!*, *Brought to Light* (with Alan Moore), numerous short stories, and *Our Cancer Year* (also with Harvey). She lives in Cleveland Heights, Ohio, and is rather more lighthearted than any of the actresses who have portrayed her in various plays or in that movie.

Mark Zingarelli

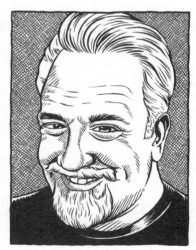

is an American comics creator, illustrator, and writer who has worked as a freelancer for the past thirty-six years. His first comics stories were published in Robert Crumb's comics anthology magazine *WEIRDO* in the mid-1980s. He worked with Harvey Pekar and Joyce Brabner on *American Splendor* and contributed to the film biopic of the same name. His illustration work and comics have appeared in many national publications, including *The New Yorker*, *Esquire*, and *Time*. He lives in a small town near Pittsburgh, Pennsylvania.